UPDATE ON HEPATITIS C

Edited by **Martina Smolić, Aleksandar Včev**
and **George Y. Wu**

Update on Hepatitis C
http://dx.doi.org/10.5772/66769
Edited by Martina Smolić, Aleksandar Včev and George Y. Wu

Contributors

Ines Bilic-Curcic, Hrvoje Roguljic, Marul Ivandic, Aleksandar Vcev, Robert Smolić, Martina Smolic, Marko Duvnjak, Nina Blazevic, Lucija Virovic-Jukic, Reham Dawood, Mostafa K. El Awadi, Damir Erceg, Tajana Filipec-Kanizaj, Kazuhiko Hayashi, Masatoshi Ishigami, Yoji Ishizu, Teiji Kuzuya, Takashi Honda, Yoshihiko Tachi, Tetsuya Ishikawa, Yoshiaki Katano, Kentaro Yoshioka, Hidenori Toyoda, Takashi Kumada, Hidemi Goto, Yoshiki Hirooka, Milan Milosevic, Lucija Kuna, Jelena Jakab, Ljiljana Peric, Dario Sabadi, Ashraf Tabll, Dominik Kralj, George Y. Wu, Alyssa Austria, Vjera Nincevic, Shaina M. Lynch, Vanja Vojnovic

Published by InTech
Janeza Trdine 9, 51000 Rijeka, Croatia

Publishing Process Manager Romina Rovan
Technical Editor SPi Global
Cover InTech Design team

First published October, 2017
Printed in Croatia
Legal deposit, Croatia: National and University Library in Zagreb

Additional hard copies can be obtained from orders@intechopen.com

Update on Hepatitis C, Edited by Martina Smolić, Aleksandar Včev and George Y. Wu
p. cm.
Print ISBN 978-953-51-3563-0
Online ISBN 978-953-51-3564-7

For EU product safety concerns:
IN TECH d.o.o., Prolaz Marije Krucifikse Kozulić 3, 51000 Rijeka, Croatia,
info@intechopen.com or visit our website at intechopen.com.

Meet the editors

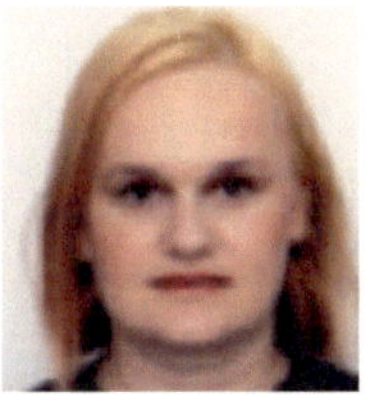

Dr. Martina Smolić is an assistant professor of Pharmacology, a program director of Postgraduate Doctoral Study of Biomedicine and Health, and also the head of the Department of Pharmacology at the University of Osijek, Faculty of Medicine. During her postdoctoral training at the University of Connecticut, she investigated the development of prospective agents for the treatment of HCV infection. Her research interests include targeted delivery to hepatocytes, mechanisms of hepatotoxicity, and mineral metabolism disorders. She has received awards from the German Research Foundation, Croatian Ministry of Science, International Society for Applied Biological Sciences, and Croatian Science Foundation and she was elected to "20 best research fellows in Croatia." She actively publishes original research work and serves as a member of the editorial board of the *Journal of Clinical and Translational Hepatology*.

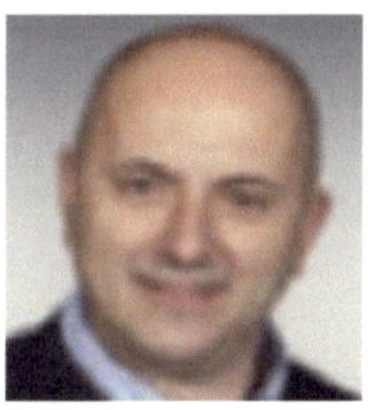

Dr. Včev is a professor of Medicine, dean of the Faculty of Medicine in Osijek, director of the National Center for Integrative Medicine, and president of the governing board of the Institute for Anthropological Research. He has published over 100 articles, several books, and book chapters and has long-standing interests in mechanisms of *Helicobacter pylori* infection and management of viral hepatitis. He mentored several master's degrees and doctoral theses focusing on chronic liver disease. He has received numerous honors and awards for his professional and scientific work, was elected to the Academy of Medical Sciences of Croatia, the Croatian Society of Gastroenterology, the World Gastroenterology Association, and the Association of Croatian medical volunteers 1990–1991, and serves as the president of the Croatian Red Cross City Branch of Osijek

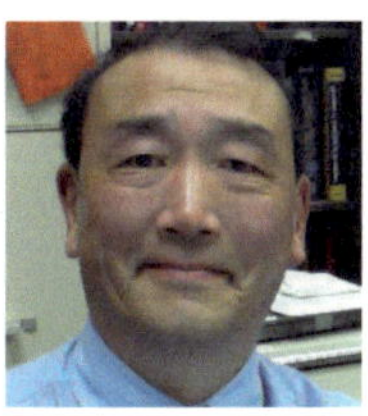

Dr. George Y. Wu has been a pioneer of targeted delivery of biological substances specifically to hepatocytes. He developed targeted gene delivery and mitochondria. He has received an American Gastroenterological Association/Industry Research Scholar Award, American Liver Foundation Research Prize, and AGA-Gastroenterology Research Group Young Scientist Award, and he was elected a fellow of the AGA and the American Association for the Study of Liver Diseases. He was elected to the American Society for Clinical Investigation and Association of American Physicians and was a Fulbright Specialist. He has published 170 articles, has edited 12 books, and is an editor in chief of the *Journal of Clinical and Translational Hepatology*.

Contents

Preface

Hepatitis C virus (HCV) is an important medical problem, affecting millions of people worldwide. HCV is one of the leading causes of chronic liver disease with one third of those affected eventually developing liver cirrhosis or hepatocellular carcinoma. Additionally, HCV infection is asymptomatic in the majority of cases, and people often do not receive necessary medical care as they are unaware of their infection. Worldwide, HCV-related complications are responsible for about 350,000 deaths annually.

In infected patients, interferon (IFN)-mediated immune response is associated with the induction of IFN-stimulated genes (ISGs) in the liver during the first 4–10 weeks of infection. To boost the immune response, in 1989, interferon alfa (IFN-α) was first developed, and in the decades that followed, IFN-α monotherapy was the standard therapy for hepatitis C virus. While developing the best regimen, various doses and durations of treatment were tested, but SVR rates remained modest (15–20%). Treatment efficacy has shown progressive improvement following the pegylation of IFN-α and its effect in combination with other antiviral drugs. Combining IFN-α with ribavirin (RBV) became the new standard therapy in 1998. However, viral escape mechanisms, IFN-α signaling in the liver, and substantial drug toxicity still restricted the efficacy of this treatment. The restricted efficacy of that treatment stimulated considerable research efforts of the academia and industry with the aim of understanding the mechanisms of nonresponse to IFN-based therapy.

In the past few years, remarkable progress has been made in our understanding of HCV biology, pathogenesis of infection, and structure-function relationships. This has led to interferon-free era, and direct-acting antivirals (DAAs) became a standard of care resulting in quantum advances in clinical efficacy and tolerability. Yet, in spite of this amazing progress, there remain obstacles to widespread successful treatment. These issues include biological failures even with direct-acting agents, lack of options for individual with organ failures, drug-drug interactions, access to medications either due to lack of availability or affordability, and psychiatric and social issues. These problems are likely to remain in the future. Therefore, this book has been created by distinguished faculties from around the world to address the progress in our understanding of HCV infection and to review new treatment options, limitations, and accessibility of new therapeutic options.

Assistant Professor Martina Smolić, MD, PhD
University of Osijek, Faculty of Medicine, Department of Pharmacology,
Osijek, Croatia

Professor Aleksandar Včev, MD, PhD
University of Osijek, Faculty of Medicine, Department of Medicine,
Osijek, Croatia

Professor George Y. Wu, MD, PhD
University of Connecticut Health Center, Department of Medicine,
Division of Gastroenterology and Hepatology,
Farmington, CT, USA

Section 1

The Era of Direct-Acting Antiviral HCV Therapies

Chapter 1

A Brief Update on the Treatment of Hepatitis C

Alyssa M. Austria, Vjera Ninčević and George Y. Wu

Additional information is available at the end of the chapter

http://dx.doi.org/10.5772/intechopen.70685

Abstract

Hepatitis C virus was discovered nearly 30 years ago, and for the first two decades, treatment was limited to agents with low response rates and substantial side effects. Since the introduction of direct-acting antivirals, there have been rapid advances made toward even higher sustained virologic responses (SVRs) and fewer side effects. This chapter provides a review of the newer agents for treatment of hepatitis C and highlights special populations, including those coinfected with HIV or hepatitis B, previously treated patients, and post-liver transplant patients.

Keywords: hepatitis C, direct-acting antivirals, protease inhibitors, HIV, hepatitis B

1. Introduction

Hepatitis C virus (HCV) infects approximately 185 million individuals worldwide and is the leading indication for liver transplant in the United States (US) [1]. In 2014, the centers for disease control and prevention (CDC) reported an estimated 30,500 new cases of HCV in the US, while the estimated number of chronic cases was approximately 2.7–3.9 million. HCV was first discovered in 1989, and there have been numerous advances in medical therapies available for the treatment and cure of HCV infection. Cure is defined as a sustained virologic response (SVR), which means undetectable levels of plasma HCV RNA for 12 or 24 weeks after completion of therapy.

The first agents available for treatment of HCV were the alfa interferons, which are immunomodulatory agents administered subcutaneously. The initial treatment regimen with interferon monotherapy resulted in SVR rates of only approximately 15% [2]. Ribavirin was subsequently added, which improved SVR rates to 33 and 41% for 24- and 48-week treatment regimens, respectively [3]. With the introduction of pegylated interferon (peg-IFN), SVR rates increased up to an estimated 50% [4]. Despite significant side effects, a suboptimal SVR rate, the need for prolonged therapy, and parenteral injections, Peg-IFN and ribavirin were the standard of care for over a decade.

The most recent development in treatment of HCV was the introduction of direct-acting antivirals (DAAs), which target various stages in the HCV life cycle. In 2014, an all-oral combination regimen was approved, and trials have demonstrated SVR rates approaching 100% [5–9]. With their unprecedented efficacy and improved tolerability, they have revolutionized the approach to treatment of chronic hepatitis C.

2. Direct-acting antivirals

2.1. First-generation NS3/4A protease inhibitors

The HCV RNA genome encodes a single polyprotein consisting of 3000 amino acids, which is cleaved by host and viral-encoded proteases to yield the functional structural and non-structural components of the virus [10]. The NS3/4A is composed of a serine protease (NS3) and cofactor (NS4A) and is involved in posttranslational processing or cleavage of the non-structural components at the NS3/NS4A, NS4A/NS4B, NS4B/NS5A, and NS5A/NS5B sites. The NS3/4A protease is essential to the processing of the HCV polypeptide and is critical for replication of the virus [10].

In 2011, boceprevir and telaprevir were the first DAAs, and the first NS3/4A inhibitors to be approved for the treatment of chronic hepatitis C, genotype 1. The mechanism of action is to inhibit the NS3/4A protease by forming a reversible covalent bond with the NS3/4A active site [11]. Both boceprevir and telaprevir were found to have significant side effects, including anemia and anemia plus rash, respectively [11]. In addition, their use was complicated by significant drug-drug interactions (both boceprevir and telaprevir are potent cytochrome p450 inhibitors), inconvenient dosing requiring multiple daily doses, and low barriers to resistance [11].

2.2. Second-generation protease inhibitors

A second generation of protease inhibitors was designed to contain macrocycles, or cyclic macromolecules, which resulted in improved antiviral potency [12]. Simeprevir was the first macrocyclic protease inhibitor to be approved for HCV treatment [13]. Simeprevir forms a noncovalent bond with the NS3/4A active site rather than the reversible covalent bond that boceprevir and telaprevir formed [14]. Paritaprevir is a protease inhibitor given in combination with three other medications (ombitasvir, paritaprevir, and dasabuvir), which comprise Viekira Pak, approved by the FDA in 2014 for HCV genotype 1. This was the second all-oral, interferon-free, fixed-dose combination for treatment of chronic HCV genotype 1 to be approved in the US [15]. Grazoprevir is another second-generation protease inhibitor that was FDA approved in 2016 in combination with an NS5A inhibitor [16]. Asunaprevir is a potent, selective NS3 protease inhibitor with activity against HCV genotypes 1, 4, 5, and 6 *in vitro* and is given in combination with daclatasvir, discussed in the next section [17]. Benefits of second-generation protease inhibitors include reduced dosing, improved side effect profiles, and fewer drug-drug interactions [18].

2.3. NS5A inhibitors

The NS5A phosphoprotein has no known enzymatic activity and its detailed function remains unclear [19]. NS5A inhibitors are thought to interact with NS5A and block formation of the "membranous web" that houses HCV RNA replication. They interfere with several functions of NS5A in the HCV life cycle, and disrupt the establishment of replication sites, which in turn prevents continued HVC RNA replication [19]. NS5A inhibitors include daclatasvir, ombitasvir, ledipasvir, elbasvir, and velpatasvir. Daclatasvir can be given in combination with sofosbuvir +/− RBV for the treatment of HCV genotypes 1–4. Ombitasvir is approved for treatment of genotype 1 in combination with paritaprevir, ritonavir, and dasabuvir. Ledipasvir is approved for genotypes 1, 3, and 4 in combination with sofosbuvir +/− RBV [20]. Velpatasvir in combination with sofosbuvir was approved in June 2016 by the FDA and became the first regimen approved for genotypes 1–6 [21].

2.4. Polymerase NS5B inhibitors

Polymerase inhibitors are another class of DAAs and are comprised of nucleoside analog and nonnucleoside analog inhibitors. Both types bind to the NS5B polymerase to terminate replication of the virus. The enzyme has a catalytic site for nucleoside binding and at least four other sites at which a nonnucleoside compound can bind and induce allosteric alterations in conformation [22].

Nucleoside analog inhibitors are incorporated into the HCV RNA chain and lead to direct chain termination. The advantage of this mechanism of action is that it is potentially active against all HCV genotypes, and the potential for viral resistance is low. This is because the NS5B active site has a low tolerance for amino acid substitutions. Any NS5B active site mutation that would potentially confer resistance to a polymerase inhibitor would likely also impair the RNA polymerase activity. Sofosbuvir is an example of a nucleoside analog inhibitor for use in treatment of HCV. It is given orally once a day, has pan-genotypic antiviral activity, and has a high barrier to viral resistance with no virologic breakthrough reported thus far [23].

Nonnucleoside analog inhibitors bind to discrete sites outside of the polymerase active center and induce a conformational protein change. Dasabuvir is an example of a nonnucleoside inhibitor of the NS5B polymerase [24].

In comparison with the nucleoside analog inhibitors, nonnucleoside polymerase inhibitors are more genotype-specific and have a lower barrier to resistance. This class of drugs is used in combination with other classes that are more potent with higher barriers to resistance.

2.5. Role of ribavirin in the era of direct-acting antivirals

Ribavirin was a critical component of hepatitis C treatment in the era of interferon-based therapy; however, its role in DAA regimens was initially unclear. At this time, guidelines do recommend the use of ribavirin in combination with DAAs, depending on genotype and presence or absence of cirrhosis. For example, there is evidence to support the use of ribavirin in specific situations, such as patients using sofosbuvir-based regimens who are either HCV genotype 1, treatment-experienced, and cirrhotic, or HCV genotype 3 with cirrhosis [25]. SVR rates tend to be lower among HCV genotype 3 patients with advanced liver disease (as low as 62% in patients with cirrhosis who were null responders to IFN-RBV therapy) [26]. In the ALLY-3+ study, ribavirin was investigated in combination with daclatasvir and sofosbuvir in patients who were HCV genotype 3, both treatment-naïve and treatment-experienced, and with advanced fibrosis or compensated cirrhosis. They achieved an overall SVR rate at 12 weeks of 90% [27]. These results, in combination with other studies, support the addition of ribavirin to achieve higher rates of SVR, allow shortening of treatment, and decrease the cost of treatment.

3. Treatment strategies

The ultimate goal of antiviral therapy for patients with chronic hepatitis C is achieving SVR. Refer to **Table 1** for additional terminology used to define treatment responses.

Monitoring viral levels during treatment with the new DAA regimens has minimal value, as the viral level is typically undetectable after 4 weeks of treatment. The more important assessment of virologic response is measuring the viral load at 12–24 weeks after therapy is completed or stopped.

When deciding on an appropriate DAA regimen, several factors must be taken into account, particularly HCV genotype, prior treatment history, stage of liver disease, presence of decompensation in patients with known cirrhosis, renal function, and other medications the patient is taking that could interact with the DAAs.

3.1. Treatment-naïve patients

Refer to **Table 2** for an overview of treatment regimens recommended based on American association for the study of liver diseases (AASLD) and infectious diseases society of America

Nonresponse	Detectable HCV RNA after 12 weeks of HCV therapy
Partial response	>2 log decline in HCV RNA but detectable HCV RNA after 12 weeks of HCV therapy
Null response	<2 log decline in HCV RNA after 12 weeks of HCV therapy
Viral breakthrough	Detectable HCV RNA after previously undetectable
Relapse	Undetectable HCV RNA on therapy with detectable HCV RNA after stopping therapy
Sustained virologic response	Undetectable HCV RNA 12 or 24 weeks after stopping therapy

Table 1. Definitions of treatment response to HCV treatment.

(IDSA) guidelines from April 2017. Compared to previous guidelines from July 2016, there is now a subcategory of patients who qualify for treatment of 8 weeks duration. Otherwise, the remainder of treatment regimens are all at least 12 weeks. This recommendation was based

Genotype 1a	Without cirrhosis	• Daily elbasvir/grazoprevir[*] • Daily ledipasvir/sofosbuvir[**] • Daily paritaprevir/ritonavir/ombitasvir plus twice-daily dosed dasabuvir with weight-based ribavirin • Daily simeprevir plus sofosbuvir • Daily sofosbuvir/velpatasvir • Daily daclatasvir and sofosbuvir
	With compensated cirrhosis	• Daily elbasvir/grazoprevir[*] • Daily ledipasvir/sofosbuvir • Daily sofosbuvir/velpatasvir
Genotype 1b	Without cirrhosis	• Daily elbasvir/grazoprevir • Daily ledipasvir/sofosbuvir[**] • Daily paritaprevir/ritonavir/ombitasvir plus twice-daily dosed dasabuvir • Daily simeprevir plus sofosbuvir • Daily sofosbuvir/velpatasvir • Daily daclatasvir plus sofosbuvir
	With compensated cirrhosis	• Daily elbasvir/grazoprevir • Daily ledipasvir/sofosbuvir • Daily paritaprevir/ritonavir/ombitasvir plus twice-daily dosed dasabuvir • Daily sofosbuvir/velpatasvir
Genotype 2	Without cirrhosis	• Daily sofosbuvir/velpatasvir
	With compensated cirrhosis	• Daily sofosbuvir/velpatasvir
Genotype 3	Without cirrhosis	• Daily daclatasvir plus sofosbuvir • Daily sofosbuvir/velpatasvir
	With compensated cirrhosis	• Daily sofosbuvir/velpatasvir • Daily daclatasvir plus sofosbuvir for 24 weeks with or without weight-based ribavirin
Genotype 4	Without cirrhosis	• Daily paritaprevir/ritonavir/ombitasvir and weight-based ribavirin • Daily sofosbuvir/velpatasvir • Daily elbasvir/grazoprevir • Daily ledipasvir/sofosbuvir
	With compensated cirrhosis	• Daily paritaprevir/ritonavir/ombitasvir and weight-based ribavirin • Daily sofosbuvir/velpatasvir • Daily elbasvir/grazoprevir • Daily ledipasvir/sofosbuvir
Genotype 5/6	With and without cirrhosis	• Daily sofosbuvir/velpatasvir • Daily ledipasvir/sofosbuvir

Dosing: elbasvir 50 mg, grazoprevir 100 mg, ledipasvir 90 mg, sofosbuvir 400 mg, paritaprevir 150 mg, ombitasvir 25 mg, dasabuvir 250 mg, simeprevir 150 mg, ritonavir 100 mg, velpatasvir 100 mg.[*]In whom no baseline NS5A RAVs for elbasvir are detected.

[**]For patients who are nonblack, HIV-uninfected, and whose HCV RNA level is <6 million IU/mL, treatment duration is 8 weeks.

Table 2. Regimens for treatment-naïve patients (dosing for 12 weeks unless specified).

on the ION-3 trial, which compared SVR rates in patients treated for 8 weeks versus 12 weeks and found no difference. However, relapse rates were higher in patients with certain characteristics. Thus, the recommendation of 8 weeks of treatment is indicated in patients with HCV genotype 1a/1b without cirrhosis who are nonblack, human immunodeficiency virus (HIV)-uninfected, and whose HCV RNA level is 6 million IU/mL.

3.2. FDA-approved regimens

While the direct-acting antivirals have been discussed up to this point as separate categories, it is clear based on the guidelines that most regimens include drugs from many categories. Pharmaceutical companies manufacture the drugs as combination pills, which makes dosing convenient.

Brand Name	Components	Year approved by FDA
Sovaldi	Sofosbuvir (NS5B)	2013
Harvoni	Ledipasvir (NS5A) Sofosbuvir (NS5B)	2014
Viekira Pak	Ombitasvir (NS5A) Paritaprevir (NS3/4A) Ritonavir (booster) Dasabuvir (NS5B)	2014
Technivie	Ombitasvir (NS5A) Paritaprevir (NS3/4A) Ritonavir (booster)	2015
Zepatier	Elbasvir (NS5A) Grazoprevir (NS3/4A)	2016
Epclusa	Sofosbuvir (NS5B) Elpatasvir (NS5A)	2016

Table 3. Hepatitis C treatment regimens and their components.

GT1	GT2	GT3	GT4	GT5	GT6
Harvoni[a]	Sovaldi/RBV	Sovaldi/Daklinza	Harvoni	Harvoni	Harvoni
Zepatier[f]	Peg-IFN/RBV[d]	Sovaldi/RBV[d]	PegIFN/Sovaldi/RBV		
Viekira +/− RBV[c]		Peg-IFN/RBV[e]	Technivie[b]		
Peg-IFN/Sovaldi/RBV			Zepatier		
Epclusa[g]	Epclusa	Epclusa	Epclusa	Epclusa	Epclusa

[a]Treatment experienced: 24-week course.

[b]Contraindicated in cirrhotics.

[c]Genotype 1a: add ribavirin, 12-week course; genotype 1a cirrhotics, add ribavirin, 24-week course.

[d]24-week course.

[e]48-week course.

[f]Genotype 1a with polymorphism: add ribavirin, 16-week course.

[g]Add ribavirin for Child-Pugh class B and C.

Table 4. FDA-approved regimens based on genotype (12-week course except where indicated).

Refer to **Table 3** for the brand names of hepatitis C treatment regimens and their components. **Table 4** provides the approved regimens based on the genotype.

4. Special populations

4.1. Coinfection with HIV

Approximately 10–30% of patients with human immunodeficiency virus (HIV) also have HCV [28], with a global prevalence estimated at 2.5–5 million people [29]. With the improved lifespan of HIV patients attributable to effective antiretroviral therapy, the focus is now shifting to treatment of concurrent infections that afflict HIV patients, with HCV-related liver complications being a leading non-HIV cause of death [30].

A meta-analysis study examined the survival benefit of achieving SVR, looking at a total of 33,360 patients with HCV and HIV/HCV coinfection [31]. Achieving HCV SVR was associated with a 50% reduction in the risk of all-cause mortality compared with not achieving SVR in the general HCV population. This result was markedly higher for the coinfected subgroup (79%), highlighting the importance and potential impact HCV cure has on patients also co-infected with HIV.

The *ION-4* study studied outcomes for patients with HIV/HCV coinfection that were given DAAs while on antiretroviral therapy for HIV [32]. There were 335 patients enrolled in the study, most of which were genotype 1 (98%). In addition, 55% of the patients were treatment experienced. They were administered ledipasvir and sofosbuvir (Harvoni). After 12 weeks of therapy, 96% were HCV RNA negative, and SVR rates of >94% were observed. None of the patients discontinued treatment due to adverse events.

Another DAA regimen combining elbasvir, an NS5A inhibitor, with grazoprevir, a second-generation NS3/4A protease inhibitor (Zepatier), was approved by the FDA for the treatment of chronic HCV genotypes 1 and 4, including those with HIV-1 coinfection. This indication was based on the C-EDGE CO-INFECTION study, which studied 218 patients with HIV/HCV coinfection who were treated with the elbasvir-grazoprevir combination [33]. Study results demonstrated an SVR rate of 96% at 12 weeks.

4.2. Coinfection with HBV

In the US, about 800,000–1.4 million people have chronic hepatitis B virus (HBV) infection. Around 2–10% of patients with chronic HCV are coinfected with HBV [34–36]. It has been shown that the presence of HBV coinfection with HCV accelerates the progression of liver damage, and is associated with a higher probability of liver cirrhosis and hepatic decompensation, higher incidence of hepatocellular carcinoma, and death [36, 37].

A potentially serious complication of stable HBV infections is the phenomenon of reactivation in which viral replication and liver damage suddenly increase. HBV reactivation can occur in patients who are hepatitis B surface antigen (HBsAg) (+), patients who have HBV DNA (+) active infection, or in patients with inactive infections, i.e., who are HBsAg (−), HBV DNA (−), but anti-HB virus core antibody (HBcAb) (+) and/or anti-HB virus surface antibody (HBsAb) (+) [38]. Reactivation can occur spontaneously, but more commonly occurs as a complication of medically induced changes in immune status. This has been clearly observed in patients with HBV infection who received antitumor necrosis factor (TNF) biologicals.

For this reason, the FDA has issued a black box warning concerning the risk of HBV reactivation in patients receiving anti-TNF and anti-CD20 monoclonal antibodies [39]. HBV reactivation has also been reported in patients with HBV/HCV coinfections treated with the combination of daclatasvir and asunaprevir. [40]. Accordingly, the FDA has issued a Drug Safety Communication about the risk of HBV reactivation in patients with current or previous infection who are to be treated with direct-acting antiviral (DAA) agents for HCV. The FDA is considering a boxed warning for nine DAAs in addition to Harvoni including Sovaldi, Viekira Pak, Viekira Pak XR, Daklinza, Epclusa, Olysio, Technivie, and Zepatier.

It is important that health-care professionals screen and monitor for HBV in all patients before initiating treatment with DAAs [41]. Coinfected HBV patients should receive anti-HBV therapy prior to and during anti-HCV treatment as prophylaxis against reactivation. Antiviral therapy started after HBV reactivation may not be effective to prevent hepatitis and/or hepatitis flares. The possible interaction of DAAs with some anti-HBV agents must also be considered [40, 42, 43].

4.3. Previously treated patients

There have been many studies that investigated retreatment strategies after lack of SVR with either an IFN-based regimen or an IFN-free regimen.

In the combination of simeprevir and sofosbuvir in HCV-infected patients (COSMOS) study (COSMOS) study trial, there were 80 HCV genotype 1 patients who were null responders to previous treatment with pegylated interferon and ribavirin. They were subsequently treated with simeprevir and sofosbuvir +/−ribavirin for 24 weeks, and achieved a mean SVR of 90%. In the ION-2 study, 440 HCV genotype 1 patients who were previously treated with an IFN-based regimen were given sofosbuvir + ledipasvir +/− RBV for 12–24 weeks, and achieved a SVR rate of greater than 94%.

In the retreatment of patients with genotype 1a and 1b who previously failed peg-interferon and ribavirin therapy, current guidelines recommend the same 12-week regimens used as initial treatment for genotype 1a and 1b patient without cirrhosis [44].

There have been a few small studies examining treatment failure with IFN-free regimens, and results have been promising, demonstrating that retreatment can successfully achieve SVR, by either prolonging the duration of treatment to 24 weeks or by adding ribavirin [45]. The retreatment regimen should include sofosbuvir with 1–3 other DAAs with different mechanisms of action.

4.4. Post-liver transplant patients

For patients with untreated recurrent hepatitis C after liver transplantation, disease progression is accelerated, with approximately 20% developing graft cirrhosis by 5 years posttransplantation [46]. DAA regimens have significantly improved SVR rates in post-transplant patients. The CORAL-I study looked at recurrent HCV genotype 1 infection in patients who had received liver transplants. These patients were treated with combination ombitasvir/paritaprevir/ritonavir plus dasabuvir with ribavirin for 24 weeks, and they achieved an SVR rate of 97% after 24 weeks of therapy [47].

5. Resistance to DAAs

NS5A inhibitors, NS3/4A protease inhibitors, and nonnucleoside polymerase inhibitors have low barriers to resistance. Prior to any antiviral treatment, resistance-associated variants (RAV) may preexist at varying frequencies and these variants may be selected rapidly during treatment with DAAs. However, with a few exceptions, HCV drug resistance testing is not recommended in naïve patients, because SVR rates were not affected by the presence of baseline NS3/4A or NS5A RAVs [45]. Moreover, the majority of treatment failures with DAAs are usually related to relapse rather than on-treatment viral breakthrough [48].

Although resistance testing is not routinely recommended for all DAAs at this time, it is an important focus of research because it could guide regimen choices if patients at high risk for treatment failure were identified early. However, there are many conditions to be met prior to the widespread use of HCV resistance testing including a standardized assay, interpretation and reporting of the data [45].

At this time, these criteria have not been met. As discussed above, not all RAVs are clinically significant, and the level of resistance conferred by a preexisting RAV needs to be further delineated.

6. Barriers to treatment

With the recent success of DAA regimens and their exceptional SVR rates demonstrated in most recent trials, the prospect of eradicating HCV infection seems near. However, there still exist multiple barriers to treatment. The most obvious barrier is the high cost associated with treatment.

Drug pricing is impacted by many factors, including market competition, presence of generic versions, existing prices of effective treatment, and business negotiations. There is very little transparency in the process, particularly in the negotiations between pharmaceutical companies and payers. However, the basis for negotiation starts with a list price set by the pharmaceutical company, called the Wholesale Acquisition Cost (WAC). Refer to **Table 5** for the wholesale acquisition costs of the current HCV regimens on the market.

In the US, sofosbuvir was approved in 2013, and the WAC was set at $84,000 for a 12-week course of treatment [49]. The more recent development of market competition has created opportunity for greater discounts and rebates. When Viekira Pak (ombitasvir/paritaprevir/ritonavir + dasabuvir)

Direct-acting antiviral	Pharmaceutical company	WAC for 12-week course
Sofosbuvir (Sovaldi)	Gilead sciences	$84,000
Ledipasvir/Sofosbuvir (Harvoni)	Gilead sciences	$94,500
Ombitasvir/paritaprevir/ritonavir + Dasabuvir (Viekira Pak)	AbbVie	$83,319
Daclatasvir (Daklinza) + Sofosbuvir (Sovaldi)	Bristol-Myers Squibb and Gilead	$147,000
Grazoprevir/Elbasvir (Zepatier)	Merck	$54,600
Sofosbuvir/Velpatasvir (Epclusa)	Gilead sciences	$74,760

Table 5. Wholesale Acquisition Cost of direct-acting antivirals.

was approved, it was made available for $51,000–$66,000 [50]. Currently, 80% of the market is exclusive to either Harvoni (Ledipasvir/Sofosbuvir) or Viekira Pak, and the average negotiated discount is 46% off of the WAC [51].

Until DAAs become widely affordable, there will be restrictions, and priority will be given to those who have failed previous IFN-based therapies with evidence of disease progression, patients ineligible for IFN-based therapy with progressive disease, patients with established cirrhosis, patients on the liver transplant waiting list, and those who have had a liver transplant.

7. Conclusions

This is a pivotal time in which there have been major advances in the treatment of hepatitis C. Patients have the option of an all-oral regimen with high tolerability and convenient dosing. With SVR nearing 100%, the prospect of limiting HCV treatment failures appears to be promising. It is important to recognize the potential of these current regimens and minimize the emergence of resistant HCV. Avoidance of development of drug resistant virus is best achieved by using HCV regimens that incorporate agents with different mechanisms of action. Some strides have been made in accessibility and affordability, but there remains a large proportion of HCV-infected patients for which treatment needs to be made available prior to disease progression. Finally, there needs to be continued screening and education to reduce the prevalence.

Author details

Alyssa M. Austria[1], Vjera Ninčević[2] and George Y. Wu[2*]

*Address all correspondence to: wu@uchc.edu

1 Department of Medicine, UConn Health, Farmington, USA

2 Department of Medicine, Division of Gastroenterology-Hepatology, UConn Health, Farmington, USA

References

[1] Mohd HK, Groeger J, Flaxman AD, Wiersma ST. Global epidemiology of hepatitis C virus infection: New estimates of age-specific antibody to HCV seroprevalence. Hepatology. 2013;**57**(4):1333-1342

[2] Di Bisceglie AM, Martin P, Kassianides C, Lisker-Melman M, Murray L, Waggoner J, Goodman Z, Banks SM, Hoofnagle JH. Recombinant interferon alfa therapy for chronic hepatitis C. A randomized, double-blind, placebo-controlled trial. The New England Journal of Medicine. November 1989;**321**(22):1506-1510

[3] Poynard T, Marcellin P, Lee SS, Niederau C, Minuk GS, Ideo G, Bain V, Heathcote J, Zeuzem S, Trepo C, Albrecht J. Randomised trial of interferon alpha2b plus ribavirin for 48 weeks or for 24 weeks versus interferon alpha2b plus placebo for 48 weeks for treatment of chronic infection with hepatitis C virus. International Hepatitis Interventional Therapy Group (IHIT). Lancet. October 1998;**352**(9138):1426-1432

[4] Manns MP, McHutchison JG, Gordon SC, Rustgi VK, Shiffman M, Reindollar R, Goodman ZD, Koury K, Ling M, Albrecht JK. Peginterferon alfa-2b plus ribavirin compared with interferon alfa-2b plus ribavirin for initial treatment of chronic hepatitis C: A randomised trial. Lancet. September 2001;**358**(9286):958-965

[5] Afdhal N, Reddy KR, Nelson DR, Lawitz E, Gordon SC, Schiff E, Nahass R, Ghalib R, Gitlin N, Herring R, et al. Ledipasvir and sofosbuvir for previously treated HCV genotype 1 infection. New England Journal of Medicine. 2014;**370**:1483-1493

[6] Afdhal N, Zeuzem S, Kwo P, Chojkier M, Gitlin N, Puoti M, Romero-Gomez M, Zarski JP, Agarwal K, Buggisch P, et al. Ledipasvir and sofosbuvir for untreated HCV genotype 1 infection. New England Journal of Medicine. 2014;**370**:1889-1898

[7] Kowdley KV, Gordon SC, Reddy KR, Rossaro L, Bernstein DE, Lawitz E, Shiffman ML, Schiff E, Ghalib R, Ryan M, et al. Ledipasvir and sofosbuvir for 8 or 12 weeks for chronic HCV without cirrhosis. New England Journal of Medicine. 2014;**370**:1879-1888

[8] Andreone P, Colombo MG, Enejosa JV, Koksal I, Ferenci P, Maieron A, Müllhaupt B, Horsmans Y, Weiland O, Reesink HW, et al. ABT-450, ritonavir, ombitasvir, and dasabuvir achieves 97% and 100% sustained virologic response with or without ribavirin in treatment-experienced patients with HCV genotype 1b infection. Gastroenterology. 2014;**147**:359-365

[9] Ferenci P, Bernstein D, Lalezari J, Cohen D, Luo Y, Cooper C, Tam E, Marinho RT, Tsai N, Nyberg A, et al. ABT-450/r-ombitasvir and dasabuvir with or without ribavirin for HCV. New England Journal of Medicine. 2014;**370**:1983-1992

[10] Hazuda DJ, Burroughs M, Howe AY, Wahl J, Venkatraman S. Development of boceprevir: A first-in-class direct antiviral treatment for chronic hepatitis C infection. Annals of the New York Academy of Sciences. July 2013;**1291**:69-76

[11] Ara AK, Paul JP. New direct-acting antiviral therapies for treatment of chronic hpatitis C virus. Gastroenterology and Hematology. July 2015;**11**(7):458-466

[12] McGivern DR, Masaki T, Lovel W, Hamlett C, Saalau-Bethell S, Graham B. Protease inhibitors block multiple functions of the NS3/4A protease-helicase during the hepatitis C virus life cycle. Journal of Virology. May 2015;**89**(10):5362-5370

[13] Rosenquist A, Samuelsson B, Johansson PO, Cummings MD, Lenz O, Raboisson P, Simmen K, Vendeville S, de Kock H, Nilsson M, Horvath A, Kalmeijer R, de la Rosa G, Beumont-Mauviel M. Discovery and development of simeprevir (TMC435), a HCV NS3/4A protease inhibitor. Journal of Medicinal Chemistry. 2014;**57**:1673-1693

[14] Tsantrizos YS. TMC-435, an NS3/4A protease inhibitor for the treatment of HCV infection. Current Opinion in Investigational Drugs. 2009;**10**(8):871-881

[15] Abramowicz M, Zuccotti G, Pflomm JM. A 4-drug combination (Viekira Pak) for hepatitis C. Journal of the American Medical Association. 2015;**313**(18):1857-1858

[16] Bell AM, Wagner JL, Barber KE, Stover KR. Elbasvir/grazoprevir: A review of the latest agent in the fight against hepatitis C. International Journal of Hepatology. 2016;**2016**:3852126

[17] McPhee F, Sheaffer AK, Friborg J, Hernandez D, Falk P, Zhai G, et al. Preclinical profile and characterization of the hepatitis C virus NS3 protease inhibitor asunaprevir (BMS-650032). Antimicrobial Agents and Chemotherapy. 2012;**56**:5387-5396

[18] Marks KM, Jacobson IM. The first wave: HCV NS3 protease inhibitors telaprevir and boceprevir. Antiviral Therapy. 2012;**17**:1119-1131

[19] Eyre NS, Beard MR. HCV NS5A inhibitors disrupt replication factory formation: A novel mechanism of action. Gastroenterology. 2014;**147**(5):959-962

[20] Seifert LL, Perumpail RB, Ahmed A. Update on hepatitis C: Direct-acting antivirals. World Journal of Hepatology. December 2015;**7**(28):2829-2833

[21] FDA Approves Epclusa for Treatment of Chronic Hepatitis C Virus Infection. U.S. Food & Drug Administration; June 2016

[22] Membreno FE, Lawitz EJ. The HCV NS5B nucleoside and non-nucleoside inhibitors. Clinics of Liver Disease. 2011;**15**:611-626

[23] Kamal S. Pharmacogenetics of hepatitis C: Transition from interferon-based therapies to direct-acting antiviral agents. Hepatic Medicine: Evidence and Research. 2014;**6**:61-77

[24] Kati W, Koev G, Irvin M, Liu Y, et al. In vitro activity and resistance profile of dasabuvir, a non-nucleoside hepatitis C virus polymerase inhibitor. American Society for Microbiology: Antimicrobial Agents and Chemotherapy. March 2015;**59**(3):1505-1511

[25] Hezode C, Bronowicki JP. Ideal oral combinations to eradicate HCV: The role of ribavirin. Journal of Hepatology. 2016;**64**:215-225

[26] Zeuzem S, Dusheiko GM, Salupere R, Mangia A, Flisiak R, Hyland RH, Illeperuma A, Svarovskaia E, Brainard DM, Symonds WT, Subramanian GM, McHutchison JG, Weiland O, Reesink HW, Ferenci P, Hézode C, Esteban R, VALENCE investigators.

Sofosbuvir and ribavirin in HCV genotypes 2 and 3. New England Journal of Medicine. May 2014;**370**(21):1993-2001

[27] Leroy V, Angus P, Bronowicki J-P, et al. Daclatasvir, sofosbuvir, and ribavirin for hepatitis C virus genotype 3 and advanced liver disease: A randomized phase III study (ALLY-3+). Hepatology. 2016;**63**(5):1430-1441

[28] Sherman KE, Rouster SD, Chung RT, Rajicic N. Hepatitis C virus prevalence among patients infected with human immunodeficiency virus: A cross-sectional analysis of the US adult AIDS Clinical Trials Group. Clinical Infectious Diseases. 2002;**34**:831-837

[29] Alter MJ. Epidemiology of viral hepatitis and HIV co-infection. Journal of Hepatology. 2006;**44**:S6-S9

[30] Morlat P, Roussillon C, Henard S. Causes of death among HIV-infected patients in France in 2010 (national survey): Trends since 2000. AIDS. 2015;**28**:1181-1191

[31] Simmons B, Saleem J, Heath K, Cooke GS, Hill A. Long-term treatment outcomes of patients infected with hepatitis C virus: A systematic review and meta-analysis of the survival benefit of achieving a sustained virological response. Clinical Infectious Diseases. September 2015;**61**(5):730-740

[32] Naggie S, Cooper C, Saag M. Ledipasvir and sofosbuvir for HCV in patients co-infected with HIV-1. New England Journal of Medicine. 2015;**373**:705-713

[33] Rockstroh JK, Nelson M, Katlama C. Efficacy and safety of grazoprevir (MK-5172) and elbasvir (MK-8742) in patients with hepatitis C virus and HIV co-infection (C-EDGE CO-INFECTION): A non-randomised, open-label trial. Lancet HIV. 2015;**2**:e319-e327

[34] Bini EJ, Perumalswami PV. Hepatitis B virus infection among American patients with chronic hepatitis C virus infection: Prevalence, racial/ethnic differences, and viral interactions. Hepatology. 2010;**51**(3):759-766

[35] Saravanan S, Velu V, Nandakumar S, et al. Hepatitis B virus and hepatitis C virus dual infection among patients with chronic liver disease. Journal of Microbiology, Immunology and Infection. 2009;**42**(2):122-128

[36] Chu CJ, Lee SD. Hepatitis B virus/hepatitis C virus coinfection: Epidemiology, clinical features, viral interactions and treatment. Journal of Gastroenterology and Hepatology. April 2008;**23**(4):512-520

[37] Gupta S, Govindarajan S, Fong TL, Redeker AG. Spontaneous reactivation in chronic hepatitis B: Patterns and natural history. Journal of Clinical Gastroenterology. 1990;**12**:562-568

[38] Fukuda W, Hanyu T, Katayama M, Mizuki S, Okada A, Miyata M, Handa Y, Hayashi M, Koyama Y, et al. Incidence of hepatitis B virus reactivation in patients with resolved infection on immunosuppressive therapy for rheumatic disease: A multicentre, prospective, observational study in Japan. Annals of the Rheumatic Diseases. December 2016;

[39] Mitka M. FDA: Increased HBV reactivation risk with ofatumumab or rituximab. The Journal of the American Medical Association. 2013;**310**:1664

[40] Takayama H, Sato T, Ikeda F, Fujiki S. Reactivation of hepatitis B virus during interferon-free therapy with daclatasvir and asunaprevir in patient with hepatitis B virus/hepatitis C virus co-infection. Hepatology Research. 2016;**46**:489-491

[41] FDA Drug Safety Communication: FDA Warns about the Risk of Hepatitis B Reactivating in Some Patients Treated with Direct-Acting Antivirals for Hepatitis C. Safety Announcement [Internet]. 2016. Available from: http://www.fda.gov/Drugs/DrugSafety/ucm522932.htm. [Accessed: 17 December 2016]

[42] Hsu C, Tsou HH, Lin SJ, Wang MC, Yao M, Hwang WL, et al. Chemotherapy-induced hepatitis B reactivation in lymphoma patients with resolved HBV infection: A prospective study. Hepatology. 2014;**59**:2092-2100

[43] Madonia S, Orlando E, Madonia G, Cannizzaro M. HCV/HBV coinfection: The dark side of DAAs treatment? Letter to the Editor. December 2016

[44] AASLD/IDSA. Recommendations for Testing, Management, and Treating Hepatitis C. Retreatment of Persons in Whom Prior Therapy has Failed.

[45] Pawlotsky J. Hepatitis C virus resistance to direct-acting antiviral drugs in interferon-free regimens. Gastroenterology. 2016;**151**:70-86

[46] Berenguer M, Ferrell L, Watson J, Prieto M, Kim M, Rayón M, Córdoba J, Herola A, Ascher N, Mir J, Berenguer J, Wright TL. HCV-related fibrosis progression following liver transplantation: Increase in recent years. Journal of Hepatology. April 2000;**32**(4):673-684

[47] Kwo PY, Mantry PS, Coakley E, Te HS, Vargas HE, Brown R Jr, Gordon F, Levitsky J, Terrault NA, Burton JR Jr, Xie W, Setze C, Badri P, Pilot-Matias T, Vilchez RA, Forns X. An interferon-free antiviral regimen for HCV after liver transplantation. New England Journal of Medicine. December 2014;**371**(25):2375-2382

[48] Buti M, Riveiro-Barciela M, Esteban F. Management of direct-acting antiviral agent failures. Journal of Hepatology. December 2015;**63**(6):1511-1522

[49] Rosenthal ES, Graham CS. Price and affordability of direct-acting antiviral regimens for hepatitis C virus in the United States. Infectious Agents and Cancer. 2016;**11**:24

[50] Pollack A. Sales of Sovaldi, New Gilead Hepatitis C Drug, Soar to $10.3 Billion. NYC, NY: The New York Times; 2015

[51] Silverman E. What the 'Shocking' Gilead Discounts on its Hepatitis C Drugs Will Mean. NYC, NY: The Wall Street Journal; 2015

Chapter 2

Hepatitis C Virus (HCV) Treatment in Croatia: Recent Advances and Ongoing Obstacles

Marko Duvnjak, Nina Blažević and
Lucija Virović Jukić

Additional information is available at the end of the chapter

http://dx.doi.org/10.5772/intechopen.70440

Abstract

The prevalence of hepatitis C virus (HCV) antibodies in Croatia is low in the general population (reported <1%), similar to the prevalence rates of many European countries, but is higher in the populations at risk, especially among intravenous drug users. With the development of new classes of direct-acting antiviral agents and interferon-free regimens, the landscape of HCV treatment has completely changed. Management of HCV infection in Croatia is in accordance with the European Association for the Study of the Liver (EASL) recommendations published in 2015, recently updated Croatian Guidelines (published in April 2016) and the recommendations of Croatian Health Insurance Fund (HZZO) which covers the costs of treatment. HZZO approved simeprevir at the beginning of 2015. By the end of the 2015 sofosbuvir, combination of sofosbuvir + ledipasvir and the combination of ombitasvir, paritaprevir and ritonavir ± dasabuvir became available. Although the drawback of these new highly effective treatments is their price, prioritization of patients on a national level offers equal opportunities to patients in need for treatment. Due to improvements in therapy and prevention, clinical care for patients with HCV in Croatia advanced significantly during the last two years.

Keywords: hepatitis C virus, Croatia, epidemiology, treatment, direct-acting antivirals (DAAs)

1. Introduction

The prevalence of hepatitis C virus (HCV) antibodies in Croatia is low in the general population (reported <1%). HCV seroprevalence in the Croatian adult general population is similar to the prevalence rates of many European countries (for example Spain, France, Belgium,

Poland, and Bulgaria) [1–5]. In comparison with other European countries, there have also been changes in the HCV epidemiology in Croatia over the past few decades. According to the published data, the estimated number of HCV-infected patients in Croatia is around 39,000, although the experts' opinion is that the real numbers are significantly smaller [6, 7]. There was no significant difference in the HCV seropositivity between males and females in the Croatian population, with the highest prevalence in the 30–39 age group (1.7%) [8]. Routine HCV screening of blood products was introduced in Croatia in 1992.

The prevalence of HCV infection in some population groups in Croatia is shown in **Table 1** [9–21]. Patients requiring multiple transfusions have a high prevalence of HCV infection, but with the implementation of mandatory anti-HCV and HCV RNA screening of blood/blood donations, the risk of transfusion-associated hepatitis C has virtually been eliminated. [22]. HCV seroprevalence in the Croatian pregnant women is comparable to data reported in Switzerland and Spain [23, 24]. In this population, injecting drug users (IDU), history of blood products transfusion before 1992 and hospitalization with surgical procedures were identified as most common risk factors [25]. Since blood donors represent a strictly controlled group, it is expected that the HCV prevalence is lower than in the general population [26]. There are no published data on the HCV prevalence in the Croatian healthcare workers who have sustained contaminated needle stick injuries (occupationally exposed groups) [27].

Population group	Prevalence of HCV infection in Croatia
General population	<1%
Injecting drug users (IDUs)	40%
Prison populations	8–44%
Human immunodeficiency virus-infected patients	15%
Persons with high-risk sexual behavior	4.6%
Alcohol abusers	2.4%
Pregnant women	0.5–1.5%
Pregnant IDUs	40–50%
Hemodialysis patients	2.3–3.2%
Children and adolescents	0.3%
First-time blood donors	0.1%
Healthcare workers (occupationally exposed groups)	No published data

Table 1. Prevalence of HCV infection in Croatia in different population groups.

Prevalence of HCV genotypes in Croatia varies by different population groups and regions. The prevalence of genotypes in Croatian population is shown in **Table 2**. In the general population, genotype 1 is the most widely distributed, while genotype 3 is predominant among IDUs. The most commonly detected subtype is 1b and it is predominant in hemodialysis patients. In prison population, genotype 1 and 3 are equally distributed and similar genotype distribution is found in groups with high-risk sexual behavior [28–31]. Similar pattern of genotype distribution is found in other European countries, where genotypes 1 and 3 also account for the majority of HCV infections with the most frequent subtype 1b [32]. The prevalence of genotype 4 is rising in Europe (in countries such as France, Germany, Greece, Italy, Poland, Portugal, Spain, Sweden, and Switzerland) due to immigration in these areas [33].

HCV genotype	Prevalence
Genotype 1	60.4–79.8%
Genotype 1, subtype 1b	41.6%
Genotype 3	12.9–47.9%
Genotype 3 (IDUs)	60.5–83.9%

Table 2. Prevalence of HCV genotypes in Croatia.

2. Indications for treatment in Europe and Croatia

Following new trends in the management of viral hepatitis, an expert panel held the first Croatian Consensus Conferences on Viral Hepatitis in 2005, and later in 2009 and 2013. With the development of new classes of direct-acting antiviral agents (DAAs) and interferon-free regimens, the landscape of HCV treatment has significantly changed. The European Association for the Study of the Liver (EASL) published its recommendations in 2015, with the latest update in September 2016, and the World Health Organization in May 2016 adopted the first-ever Global Health Sector Strategy on viral hepatitis with the longer-term aim to reduce new viral hepatitis infection by 90% by 2030. Management of HCV infection in Croatia is in accordance with the EASL Guidelines published in 2015, Croatian Guidelines (published by the Croatian Referral Centre for the Diagnostics and Treatment of Viral Hepatitis at University Hospital for Infectious diseases 'Dr. Fran Mihaljević' and updated in April 2016), and the recommendations of the Croatian Health Insurance Fund (HZZO) which covers the costs of treatment for all patients in accordance with the recommended guidelines. These recommendations are based on currently licensed drugs and updated regularly, following approval of new drug regimens.

There are some differences comparing EASL and Croatian Guidelines, which are listed as following. According to EASL Guidelines from 2015 and Croatian Guidelines, treatment should be prioritized (considered without delay) in patients with significant fibrosis or cirrhosis (METAVIR Score F3 or F4), including decompensated (Child-Pugh B or C) cirrhosis, in patients with clinically significant extra-hepatic manifestations, in patients with HCV recurrence after liver transplantation, and in HBV/HIV-coinfected patients (not in latest EASL Guidelines in 2016). Compared with EASL Guidelines, in Croatia, treatment is also prioritized in patients before or after solid organ transplantation and justified for individuals at risk of transmitting HCV (IDU, men who have sex with men with high-risk sexual practices, women of child bearing age who wish to get pregnant, hemodialysis patients, and incarcerated patients); in EASL Guidelines, they are in prioritized category. In Croatia, treatment is justified in patients with moderate cirrhosis (METAVIR F2) and in patients with long disease duration (>20 years), regardless of fibrosis (not in EASL recommendations; indication of moderate cirrhosis was in previous EASL recommendations from 2015.). Treatment can be deferred in Croatian patients (not in EASL Guidelines) with no or mild disease (METAVIR Score F0 and F1) and in patients with none of the clinically significant extra-hepatic manifestations. The latest EASL recommendations from 2016 (not in Croatian Guidelines) say that treatment should be considered without delay in patients with significant fibrosis or cirrhosis (METAVIR score F2, F3, or F4), including decompensated (Child-Pugh B or C) cirrhosis, in patients with clinically significant extra-hepatic manifestations (e.g., symptomatic vasculitis associated with HCV-related mixed cryoglobulinemia, HCV immune complex-related nephropathy, and non-Hodgkin B cell lymphoma), in patients with HCV recurrence after liver transplantation, and in individuals at risk of transmitting HCV (active injection drug users, men who have sex with men with high-risk sexual practices, women of child-bearing age who wish to get pregnant, hemodialysis patients, and incarcerated individuals). In all recommendations, treatment is not recommended in patients with limited life expectancy due to non-liver-related comorbidities [34–38].

3. Therapeutic protocol

The goal of therapy is to cure HCV infection to prevent hepatic cirrhosis, decompensation of cirrhosis, hepatocellular carcinoma, severe extrahepatic manifestations, and death. The endpoint of therapy is undetectable HCV RNA in blood by a sensitive assay 12 weeks (SVR12—sustained virologic response) and/or 24 weeks (SVR24) after the end of treatment [37].

For decision-making related to therapies/drug selection, various factors are important: age, duration of infection, stage of fibrosis/cirrhosis, response to previous antiviral therapy, extrahepatic manifestations, comorbidities (HBV/HIV coinfection, autoimmune disease), concomitant therapy, genotype (1, 2, 3, 4), subgenotype (1a, 1b), HCV RNA viral load, presence of mutations that confer resistance to certain antiviral drugs and IL-28B genotype (CC, CT, TT) if interferon-based therapies are being considered.

With the introduction of the first two protease inhibitors (PI) in 2011, the new era of HCV therapy began. Boceprevir and telaprevir as the first-generation of oral direct-acting antiviral agents (DAAs) became available in Croatia in 2013, for the treatment of genotype 1 HCV patients who failed PegIFN and ribavirin therapy.

Croatia is a member of the European Union and all drugs registered by European Medicines Agency are also approved for use in Croatia. Available drugs for the treatment of HCV in Croatia (with costs covered directly by Croatian Health Insurance Fund—HZZO) in 2016 are: PegIFN, ribavirin, simeprevir, sofosbuvir, combination of ombitasvir + ritonavir-boosted paritaprevir ± dasabuvir, and sofosbuvir + ledipasvir. In the European Union, there are some drugs that are not yet available in Croatia: velpatasvir, daclatasvir, grazoprevir, and elbatasvir.

Croatian Guidelines for the treatment are based on EASL and AASLD recommendations, but are somewhat more restrictive. For the treatment of naive patients with genotype 1 in 2016, it was still recommended to use the combination therapy with PegIFN and ribavirin (24–48 weeks) for patients with mild fibrosis and favorable predictors of response. For those patients with unfavorable predictors, if they achieve rapid virologic response (RVR), standard PegIFN and ribavirin combination is also recommended, otherwise a protease inhibitor (PI)—simeprevir or sofosbuvir should be added. In those with advanced fibrosis (F3), simeprevir or sofosbuvir should be added to PegIFN + ribavirin. Patients with significant (F4) fibrosis, who have contraindications to IFN therapy, presence of extrahepatic manifestations, HIV-coinfection or in transplanted patients, IFN-free regimens should be used for 12 weeks (ombitasvir, ritonavir-boosted paritaprevir, dasabuvir ± ribavirin; sofosbuvir and ledipasvir ± ribavirin; sofosbuvir and simeprevir ± ribavirin). For patients with decompensated cirrhosis, the combination of sofosbuvir and ledipasvir with or without ribavirin should be used, which is the same as recommended by the EASL and AASLD Guidelines. The main difference to EASL Guidelines is that, according to EASL, naive patients with or without compensated cirrhosis are treated with fixed-dose combination of sofosbuvir and ledipasvir without ribavirin.

For the treatment of experienced patients with genotype 1, triple combination of PegIFN, ribavirin, and a PI (simeprevir or sofosbuvir) is recommended in those with previous relapse or partial response (F1-F3 fibrosis). For nonresponders to PegIFN-ribavirin treatment (regardless of fibrosis) and for patients with F4 fibrosis (regardless of type of response), as well as for patients with TT IL-28B genotype, contraindications to IFN therapy, presence of extrahepatic manifestations, HIV-coinfection and transplanted patients, IFN-free regimens are offered (previously mentioned for treatment of naive patients). For patients with decompensated cirrhosis, the only treatment option currently available is the combination of sofosbuvir and ledipasvir with ribavirin for 12 weeks or without ribavirin for 24 weeks. This is also the only available option for patients previously treated with the triple combination of PegIFN + ribavirin + first-generation PIs (boceprevir or telaprevir) (in Croatia, there are only a few patients that have not responded to treatment with new-generation DAAs, as they have recently become available). According to EASL, experienced, DAA-naive patients with genotype 1b with or without compensated cirrhosis should be treated with fixed-dose combination of sofosbuvir and ledipasvir without ribavirin, and with ribavirin in those patients with genotype 1a. In EASL Guidelines, for the treatment of naive and experienced patients with genotype 1, there are two more options (not available in Croatia): fixed-dose combination of sofosbuvir and velpatasvir without ribavirin, ritonavir-boosted paritaprevir, ombitasvir and dasabuvir with or without ribavirin, grazoprevir and elbasvir with or without ribavirin, and sofosbuvir and daclatasvir with or without ribavirin.

For the treatment of patients with genotype 4, the same recommendations as for genotype 1 apply, with the exception of fixed combination of ombitasvir, paritaprevir, and ritonavir, which is used without dasabuvir. In patients with cirrhosis, duration of treatment is 24 weeks.

In EASL Guidelines, for the treatment of these patients, there are few more options available: sofosbuvir and velpatasvir without ribavirin, grazoprevir and elbasvir with or without ribavirin, and sofosbuvir and daclatasvir with or without ribavirin.

For the treatment of naive patients with genotype 2, with F1-F3 fibrosis, the use of standard combination treatment with PegIFN and ribavirin for 24 weeks is still recommended. Naive patients with F4 fibrosis, nonresponders (regardless of fibrosis), patients with contraindications to IFN therapy, with presence of extrahepatic manifestations, HIV-coinfection and transplanted patients are treated with combination of sofosbuvir and ribavirin (12 weeks without cirrhosis and 16–20 weeks with cirrhosis). In EASL recommendations, for the treatment of these patients there are two options: sofosbuvir and velpatasvir without ribavirin and sofosbuvir and daclatasvir without ribavirin.

For the treatment of naive patients with genotype 3, with F1-F3 fibrosis, it is still recommended to use PegIFN and ribavirin for 24 weeks. Naive patients with F4 fibrosis and nonresponders to PegIFN + ribavirin therapy (regardless of fibrosis) are treated with combination of sofosbuvir, PegIFN, and ribavirin for 12 weeks. Patients with F1-F3 fibrosis and with contraindication to IFN therapy are treated with combination of sofosbuvir and ribavirin for 24 weeks. Those patients with F4 fibrosis and with contraindication to IFN therapy are treated with combination of sofosbuvir and daclatasvir for 12 weeks or combination of sofosbuvir, ledipasvir, and ribavirin for 24 weeks. In EASL Guidelines, for treatment of naive and experienced patients there are two options: sofosbuvir and velpatasvir with or without ribavirin and sofosbuvir and daclatasvir with or without ribavirin [37, 38].

4. Croatian Health Insurance Fund (HZZO)—reimbursement requirements

Croatian Health Insurance Fund (HZZO) is covering over 99% of the population. HCV treatments are funded from a separate budget for expensive medicines [39]. HZZO has listed conditions that patients have to fulfill in order for HCV treatment to be covered from the before-mentioned fund: age between 18 and 70 years, HCV RNA positive, with a specified genotype, histologic evidence of chronic inflammation (biopsy finding) or fibroscan result larger than 8 kPa, and abstinence of IDU and significant alcohol consumption for the past 12 months. In patients with normal alanine aminotransferase (ALT) level, treatment is indicated with fibrosis $F \geq 2$ or fibroscan finding >8 kPa. Patients who are IDUs need to have evidence of abstinence from illegal substances for at least one year and documented psychiatrist's finding and results of toxicology testing every 3 months during medical treatment. Treatment reimbursement requirements in Croatia include: specialist recommendation for treatment, Hospital's drug committee approval, and request for treatment sent to Expert committee for the treatment of hepatitis C of HZZO for final approval of treatment modality and duration (respect priorities among patients). All other Croatian patients with chronic hepatitis C (not fulfilling the above-mentioned requirements) can also be treated based on the judgment of the treating physician, but with a more restricted reimbursement options.

http://dx.doi.org/10.5772/intechopen.70440

5. Conclusion

Regarding improvements in therapy and prevention, clinical care for patients with HCV in Croatia has advanced significantly during the past two years. Comparing epidemiology, indications for the treatment, available drugs, and therapeutic protocols, it is clear that Croatia accompanies European trends in HCV treatment. In future, rapid changes in the treatment of chronic HCV infection with the innovation of new drugs will lead to more effective, shorter treatment courses and PegIFN-free modalities.

Author details

Marko Duvnjak[1,2]*, Nina Blažević[1] and Lucija Virović Jukić[1,2]

*Address all correspondence to: marko.duvnjak1@gmail.com

1 Division of Gastroenterology and Hepatology, Department of Internal Medicine, Sestre Milosrdnice University Hospital Center, Zagreb, Croatia

2 University of Zagreb School of Medicine, Zagreb, Croatia

References

[1] Muñoz-Gámez JA, Salmerón J. Prevalence of hepatitis B and C in Spain – further data are needed. Revista Española de Enfermedades Digestivas. 2013;105:245-248

[2] Meffre C, Le Strat Y, Delarocque-Astagneau E, et al. Prevalence of hepatitis B and hepatitis C virus infections in France in 2004: Social factors are important predictors after adjusting for known risk factors. Journal of Medical Virology. 2010;82:546-555

[3] Van Damme P, Thyssen A, Van Loock F. Epidemiology of hepatitis C in Belgium: Present and future. Acta Gastro-Enterologica Belgica. 2002;65:78-79

[4] Gańczak M, Szych Z. Rationale against preoperative screening for HIV in Polish hospitals: A prevalence study of anti-HIV in contrast to anti-hepatitis C virus and hepatitis B surface antigen. Infection Control and Hospital Epidemiology. 2009;30:1227-1229

[5] Atanasova MV, Haydouchka IA, Zlatev SP, et al. Prevalence of antibodies against hepatitis C virus and hepatitis B coinfection in healthy population in Bulgaria. A seroepidemiological study. Minerva Gastroenterologica e Dietologica. 2004;50:89-96

[6] Civljak R, Kljakovic-Gaspic M, Kaic B, Bradaric N. Viral hepatitis in Croatia. Journal of Viral Hepatitis. 2014;20:49-56

[7] Kaić B, Vilibić-Cavlek T, Filipović SK, et al. Epidemiology of viral hepatitis. Acta Medica Croatica. 2013;67:273-279

[8] Vilibić-Cavlek T, Kucinar J, Ljubin-Sternak S, et al. Prevalence of viral hepatitis in Croatian adult population undergoing routine check-up, 2010-2011. Central European Journal of Public Health. 2014;22:29-33

[9] Kolarić B, Stajduhar D, Gajnik D, et al. Seroprevalence of blood-borne infections and population sizes estimates in a population of injecting drug users in Croatia. Central European Journal of Public Health. 2010;18:104-109

[10] Medić A, Dzelalija B, Sonicki Z, Zekanović D. Characteristics of hepatitis C infection in injecting drug users in Zadar County, Croatia. Collegium Antropologicum. 2008;32:697-702

[11] Kolovrat A, Jurisić I, Marić Z, Cvitković A. Prevalence of hepatitis B, hepatitis C and HIV among injecting drug users treated outpatiently and in therapeutic community in Brod-Posavina County, Croatia. Acta Medica Croatica. 2010;64:287-296

[12] Cavlek TV, Marić J, Katicić L, Kolarić B. Hepatitis C virus antibody status, sociodemographic characteristics, and risk behaviour among injecting drug users in Croatia. Central European Journal of Public Health. 2011;19:26-29

[13] Trisler Z, Seme K, Poljak M, et al. Prevalence of hepatitis C and G virus infections among intravenous drug users in Slovenia and Croatia. Scandinavian Journal of Infectious Diseases. 1999;31:33-35

[14] Vilibic-Cavlek T, Gjenero-Margan I, Retkovac B, et al. Sociodemographic characteristics and risk behaviors for HIV, hepatitis B and hepatitis C virus infection among Croatian male prisoners. International Journal of Prisoner Health. 2011;7:28-31

[15] Burek V, Horvat J, Butorac K, Mikulić R. Viral hepatitis B, C and HIV infection in Croatian prisons. Epidemiology and Infection. 2010;138:1610-1620

[16] Seme K, Poljak M, Begovac J, et al. Low prevalence of hepatitis C virus infection among human immunodeficiency virus type 1-infected individuals from Slovenia and Croatia. ActaVirologica. 2002;46:91-94

[17] Cavlek TV, Margan IG, Lepej SZ, et al. Seroprevalence, risk factors, and hepatitis C virus genotypes in groups with high-risk sexual behavior in Croatia. Journal of Medical Virology. 2009;81:1348-1353

[18] Crnjaković-Palmović J, Jeren-Strujić B, Gudel-Gregurić J, et al. Hepatitis virus infection among hemodialysis patients. Acta Medica Croatica. 2005;59:113-116

[19] Istria County Institute of Public Health. Data on the Health Status of the Population and the Work of Health Care Services in the Istria County in 2013 [Internet]. 2013. Available from: http://www.zzjziz.hr/uploads/media/2013_uvod.pdf. [Accessed: December 30, 2016]

[20] Indolfi G, Bartolini E, Casavola D, Resti M. Chronic hepatitis C virus infection in children and adolescents: Epidemiology, natural history, and assessment of the safety and efficacy of combination therapy. Adolescent Health, Medicine and Therapeutics. 2010;1:115-128

[21] Gerner P, Wirth S, Wintermeyer P, et al. Prevalence of hepatitis C virus infection in children admitted to an urban hospital. The Journal of Infection. 2006;52:305-308

[22] Busch MP. Closing the windows on viral transmission by blood transfusion. In: Stramer SL, editor. Blood Safety in the New Millennium. Bethesda: American Association of Blood Banks; 2001. pp. 33-54

[23] Santiago B, Blázquez D, López G, et al. Serological profile of immigrant pregnant women against HIV, HBV, HCV, rubella, *Toxoplasma gondii, Treponema pallidum,* and *Trypanosoma cruzi*. Enfermedades Infecciosas Y Microbiologica Clinica. 2012;30:64-69

[24] Suárez González A, Viejo De La Guerra G, Oterro Guerra L, Solís Sánchez G. Antibody determination for the human immunodeficiency virus in pregnant women in the public health care area of Gijón, Spain. Medicina Clínica (Barcelona). 2001;116:517-519

[25] Aniszewska M, Kowalik-Mikołajewska B, Pokorska-Lis M, et al. Seroprevalence of anti-HCV in pregnant women. Risk factors of HCV infection. Przegląd Epidemiologiczny. 2009;63:293-298

[26] Transfusion Medicine Newsletter. (In Croatian). No. 53, 2013 [Internet]. 2013. Available from: http://www.hztm.hr/glasilo/53/index.html

[27] Vilibic-Cavlek T, Kucinar J, Kaic B, et al. Epidemiology of hepatitis C in Croatia in the European context. The World Journal of Gastroenterology. 2015;21(32):9476-9493

[28] Vince A, Iscić-Bes J, ZidovecLepej S, et al. Distribution of hepatitis C virus genotypes in Croatia – A 10 year retrospective study of four geographic regions. Collegium Antropologicum. 2006;30(Suppl 2):139-143

[29] Davila S. Comparison of hepatitis C virus genotypes distribution in prison population and injecting drug users in northwest Croatia [thesis in Croatian]. Zagreb: School of Medicine University of Zagreb; 2013

[30] Bingulac-Popović J, Babić I, Dražić V, Grahovac B. Distribution of hepatitis C virus genotypes in the Croatian population. Biochemia Medica. 2000;3-4:175-180

[31] Golubić D, Vurusić B, Kessler HH. Prevalence and significance of hepatitis C virus (HCV) genotypes in anti-HCV positive patients in northwest Croatia. Acta Medica Croatica. 1997;51:79-82

[32] MohdHanafiah K, Groeger J, Flaxman AD, Wiersma ST. Global epidemiology of hepatitis C virus infection: new estimates of age-specific antibody to HCV seroprevalence. Hepatology. 2013;57:1333-1342

[33] Quer J and Esteban Mur JI. Epidemiology and prevention. In: Thomas HC, Lok ASF, Locarnini A, Zuckerman A, editors. Viral Hepatitis. 4th ed. Chichester: John Wiley & Sons; 2014. pp. 256-265

[34] Vince A, Hrstić I, Begovac J, et al. Viral hepatitis – Croatian Consensus Statement 2013. Acta Medica Croatica. 2013;67: 273-279

[35] World Health Organization. Guidelines for Screening, Care and Treatment of Persons with Hepatitis C Infection [Internet]. 2016. Available from: http://www.who.int/hepatitis/publications/hepatitis-c-guidelines-2016/en/. [Accessed: December 30, 2016]

[36] World Health Organization. Global Health Sector Strategy on Viral Hepatitis 2016-2021 [Internet]. 2016. Available from: http://www.who.int/hepatitis/strategy2016-2021/ghss-hep/en/. [Accessed: December 30, 2016]

[37] European Association for the Study of the Liver. EASL recommendations on treatment of hepatitis C 2016. Journal of Hepatology. 2017;66:153-194

[38] Ministry of Health Referral Centre for Diagnosis and Treatment of Viral Hepatitis. Hepatitis C Treatment Recommendations [Internet]. 2016. Available from: www.bfm.hr/page/hepatitis-c [Accessed: December 30, 2016]

[39] De Bruijn W, Ibanez C, Frisk P, et al. Introduction and utilization of high priced HCV medicines across Europe: Implications for the future. Frontiers in Pharmacology. 2016;7:197

Chapter 3

Liver Transplantation in Patients with Hepatitis C

Tajana Filipec Kanižaj

Additional information is available at the end of the chapter

http://dx.doi.org/10.5772/intechopen.70438

Abstract

As a leading indication for liver transplantation in Western countries, hepatitis C virus (HCV) poses a significant burden both before and after transplantation. Post-transplant disease recurrence occurs in nearly all patients with detectable pre-transplant viremia, therefore compromising the lifesaving significance of transplantation. Many factors involving the donor, recipient and virus have been evaluated throughout the literature, although few have been fully elucidated and implemented in actual clinical practice. Antiviral therapy has been recognized as a cornerstone of HCV infection control; however, experience and success are limited following transplantation in a challenging cohort of patients with liver cirrhosis. Current therapeutic protocols surpass those that were used previously, both in regards to sustained viral response (SVR) and the side-effect profile.

Keywords: hepatitis C, liver transplantation, antiviral treatment, direct-acting drugs, adverse events

1. Introduction

Complications of chronic hepatitis C, mainly decompensated liver cirrhosis and hepatocellular carcinoma (HCC), are leading indications for liver transplantation (LT) in the Western world [1]. Viremic patients at the time of LT have almost a universal recurrence of the disease. The aging of the population with chronic hepatitis C virus (HCV) infection and longer infection duration influence the higher prevalence of advanced liver disease; HCC and the need for LT have doubled over the last decade.

HCV infection significantly impairs patient and allograft survival after liver transplantation. The clinical course of HCV recurrence is highly variable. Compared to the course of HCV disease in patients who underwent transplantation in previous years, with advancement of transplant medicine and the usage of marginal donors and potent immunosuppression,

HCV-related disease progression to cirrhosis is becoming faster and is accompanied by a higher number of complications. Recurrent HCV-related graft failure remains the leading cause of death in these patients. The overall 5-year survival of HCV-positive recipients is slightly lower than that for other indications (60–80%) [2–5].

2. Pathogenesis of disease recurrence

The progression of hepatitis C is accelerated in immunocompromised liver transplant recipients compared with immunocompetent patients both before and after the development of compensated cirrhosis. During reperfusion, the allograft is overwhelmed with HCV that is mainly present in recipient blood and monocytes. The initial decrease of viral titre (linked to the removal of the main viral reservoir) is followed by an exponential increase, reaching pre-transplant levels in a few days [6].

In the first 3 months, most patients (70%) develop acute hepatitis, which is followed by chronic hepatitis (up to 60%) in next 6 months. If untreated, 10–30% of patients develop cirrhosis within 5 years. The majority of other HCV-positive recipients develop graft cirrhosis by 9–12 years post-transplant. In contrast, the median time to cirrhosis in the non-transplanted population is >30 years. The rate of decompensation is >40% at 1 year and >70% at 3 years in LT recipients versus <5 and <10%, respectively, in immunocompetent patients [7].

The variables leading to different patterns of disease recurrence in individual patients are not well understood. Up to 50% of recipients develop mild to moderate inflammation on liver biopsy; 20% results in minimal changes and 20–40% leads to progressive inflammatory changes with high-grade histological damages [8]. Due to the direct effects of the virus on liver cells, up to 15% of graft recipients develop the most detrimental pattern of disease recurrence with unfavorable prognosis—fibrosing cholestatic hepatitis (FCH). The development of FCH may be more common in patients with higher HCV viral titre and higher levels of immunosuppressive medications, usually due to treatment of acute cellular rejection [9]. If untreated, FCH rapidly proceeds to liver failure.

Several variables, including donor characteristics (donor age and type), recipient characteristics (female gender, HIV co-infection), viral characteristics (genotype (G) 1b, higher viral titre and IL28B non-CC polymorphism), a higher degree and type of immunosuppression, earlier timing of recurrence and early severe histological findings are implicated in the outcome of hepatitis C patients post-transplantation [10]. None of previously mentioned factors have been extensively validated, achieved universal consensus among the literature or permitted clinically important intervention.

2.1. The role of immunosuppression

There is much interest in the influence, level and type of immunosuppression following LT on the severity of disease recurrence. The impact is most pronounced when high-intensity regimens are used to treat acute rejection, particularly with high-dose steroid boluses and anti-lymphocyte antibody preparations [11–13]. There are no convincing data to support the use of any specific induction or maintenance regimen, and it is likely that the choice of initial calcineurin inhibitor (tacrolimus or cyclosporine) does not significantly impact overall outcomes in HCV-positive liver transplant recipients [14].

3. Diagnosis of HCV recurrence post-transplant

The initial drop in transaminase level during the early post-transplant setting is usually followed by only minimally to mildly elevated alanine aminotransferase (ALT) levels in later post-transplant periods. Further increases of liver enzymes are influenced not only by the degree of HCV recurrence but also the wide spectrum of other post-transplant complications such as acute cellular rejection, reperfusion or drug-induced liver injury, vascular and biliary complications.

Consequently, the diagnosis of graft HCV infection is based on the combined analysis of polymerase chain reaction (PCR) and liver biopsy findings. Liver biopsy remains the gold standard in the detection of the severity of disease progression and the differentiation of liver pathology (the exclusion of other diseases). Except in the setting of FCH liver biopsy, findings are mostly mild and nonspecific. They include periportal inflammation, lobular hepatocytes ballooning, acidophilic bodies or lobular apoptosis. Some of these features are also seen in acute cellular rejection. High blood levels of cholestatic enzymes are characteristic of FCH, including extensive dense portal fibrosis immature fibrous bands extending into the sinusoidal spaces, ductular proliferation, cholestasis and moderate mononuclear inflammation on liver graft biopsies. Differentiating rejection from hepatitis C based only on pathology can be difficult, in real clinical practice, final clinical judgment is reconsidering also the timing after transplantation and clinical features (e.g., the degree of baseline immunosuppression and prior rejection episodes) [15]. Substantial periportal sinusoidal fibrosis in early biopsies (<6 months) has been shown to be a good predictor of severe HCV recurrence.

Even in situations of typical HCV recurrence, final clinical judgment is performed after the exclusion of other possible causes of post-transplant liver injury (usually based on the combination of clinical examination, various laboratory tests, liver ultrasound and liver biopsy findings).

Methods of non-invasive fibrosis measurement were investigated in HCV recurrence after LT. In a systematic review that pooled five studies of patients with recurrent HCV, the sensitivity and specificity for ultrasound-based elastography for predicting significant fibrosis were both 83%, and its sensitivity and specificity for predicting cirrhosis were 98 and 84%, respectively [16].

4. Approaches to the treatment of HCV recurrence following liver transplantation

Along with the impact of the previously mentioned factors on disease recurrence and overall patient and graft survival, antiviral therapy success rates appear to be one of the most important factors.

Several strategies for HCV treatment in the setting of LT have been attempted: treatment prior to LT, immediate or perioperative prophylaxis of HCV graft infection, early pre-emptive HCV therapy and treatment of established recurrent graft disease.

There is an open debate regarding which of the previously stated options are preferable following liver transplantation. Thus far, a consensus has not been reached because these four approaches have not been prospectively compared in appropriately powered randomized trials using clinical endpoints. Unfortunately, due to the heterogeneity of end-stage liver disease, the small number of patients, and the highly complex treatment of liver transplant candidates and recipients, it is unlikely that such trials will be performed in a randomized controlled fashion. In their absence, the recommendations are guided by the results of clinical trials that assess each approach separately as well as data from the real-world and the panel members' experiences.

4.1. Treatment prior to LT

Strategies to eradicate HCV infection before LT is directed at preventing disease recurrence, leading to significant improvement in liver function and prolongation or avoidance of the need for LT (delisting of selected patients). Interferon (IFN)-based regimens are contraindicated in decompensated patients due to the high rate of side effects (mainly infections and further liver disease deterioration). In the IFN era, less than 25% of LT candidates were eligible for treatment. The accomplished eradication rate (sustained viral response, SVR) was 8–30%. The main reason for the generally lower SVR rates in patients with liver cirrhosis was poor treatment tolerability with substantially high rates of serious adverse events (SAE), leading to dose reductions (70%) and therapy discontinuation (30%). With the availability of new generations of direct-acting agents (DAA) with an improved safety profile, more LT candidates are eligible for treatment. SVR rates greater than 95% can now be reached in patients with compensated cirrhosis who are undergoing transplantation for coexistent HCC. Although very good, slightly lower SVR rates (approximately 80%) are expected with the use of currently available DAA in case of decompensated cirrhosis (**Figure 1**) [17–21].

Regarding this treatment approach, there are many open questions. While deciding to treat liver transplant candidates on the waiting list, we must keep in mind that the time of LT and the duration of antiviral therapy cannot be predicted. Consequently, some of the patients may be transplanted before the virus has been cleared. In addition, there remain uncertainties regarding the safety of DAA therapy and the outcomes among those with advanced liver insufficiency. Is there indeed a point after which antiviral therapy is futile? It is unknown whether meaningful functional hepatic recovery is possible in most eradicated HCV patients with advanced cirrhosis, how long such recovery would take, whether short-term positive effects on Model of End-Stage Liver Disease (MELD) will indeed translate into long-term clinical benefits with a reduced occurrence of HCC, decompensation or all-cause mortality following DAA therapy. Most of the patients will keep a diseased liver with the risk of subsequent decompensations, HCC occurrence and death and thus could lose an opportunity to cure both the liver disease and the infection with LT (MELD purgatory). So far, it is yet to be explored whether DAA therapy can reduce the risk of subsequent decompensations, HCC occurrence and death, or, even in patients with previous HCC or increased risk of HCC occurrence.

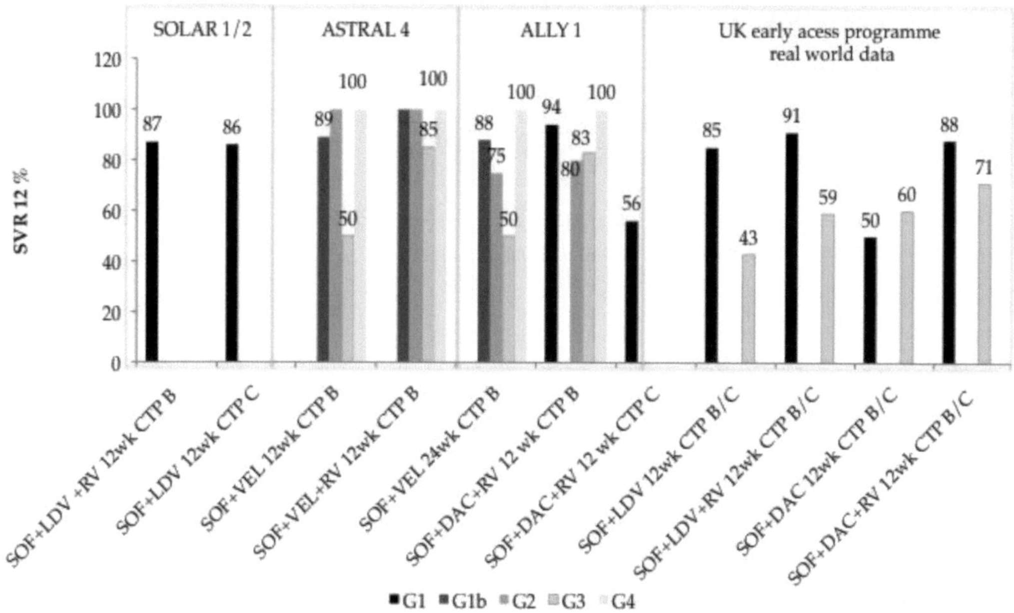

Figure 1. Twelve week sustained viral response (SVR12) in patients with decompensated cirrhosis (adapted from Refs. [18–22]).

Due to a favorable side-effect profile, treatment of decompensated patients with new DAA drugs such as sofosbuvir (SOF), ledipasvir (LDV), velpatasvir (VEL) or daclatasvir (DAC)-based regimens, is recommended (**Table 1**). Recently, many new data from clinical studies are emerging with more potent DAA combinations.

4.1.1. Clinical study data on DAA treatment in LT candidates

The proof of concept of DAA treatment for LT candidates came from a phase 2, open-label study on 61 patients with (all genotypes) HCV liver cirrhosis (Child-Turcotte-Pugh score, CTP ≤ 7; Model of End-Stage Liver Disease, MELD < 22) who were on waiting lists for liver transplantation. Patients received up to 48 weeks of SOF + RV. Among 46 patients who underwent LT, 43 had negative viremia at the time of LT and 70% remained negative 12 weeks after LT. Overall, 63% of transplanted patients had a virological response at 12 weeks post-transplant. Recurrence was inversely related to the number of days of undetectable HCV viremia prior to LT. None of the patients who were negative for more than 4 weeks before LT experienced HCV recurrence [17]. However, with the development of new drugs, this combination is suboptimal and is, thus, not recommended.

The SOLAR I study assessed treatment with the SOF + LDV + RV for 12–24 weeks in patients infected with HCV genotypes 1 (99%) or 4 (1%). Patients were stratified to two cohorts depending on the time of treatment: cohort A (decompensated cirrhosis and CTP B/C) treated before LT or cohort B treated after LT. Patients in cohort A achieved SVR12 rates of 87–89% in CTP B patients and 86–87% in CTP C patients, respectively, after treatment for 12–24 weeks [17]. The SOLAR II study had an identical design. Data revealed SVR12 rates of 87–96% in CTP

Genotype	Compensated cirrhosis regimen*	Decompensated cirrhosis (CTP B/C) regimen*
G1	SOF + LDV 12 wk; G1a experienced 24 wk or + RV 12 wk	SOF + LDV + RV 12 wk
	3D G1b 12 wk, G1a + RV 24 wk	SOF + DAC + RV 12 wk
	SOF + DAC 12 wk; G1a experienced 24 wk or + RV 12 wk	SOF + VEL + RV 12 wk
	SOF + VEL 12 wk	
	GRA + ELB G1b 12 wk; G1a 12 wk if HCV RNA ≤800,000 (5.9 log) IU/ml or + RV 16 wk HCV RNA >800,000 (5.9 log) IU/ml	
G2	SOF + VEL 12 wk	SOF + DAC + RV 12 wk
	SOF + DAC 12 wk	SOF + VEL + RV 12 wk
G3	SOF + DAC + RV 24 wk	SOF + DAC + RV 24 wk
	SOF + VEL 24 wk, + RV 12 wk	SOF + VEL + RV 24 wk
G4	SOF + LDV 12 wk; experienced 24 wk or + RV 12 wk	SOF + LDV + RV 12 wk
	2D + RV 12 wk	SOF + DAC + RV 12 wk
	SOF + DAC 12 wk, experienced 24 wk or + RV 12 wk	SOF + VEL + RV 12 wk
	SOF + VEL 12 wk	
	GRA + ELB 12 wk, experienced 12 wk if HCV RNA ≤800,000 (5.9 log) IU/ml or + RV 16 wk HCV RNA >800,000 (5.9 log) IU/ml	
	SOF + SIM 12 wk, experienced 24 wk or + RV 12 wk	
G5,6	SOF + LDV 12 wk, experienced 24 wk or + RV 12 wk	SOF + LDV + RV 12 wk
	SOF + DAC 12 wk, experienced 24 wk or + RV 12 wk	SOF + DAC + RV 12 wk
	SOF + VEL 12 wk	SOF + VEL + RV 12 wk

SOF, sofosbuvir (400 mg/day); LDV, ledipasvir (90 mg/day); DAC, daclatasvir (60 mg/day); 3D, ombitasvir (25 mg/day)/paritaprevir (150 mg/day)/ritonavir (100 mg/day) + dasabuvir (250 mg twice daily); 2D, ombitasvir (25 mg/day)/paritaprevir (150 mg/day)/ritonavir (100 mg/day); VEL, velpatasvir (100 mg/day); GRA, grazeoprevir (100 mg/day); ELB, elbasvir (50 mg/day); RV, ribavirin (when ribavirin is used, especially in patients with advanced recurrent disease, it may need be started at a dose of 600 mg daily, with subsequent increase in the dose as tolerated until reaching a dose of 1000 mg daily (for patients <75 kg) or 1200 mg daily (for patients ≥ 75 kg). The dosing of ribavirin should take into account the patient's creatinine clearance and hemoglobin level); wk, weeks; CTP, Child-Turcotte-Pugh score.

*If no RV eligible 24 weeks.

Table 1. Recommended HCV treatment options for liver transplant candidates and patients with liver cirrhosis (adapted from Ref. [26]).

B patients and 85–88% in CTP C patients, respectively, after treatment for 12–24 weeks. The MELD and CTP scores improved in approximately half of the treated patients. Up to 88% of patients with baseline CTP B/C scores exhibited improved CTP scores (35% CTP B to A, 48% CTP C to B, but only 5% CTP C to A) [19]. About 4% of patients with CTP score A deteriorated to CTP B; 95% experienced adverse events (AE); 14–28% experienced SAE, but only 1–5% of SAE were related to DAA. No deaths were proven to be treatment related.

The ASTRAL 4 study evaluated the efficacy, safety and tolerability of SOF + velpatasvir (VEL) ± RV for 12 weeks and SOF/VEL for 24 weeks in genotype 1–6 patients with CTP B cirrhosis. The overall SVR12 rates were 83% among patients who received 12 weeks of SOF + VEL, 94%

among those who received 12 weeks of SOF + VEL + RV, and 86% among those who received 24 weeks of SOF + VEL. Post hoc analysis did not detect any significant differences in the rates of SVR among the three study groups. Among genotype three patients, 85% achieved SVR12 with the SOF + VEL + RV 12-week treatment. SAE occurred in 19% of the patients who received SOF + VEL for 12 weeks, 16% of the patients who received SOF + VEL + RV for 12 weeks, and 18% of the patients who received SOF + VEL for 24 weeks. The most common AE were fatigue (29%), nausea (23%), headache (22%) and anemia (31%) in the patients receiving RV. A total of 51% of patients with a baseline MELD score <15 exhibited improved MELD scores at week 12 post-treatment and 27% of patients exhibited worsened MELD scores. A total of 81% of the patients with a baseline MELD score ≥15 exhibited improved MELD scores, and 7% of patients exhibited worsened MELD scores [20].

In a multicentre, prospective, open-label, phase-3 study (ALLY I), a combination therapy of DAC + SOF + RV for 12 weeks was evaluated in 60 (genotypes 1–6) patients with advanced cirrhosis (80% CTP B/C) or post-liver transplant HCV recurrence. In patients with advanced cirrhosis, the overall SVR12 rate was 94% (92% for CTP A, 94% CTP B and 56% CTP C). The overall SVR12 rate in genotype (G) 1 was 82% (76% G1a and 100% G1b), and based on the baseline cirrhosis stage, the overall SVR12 rate was 91% for CTP A, 92% for CTP B and 50% for CTP C patients. The corresponding SVR12 rates in patients with genotypes 2, 3 and 4 were 80, 83 and 100%, respectively. SAE occurred in 17% of patients. There were no treatment-related SAE and no deaths due to treatment. The overall CTP scores improved in 60% of patients and worsened in 15% of patients. Among patients with baseline CTP B and C scores, 50% improved to class A and B, respectively. MELD scores improved in 47% of patients and worsened in 35% of patients [21].

Experience from the United Kingdom Expanded Access Programme in real-world patients with advanced stages of liver cirrhosis (CTP B/C) who were treated with SOF + DAC or LDV + RV for 12 weeks revealed an overall SVR12 rate of 82%. The SVR12 rates for G1 patients were 85% for SOF + LDV, 91% for SOF + LVD + RV, 50% for SOF + DAC and 88% for the SOF + DAC + RV regimen. In patients with decompensated cirrhosis infected with genotype 3, the SVR12 rates were 60% for SOF + DAC and 71% SOF + DAC + RV 12-week regimens. Viral clearance was associated with improvement in liver function within 6 months compared to untreated patients. Patients with initial serum albumin levels <35 g/L, aged >65 or with low (<135 mmol/L) baseline serum sodium concentrations were least likely to benefit from therapy [22]. When compared to the outcome in first 6 months from the start of treatment and to untreated patients, after 6 months of treatment, there was a reduction in the incidence of decompensation (7% in months 6–15 versus 18% in months 0–6 for treated patients and 28% in untreated patients) and in the incidence of MELD score worsening by >2 points (23% in months 0–6 for treated patients versus 38% in untreated patients). There was no significant difference in HCC incidence (2.5% in months 6–15 versus 4% in months 0–6 for treated patients and 4% in untreated patients). The long-term impact of HCV treatment in patients with decompensated cirrhosis remains to be determined since in longer follow-up studies (15 months), AE-free survival among treated patients with CTP C or a MELD score >14 at baseline remained poor [23].

Data about the possibility of delisting patients with improved liver function from the LT list are scarce. In a multicentre, European, retrospective real-world study on 103 LT candidates in 11 transplant centers, DAA-based therapy reversed liver dysfunction in approximately one patient out of three patients who were put on hold, and enabled delisting in approximately 1 patient out of 5 in 60 weeks. Patients with lower MELD scores (<16) had higher chances of being delisted. The short-term benefits observed must be balanced with the respective risks of LT and of not undergoing LT. The long-term clinical benefit of therapy was not assessed [24].

According to all of the presented data, the severity of liver disease at the time of antiviral treatment initiation seems to be a more relevant determinant of early mortality than the virological response and should thus be considered to guide patient prioritization for LT. According to European guidelines, patients with decompensated cirrhosis and an indication for LT with a MELD score ≥18–20 should be transplanted first and then treated after transplantation [25, 26].

4.2. Perioperative treatment

There is limited data about the benefits of perioperative treatment of HCV-positive recipients. In a small study on 16 patients treated with LED + SOF for 4 weeks (starting at day of LT), an SVR12 rate of 88% was achieved [27].

4.3. Early pre-emptive HCV therapy

The use of DAA combinations in this setting has not yet been studied, and many centers now treat recurrent HCV with the regimens detailed below during the early post-operative period once the patient is stable. Studies regarding the safety and optimal timing of treatment in this setting are needed [26]. Meta-analyses of the IFN-based studies did not identify benefits for patients who received early pre-emptive antiviral therapy following LT and those who did not [28].

4.4. Treatment of post-transplant HCV disease recurrence

In the post-liver transplant setting, IFN-based therapies could be used, but they induced numerous and often severe side effects; additionally, their results were disappointing (SVR12 30–40%). The latest European guidelines recommend DAA as the most suitable in the post-transplant setting, including combinations of SOF with LDV, VEL and DAC with or without RV (**Table 2**) [26]. All patients should be considered for therapy. Treatment should be initiated early after LT, ideally as early as possible when the patient is stabilized (generally after the first 3 months) because the SVR12 rates decrease in patients with advanced post-transplant liver disease. Patients with FCH, the presence of moderate to extensive fibrosis or portal hypertension 1 year after LT are associated with rapid disease progression and graft loss and require more urgent antiviral treatment [26]. An SVR12 rate higher than 95% can be accomplished with new DAA drugs in LT recipients (**Figure 2**). Due to possible drug-to-drug interactions and post-transplant complications, therapy should be performed only at centers with considerable experience in managing transplanted patients.

Genotype	Regimen*
G1	SOF + LDV + RV 12 wk
	SOF + DAC + RV 12 wk
	SOF + VEL + RV 12 wk (24 wk CTP B/C)
G2	SOF + DAC + RV 12 wk
	SOF + VEL + RV for 12 weeks (24 wk CTP B/C)
G3	SOF + DAC + RV 24 wk
	SOF + VEL + RV 24 wk
G4	SOF + LDV + RV 12 wk
	SOF + DAC + RV 12 wk
	SOF + VEL + RV 12 wk (24 wk CTP B/C)
G5,6	SOF + LDV + RV 12 wk
	SOF + DAC + RV 12 wk
	SOF + VEL + RV 12 wk (24 wk CTP B/C)

SOF, sofosbuvir (400 mg/day); LDV, ledipasvir (90 mg/day); DAC, daclatasvir (60 mg/day); VEL, velpatasvir (100 mg/day); RV, ribavirin (when RV is used, especially in patients with advanced recurrent disease, it may need be started at a dose of 600 mg daily, with subsequent increase in the dose as tolerated until reaching a dose of 1000 mg daily (for patients <75 kg) or 1200 mg daily (for patients ≥ 75 kg). The dosing of RV should take into account the patient's creatinine clearance and hemoglobin level); wk, weeks; CTP, Child-Turcotte-Pugh score.

*If no RV eligible 24 weeks.

Table 2. Recommended treatment options for patients with transplanted liver and HCV infection (adapted from Ref. [26]).

4.4.1. Clinical study data on DAA treatment of transplanted patients

Fixed combination therapy of SOF + LDV + RV for 12–24 weeks has been studied (SOLAR I and II) in transplanted patients with genotypes 1 and 4 and a wide range of liver disease stages (METAVIR fibrosis stage 1–3 (F0–3) and CTP A-C). In the 12- and 24-week treatment groups, SVR12 rates of 96 and 98% were achieved in patients with baseline F0–3. In both treatment duration groups, the SVR12 rate was 96% for CTP A patients. The efficacy was lower in patients with CTP B cirrhosis (85 and 88% SVR12) or CTP C cirrhosis (60 and 75% SVR12) in the 12- and 24-week groups, respectively [18]. Similar results were obtained in the SOLAR II study. SVR12 was achieved in 98 and 100% of patients with F0–3, in 100 and 96% of patients with CTP A, in 95 and 100% of patients with CTP B and in 50 and 80% of patients with C cirrhosis with 12 and 24 weeks of treatment, respectively. SVR among patients with FCH was 100% [19]. In both studies, unsatisfactory viral eradication was observed for patients with CTP C liver cirrhosis. This could be explained by the small number of patients within the CTP C groups in both studies, consequently additional data are needed for final conclusions. In summary, 95% of patients experienced AE, and 15–28% of patients experienced SAE depending on the severity of the liver disease (F0–3/CTP A: 15% and CTP B/C: 28%). Up to 5% of patients discontinued the study due to SAE [18, 19].

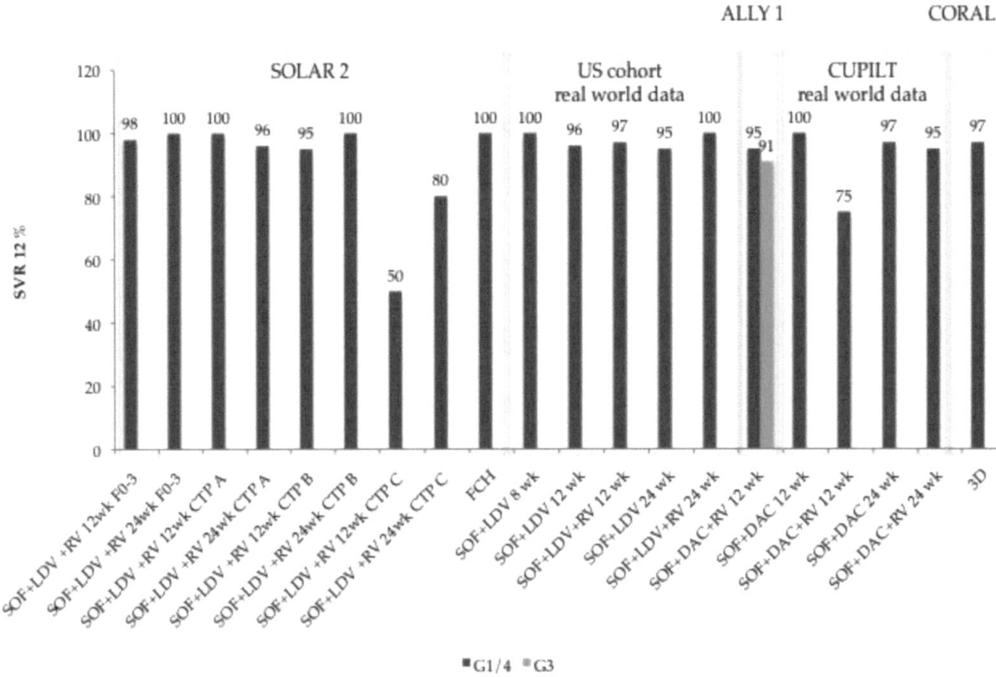

Figure 2. Twelve week sustained viral response (SVR12) in patients with pos-transplantation HCV recurrence (adapted from Ref. [19, 21, 29–31]).

The same conclusions were revealed in real-world studies. In a large retrospective US cohort study, 204 patients (21% advanced fibrosis, 49% treatment-experienced and 66% genotype 1) were treated with SOF + LDV ± RV for 8, 12 or 24 weeks. The overall SVR12 rate was 96% (100% for 8 weeks of SOF + LDV, 96% for 12 weeks of SOF + LDV, 97% for 12 weeks of SOF + LDV + RV, 95% for 24 weeks of SOF + LDV and 100% for 24 weeks of SOF + LDV + RV) [29]. Excellent results in groups without RV treatment raise the question of its universal need in all transplanted patients. Since all controlled studies have been done using RV-based regimens, prospective studies are required for a final conclusion.

In a phase-3 ALLY I study, a combination of SOF + DAC + RV was administered to 53 transplanted patients (77% genotype 1); 95 and 91% patients with genotypes 1 and 3 infection achieved SVR12, respectively. Overall, 99% of patients experienced AE, 9% of patients experienced SAE and 2% of patients discontinued the drug therapy due to drug-related AE [21].

Real-world data from the CUPILT study revealed similar results. A total of 137 transplanted patients (81% genotype 1 and 31% cirrhosis) were treated with SOF + DAC ± RV for 12 weeks. Overall the SVR12 rate was 96% under the intention-to-treat analysis, and it was 99% when non-virological failures were excluded (75% for 12 weeks of SOF + DAC + RV, 100% for 12 weeks of SOF + DAC, 95% for 24 weeks of SOF + DAC + RV and 97% for 24 weeks of SOF + DAC). The rate of SAE reached 17.5% with 3% of patients discontinuing treatment prematurely because of SAE. A slight but significant reduction in creatinine clearance was reported. No clinically relevant drug-drug interactions were noted, although 52% of patients required a change in the dosage of immunosuppressive drugs [30].

A trial with SOF + VEL combination therapy is ongoing for transplanted patients.

In a study of 34 patients with HCV G1 recurrence following liver transplantation and METAVIR stage F0–F2 fibrosis, patients were given ombitasvir/ritonavir-boosted paritaprevir + dasabuvir + RV (3D therapy). Patients were treated for 24 weeks. An SVR at 12 and 24 weeks post-treatment was achieved by 97% of patients. Overall, 97% of patients experienced adverse events with only 6% of patients experiencing serious adverse events. Common adverse events included fatigue, headache and cough. One patient (3%) discontinued the study drugs due to adverse events. There were no episodes of graft rejection [31]. The 3D treatment required dosing modifications for calcineurin inhibitors tacrolimus and ciclosporin. The recommended dose of tacrolimus should be reduced to 0.5 mg per week or 0.2 mg every 3 days, and cyclosporine should be reduced to one-fifth of the daily pre-3D therapy dose and given once a day with regular immunosuppressive drug level monitoring. This combination should not be administered with everolimus. SOF, LDV and DAC do not seem to interact with calcineurin inhibitors. However, close monitoring before, during and after DAA therapy is essential. In the CUPILT study, 59% of the patients treated with SOF and DAC after LT had to change the dose of one immunosuppressive drug during therapy.

Even in patients with decompensated graft cirrhosis, treatment with DAA could improvement MELD and CTP scores. In the SOLAR II study, 28% of baseline CTP B patients reversed to CTP A and 68% of the CTP C patients reversed to CTP B [19]. In the ALLY I study, these percentages were 50 and 46%, respectively [21].

The optimum timing for the initiation of therapy post-transplantation remains to be determined. Based on the tolerability of the classic IFN-based regimen, the most common initial approach was to treat graft hepatitis after histological damage was confirmed (fibrosis stage 2 or higher on the METAVIR score or severe and rapid progression of fibrosis as observed in FCH) and before clinical decompensation had developed. With the DAAs, there are no limitations on treating post-transplant recurrence early after LT, including patients with decompensated cirrhosis or those with fibrosing cholestatic hepatitis (FCH)—a life-threatening form of HCV recurrence. This strategy is even more reasonable when considering that treatment in patients with decompensated graft cirrhosis is related to reduced SVR12 rates [32].

5. Conclusions

HCV-associated cirrhosis is the most common indication for LT in the Western world. Recurrent HCV infection still remains a major cause of morbidity and mortality post-transplantation. The clinical course of HCV infection appears to be accelerated compared with the pre-transplant setting, and several patterns of recurrence have been described. Many predictors of outcome following LT have been described, but their accuracy in predicting the course of recurrence in individual patients or in guiding interventions is uncertain. With the evolution of new antiviral drugs and more precise and clear knowledge of HCV disease recurrence, promising results have begun to emerge in the complex field of liver LT. Treatment regimens based on DAAs are highly effective and well tolerated in both pre- and post-transplant patients, including patients with decompensated cirrhosis or those with FCH. All patients who do not achieve an SVR pre-transplant should be treated post-transplant. The optimal timing is uncertain, and the decision of when to treat must be made on an individual basis. SVR rates greater than 95% could be achieved. From a safety point of view, very few severe adverse events have been reported among studies. Therapy should only be attempted at centers with considerable experience in managing post-transplantation patients.

Author details

Tajana Filipec Kanižaj

Address all correspondence to: tajana.filipec@gmail.com

Department of Gastroenterology, University Hospital Merkur, School of Medicine, University of Zagreb, Zagreb, Croatia

References

[1] Kanwal F, Hoang T, Kramer JR, et al. Increasing prevalence of HCC and cirrhosis in patients with chronic hepatitis C virus infection. Gastroenterology. 2011;140:1182-1188. DOI: 10.1053/j.gastro.2010.12.03

[2] Thuluvath PJ, Guidinger MK, Fung JJ, et al. Liver transplantation in the United States, 1999-2008. American Journal of Transplantation. 2010;10(4):1003-1019. DOI: 10.1111/j.1600-6143.2010.03037.x

[3] Böker KH, Dalley G, Bahr MJ, et al. Long-term outcome of hepatitis C virus infection after liver transplantation. Hepatology. 1997;25(1):203-210. DOI: 10.1002/hep.510250137

[4] Féray C, Caccamo L, Alexander GJ, et al. European collaborative study on factors influencing outcome after liver transplantation for hepatitis C. European Concerted Action on Viral Hepatitis (EUROHEP) Group. Gastroenterology. 1999;117(3):619-625. DOI: 10.1016/0016-5085(95)90207-4

[5] Forman LM, Lewis JD, Berlin JA, Feldman HI, Lucey MR. The association between hepatitis C infection and survival after orthotopic liver transplantation. Gastroenterology. 2002;122(4):889-896. DOI: 10.1053/gast.2002.32418

[6] Garcia-Retortillo M, Forns X, Feliu A, et al. Hepatitis C virus kinetics during and immediately after liver transplantation. Hepatology. 2002;35(3):680-687. DOI: 10.1053/jhep.2002.31773

[7] Berenguer M, Prieto M, Rayon JM, et al. Natural history of clinically compensated hepatitis C virus-related graft cirrhosis after liver transplantation. Hepatology. 2000;32:852-858. DOI: 10.1053/jhep.2000.17924

[8] Gane EJ, Portmann BC, Naoumov NV, et al. Long-term outcome of hepatitis C infection after liver transplantation. The New England Journal of Medicine. 1996;334(13):815-820. DOI: 10.1056/NEJM199603283341302

[9] Graziadei IW, Zoller HM, Schloegl A, et al. Early viral load and recipient interleukin-28B rs12979860 genotype are predictors of the progression of hepatitis C after liver transplantation. Liver Transplantation. 2012;18(6):671-679. DOI: 10.1002/lt.23402

[10] Berenguer M. Natural history of recurrent hepatitis C. Liver Transplantation. 2002;8(10 Suppl 1):S14-S18. DOI: 10.1053/jlts.2002.35781

[11] Nelson DR, Soldevila-Pico C, Reed A, et al. Anti-interleukin-2 receptor therapy in combination with mycophenolate mofetil is associated with more severe hepatitis C recurrence after liver transplantation. Liver Transplantation. 2001;7(12):1064-1070. DOI: 10.1053/jlts.2001.29414

[12] Neumann UP, Berg T, Bahra M, et al. Fibrosis progression after liver transplantation in patients with recurrent hepatitis C. Journal of Hepatology. 2004;41(5):830-836. DOI: 10.1016/j.jhep.2004.06.029

[13] Berenguer M, Crippin J, Gish R, Bass N, et al. A model to predict severe HCV-related disease following liver transplantation. Hepatology. 2003; 38(1):34-41. DOI: 10.1053/jhep.2003.50278

[14] Liu Z, Chen Y, Tao R, et al. Tacrolimus-based versus cyclosporine-based immunosupression in hepatitis C virus-infected patients after liver transplantation: A meta analysis and systemic review. PLoS ONE. 2014;9:e107057. DOI: 10.1371/journal.pone.0107057

[15] Araya V, Rakela J, Wright T. Hepatitis C after orthotopic liver transplantation. Gastroenterology. 1997;112(2):575-582

[16] Adebajo CO, Talwalkar JA, Poterucha JJ, Kim WR, Charlton MR. Ultrasound-based transient elastography for the detection of hepatic fibrosis in patients with recurrent hepatitis C virus after liver transplantation: A systematic review and meta-analysis. Liver Transplantation. 2012;18(3):323-331. DOI: 10.1002/lt.22460

[17] Curry MP, Forns X, Chung RT, et al. Sofosbuvir and ribavirin prevent recurrence of HCV infection after liver transplantation: An open-label study. Gastroenterology. 2015;148(1):100-107. DOI: 10.1053/j.gastro.2014.09.023

[18] Charlton M, Everson GT, Steven L, et al. Ledipasvir and sofosbuvir plus ribavirin for treatment of HCV infection in patients with advanced liver disease. Gastroenterology. 2015;149(3):649-659. DOI: 10.1053/j.gastro.2015.05.010

[19] Manns M, Samuel D, Gane EJ et al. Ledipasvir and sofosbuvir plus ribavirin in patients with genotype 1 or 4 hepatitis C virus infection and advanced liver disease: A multicentre, open-label, randomised, phase 2 trial. The Lancet Infectious Diseases. 2016;16(6):685-697. DOI: 10.1016/S1473-3099(16)00052-9

[20] Curry MP, OLery JG, Bzowej N, et al. Sofosbuvir and velpatasvir for HCV in patients with decompensated cirrhosis. The New England Journal of Medicine. 2015;373(27):2618-2628. DOI: 10.1056/NEJMoa1512614

[21] Poordad F, Schiff ER, Vierling JM, et al. Daclatasvir with sofosbuvir and ribavirin for hepatitis C virus infection with advanced cirrhosis or post-liver transplantation recurrence. Hepatology. 2016;63(5):1493-1505. DOI: 10.1002/hep.28446

[22] Foster GR, Irving WL, Cheung MC, et al. Impact of direct acting antiviral therapy in patients with chronic hepatitis C and decompensated cirrhosis. Journal of Hepatology. 2016;64(6):1224-1231. DOI: 10.1016/j.jhep.2016.01.029

[23] Cheung MC, Walker AJ, Hudson BE, et al. Outcomes after successful direct-acting antiviral therapy for patients with chronic hepatitis C and decompensated cirrhosis. Journal of Hepatology. 2016;65(4):741-747. DOI: 10.1016/j.jhep.2016.06.019

[24] Belli LS, Berenguer M, Cortesi PA, et al. Delisting of liver transplant candidates with chronic hepatitis C after viral eradication: A European study. Journal of Hepatology. 2016;65(3):524-531. DOI: 10.1016/j.jhep.2016.05.010

[25] Van der Meer A, Berenguer M. Reversion of disease manifestations after HCV eradication. Journal of Hepatology. 2016;65:95-108. DOI: 10.1016/j.jhep.2016.07.039

[26] European Association for the Study of the Liver. EASL recommendations on treatment of hepatitis C 2016. Journal of Hepatology. 2017;66(1):153-194. DOI: 10.1016/j.jhep.2016.09.001

[27] Levitsky J, Verna EC, O'Leary JG, Bzowej NH, et al. Perioperative ledipasvir-sofosbuvir for HCV in liver-transplant recipients. The New England Journal of Medicine. 2016;375(21):2106-2108. DOI: 10.1056/NEJMc1611829

[28] Gurusamy KS, Tsochatzis E, Toon CD, Davidson BR, Burroughs AK. Antiviral prophylaxis for the prevention of chronic hepatitis C virus in patients undergoing liver transplantation. The Cochrane Database of Systematic Reviews. 2013, Dec 2;12:CD00657. DOI: 10.1002/14651858.CD006573.pub3

[29] Kwok RM, Ahn J, Schiano TD, et al. Sofosbuvir plus ledispasvir for recurrent hepatitis C in liver transplant recipients. Liver Transplantation. 2016;22(11):1536-1543. DOI: 10.1002/lt.24614

[30] Coilly A, Fougerou-Leurent C, deLedinghen V, et al. Multicentre experience using daclatasvir and sofosbuvir to treat hepatitis C recurrence. The ANRS CUPILT study. Journal of Hepatology. 2016;65(4):711-718. DOI: 10.1016/j.jhep.2016.05.039

[31] Kwo PY, Mantry PS, Coakley E, et al. An interferon-free antiviral regimen for HCV after liver transplantation. The New England Journal of Medicine. 2014;371(25):2375-2382. DOI: 10.1056/NEJMoa1408921

[32] Felmlee D, Coilly A, Chung RT, Samuel D, Baumret TF. New perspectives for preventing hepatitis C virus liver graft infection. The Lancet Infectious Diseases. 2016;16:735-745. DOI: 10.1016/S1473-3099(16)00120-1

Chapter 4

Impact of HBV Infection on Outcomes of Direct-Acting Antiviral Therapy of Chronic Hepatitis C

Kazuhiko Hayashi, Masatoshi Ishigami, Yoji Ishizu, Teiji Kuzuya, Takashi Honda, Yoshihiko Tachi, Tetsuya Ishikawa, Yoshiaki Katano, Kentaro Yoshioka, Hidenori Toyoda, Takashi Kumada, Hidemi Goto and Yoshiki Hirooka

Additional information is available at the end of the chapter

http://dx.doi.org/10.5772/intechopen.70436

Abstract

Background: Most clinical trials of direct-acting antiviral (DAA) therapy for hepatitis C virus (HCV) infection have excluded hepatitis B virus (HBV) coinfection, and little is known about the effects of DAA on chronic hepatitis C patients with HBV coinfection. Recent studies have reported that DAA therapy for HCV can also cause HBV reactivation in patients with HBV and HCV coinfection. The aim of this study was to assess the effects of DAA on sustained virologic response (SVR) and HBV reactivation in patients with chronic hepatitis C. **Methods:** Participants comprised 199 chronic hepatitis C patients who received DAA therapy (96 men, 103 women; mean age, 66.7 ± 12.0 years). **Results:** Twelve patients were coinfected with HCV and HBV. Sixty patients were HBV surface antigen negative but positive for hepatitis B core antibody and/or hepatitis B surface antibody, and one hundred and twenty-seven patients had not been exposed to HBV. Rates of SVR in HBV and HCV coinfected patients, HBV prior infection, and no exposure to HBV were 100, 95, and 97%, respectively. Significant differences were seen between each group. No case showed HBV reactivation. **Conclusions:** DAA treatments were effective in patients with HBV coinfection or HBV prior infection, as well as HCV monoinfection. As the number of cases was small, we still suggest caution regarding HBV reactivation in HCV and HBV coinfected patients undergoing treatment with DAA.

Keywords: HBV reactivation, hepatitis C virus, hepatitis B virus, sustained virologic response, direct-acting antiviral

1. Introduction

An estimated 170 million individuals worldwide are infected with hepatitis C virus (HCV), causing chronic hepatitis that can develop into potentially fatal cirrhosis and hepatocellular carcinoma [1]. HCV infection is therefore a major global health problem. Since 1992, interferon (IFN)-based therapies have represented the gold standard of treatment for HCV infection. However, sustained virologic response (SVR) from IFN-based therapy is insufficient for all patients, especially those with HCV genotype 1 or cirrhosis and the elderly. In addition, IFN-based therapy is associated with numerous adverse events, such as fatigue, headache, nausea, insomnia, loss of appetite, influenza-like illness, chills, pyrexia, rash, pruritus, anemia or neutropenia, mental disorder, and thyroid dysfunction. To overcome these problems, IFN-free regimens have been developed and are now becoming the standard of care. Daclatasvir plus asunaprevir was the first IFN-free regimen to become commercially available in Japan for patients with HCV genotype 1b, from 2014 [2]. Several IFN-free regimens have become available for daily practice, and most studies have demonstrated high SVR rates and good safety outcomes [3, 4]. Some IFN-free regimens have demonstrated favorable safety and high efficacy within clinical trials among difficult-to-treat patients such as patients who have experienced DAA treatment, cirrhosis, chronic kidney disease, Human immunodeficiency virus co-infection, those on opiate agonist therapy, and patients with liver transplant [5–10]. However, most clinical trials of IFN-free therapy for chronic hepatitis C have excluded hepatitis B virus (HBV) coinfection. Few questions remain unanswered for IFN-free regimens, but little is known about the effects of DAA on SVR and HBV reactivation among chronic hepatitis C patients with HBV coinfection. Reactivation of HBV in HBV surface antigen (HBsAg)–positive patients treated with immunosuppressive or cytotoxic chemotherapy is well known and has emerged as an important clinical issue [11, 12]. HBV reactivation can be caused not only by immunosuppressive or cytotoxic chemotherapy but also by DAA, with some studies reporting HBV reactivation in patients with HBV and HCV coinfection treated by DAA therapy for HCV [13–16]. In addition, although the risk is low, HBV reactivation in patients with resolved HBV infection—that is, in patients negative for HBsAg but positive for hepatitis B core antibody (HBcAb) and/or hepatitis B surface antibody (HBsAb)—can also occur [17]. HBV reactivation should thus be considered in HCV patients with not only HBV infection but also HBV prior infection treated using DAA therapy. However, little is known about HBV reactivation in chronic hepatitis C patients who have received DAA therapy or the relationship between SVR and HBV coinfection. The aim of this study was to assess the effects of DAA on HBV reactivation in patients with HBsAg-positive status or HBV prior infection, and whether HBV infection affects SVR.

2. Methods

2.1. Subjects

A total of 199 patients with chronic hepatitis C who had received DAA therapy were enrolled retrospectively, comprising 96 men and 103 women (mean age, 66.7 ± 12.0 years). Patients with Child Pugh classification B and C were excluded. No patient had autoimmune disease or chronic alcohol abuse. Prior to DAA therapy, HBsAg was measured for all patients. Patients showing

HBsAg also underwent measurement of HBsAb and HBcAb. Patients were classified by HBV infection status. Patients with HBs Ag were regarded as HBV + HCV group, and patients were positive for HBcAb and/or HBsAb were regarded as prior infection group, and patients without any of HBsAg, HBcAb, or HBsAb were regarded as no exposure group. Eighty patients were treated with ledipasvir-sofosbuvir, 100 patients were treated using asunaprevir and daclatasvir, and 19 patients were treated with sofosbuvir and ribavirin. Patients who were persistently negative for serum HCV-RNA at 12 weeks after withdrawal of DAA treatment were considered to have shown SVR. Investigation of HBV reactivation was performed during and 12 months after the end of DAA treatment. This study was approved by the Nagoya University Hospital ethics committee. Written informed consent was obtained from each patient, and the study protocol conformed to the ethical guidelines of the Declaration of Helsinki.

2.2. Statistical analyses

Data are expressed as mean ± standard deviation. Contingency table analysis with Fisher's exact probability test was used for comparisons between groups. Values of $p < 0.05$ were considered statistically significant. Analyses were conducted using SPSS version 23 software (IBM, New York, NY).

3. Results

Twelve patients were positive for HBsAg and defined as showing chronic hepatitis C with HBV coinfection. A total of 187 patients were negative for HBsAg, but 65 patients were positive for HBcAb and/or HBsAb. Five of the sixty-five patients had received HBV vaccination

	HBV + HC	**Prior infection**	**No exposure**
	N = 12	**N = 60**	**N = 127**
Age (y.o.)	64.2 ± 6.8	68.7 ± 9.5	65.7 ± 13.0
Sex: M/F	10/2	30/30	56/71
AST (IU/L)	45.6 ± 36.7	44.3 ± 21.1	49.3 ± 27.0
ALT (IU/L)	56.2 ± 44.1	38.8 ± 19.9	49.4 ± 36.5
Platelet (104/uL)	12.5 ± 5.0	15.2 ± 5.2	15.5 ± 7.1
HCV-RNA level (log IU/mL)	5.9 ± 0.8	6.1 ± 1.1	6.2 ± 0.9
HCV genotype (1/2)	(11/1)	(54/6)	(115/12)
DAA (ASV + DCV/SOF + RBV/LDV + SOF)	(5/1/6)	(28/6/26)	(67/12/48)
SVR	12 (100%)	57 (95%)	123 (97%)
HBV reactivation	none	none	none

HBV, hepatitis B virus; HCV, hepatitis C virus; AST, aspartate aminotransferase; ALT, alanine aminotransferase; DAA, direct-acting antiviral; ASV, asunaprevir; DCV, daclatasvir; SOF, sofosbuvir; RBV, ribavirin; LDV, ledipasvir; SVR, sustained virologic response.

Table 1. Clinical characteristics.

	Case 1	Case 2	Case 3	Case 4	Case 5	Case 6	Case 7	Case 8	Case 9	Case 10	Case 11	Case 12
Age	66	54	70	61	70	56	70	55	66	69	59	74
Sex	M	M	F	M	M	M	M	F	M	M	M	M
ALT(IU/L)	27	38	164	29	31	87	70	111	19	28	39	31
HCV RNA (log IU/ml)	7.0	5.8	5.7	5.3	5.7	7.1	5.3	4.1	6.3	6.6	5.6	6.2
HCV genotype	2a	1b	1b	1b	1b	1b	1b	1b	1b	1b	1b	1b
Treat for HCV	SOF RBV	ASV DCV	LDV SOF	LDV SOF	LDV SOF	LDV SOF	ASV DCV	LDV SOF	LDV SOF	ASV DCV	ASV DCV	ASV DCV
HBV DNA (log copy/mL)	2.1	0	2.1	2.1	2.8	4.5	0	4.7	3.3	ND	ND	ND
HBs Ag titer (IU/mL)	23	3	43	100	250	3.5	539	63	6	11	11	14
HBeAb	Positive	Positive	Positive	Positive	Positive	Positive	Positive	Positive	Positive	Positive	Positive	Positive
Treat for HBV	None	ETV	ETV	None	None	ETV	ETV	None	None	None	None	None
HBV genotype	ND	C	ND	ND	ND	B	ND	C	ND	ND	ND	ND
SVR	Yes	Yes	Yes	Yes	Yes	Yes	Yes	Yes	Yes	Yes	Yes	Yes
Reactivation	None	None	None	None	None	None	None	None	None	None	None	None

HBV, hepatitis B virus; HCV, hepatitis C virus; AST, aspartate aminotransferase; ALT, alanine aminotransferase; DAA, direct-acting antiviral; ASV, asunaprevir; DCV, daclatasvir; SOF, sofosbuvir; RBV, ribavirin; LDV, ledipasvir; SVR, sustained virologic response; ND, not done; ETV, entecavir.

Table 2. Clinical characteristics of patients with HBV and HCV coinfection.

and were thus excluded from being considered as showing previous HBV infection; as a result, sixty patients were defined as having prior infection with HBV. The remaining 122 patients were not positive for any of HBsAg, HBcAb, or HBsAb. With the addition of the 5 vaccinated patients, a total of 127 patients were defined as showing no exposure to HBV. Clinical characteristics at baseline and outcomes such as SVR and incidence of HBV reactivation according to HBV infection status are shown in **Table 1**. No significant differences in clinical characteristics including age, sex, alanine aminotransferase, platelet count, HCV genotypes, and HCV viral load were evident between these three groups. SVR rate in HBV and HCV coinfected patients, HBV prior infection, and no exposure to HBV were 100, 95, and 97%, respectively. No significant differences in SVR were seen between groups. No cases representing definitive HBV reactivation were seen during and after DAA treatment. Clinical characteristics of the 12 patients with HBV and HCV coinfection are shown in **Table 2**. Concentrations of HBsAg were less than 100 IU/mL in most cases, and all titers of HBV-DNA were less than 5 log copies/mL. All patients were positive for hepatitis B e antibody (HBeAb). Four patients received entecavir (ETV) before DAA therapy.

4. Discussion

With the advent of novel agents for chemotherapy and immunotherapy, insufficient data have been accumulated regarding the incidence of HBV reactivation. The association between novel agents and HBV reactivation was noteworthy. At first glance, DAA therapy appears safe, since no HBV reactivation has been observed in several clinical trials. However, most clinical trials of DAA therapy for HCV infection have excluded patients with HBV coinfection, and this bias would obviously mask the incidence of HBV reactivation due to DAA therapy. Real-world experience has revealed HBV reactivation in patients with chronic hepatitis C treated using all-oral direct-acting antiviral regimens [13–16]. In the era of IFN-based therapy against HCV infection, HBV reactivation was not a noteworthy phenomenon for chronic hepatitis C. However, in the era of DAA therapy against HCV infection, HBV reactivation should be a concern in the treatment of patients with HCV infection. IFN rarely induces HBV reactivation, because IFN acts on both HBV and HCV, whereas DAAs act only on HCV. Viral interference between HCV and HBV is known to occur and HCV infection may suppress HBV replication. Rapid eradication of HCV by DAA would thus promote HBV replication and subsequent HBV reactivation. The small number of the total cohort and lack of incidence of HBV reactivation is of major concern for this study. Twelve patients infected with HBV and HCV were observed, and no cases showed definitive HBV reactivation during or after DAA treatment. Wang et al. reported that of 317 patients enrolled, 3 of the 10 patients with HBsAg showed HBV reactivation [18]. However, another study reported no evidence of HBV reactivation among patients treated with ledipasvir-sofosbuvir [19]. HBV reactivation thus remains controversial. Wang et al. speculated that DAAs, particularly NS3 polymerase inhibitors, carry a high risk of HBV reactivation because most reports of HBV reactivation related to DAA involved NS3 polymerase inhibitors [13, 14, 16, 18]. Ledipasvir is a NS5A replication complex inhibitor, and sofosbuvir is a NS5B polymerase inhibitor. The regimen with ledipasvir-sofosbuvir did not use NS3 polymerase inhibitors, which may be why their study found no cases of HBV reactivation. HBV reactivation induced by ledipasvir-sofosbuvir has been reported, in a patient infected with HIV who was receiving antiretroviral therapy including tenofovir [15]. However, that patient discontinued tenofovir because of osteoporosis 14 months before the onset of HBV reactivation. The effects of discontinuing tenofovir would thus have been relevant in that case. Further studies are needed to clarify whether HBV reactivation may occur irrespective of the class of DAA used. Another hypothesis that could explain the lack of HBV reactivation in this study was that the efficacy of prophylactic treatment with a nucleotide analog in preventing HBV reactivation among patients with HBV infection during and after chemotherapy and immunotherapy is well known. Four of twelve patients had received ETV before DAA therapy in our study and ETV would work as pre-emptive therapy in reducing the incidence of HBV reactivation. A second hypothesis for the absence of HBV reactivation in this study involves HBV status. All patients were negative for hepatitis B e antigen (HBeAg) and HBV-DNA titers were less than 5 log copies/mL. Several risk factors for HBV reactivation have been identified, including HBeAg positivity and high HBV DNA levels [20–22]. Thus, the majority of patients enrolled in our study were low-risk patients with HBeAg-negative status and low titers of HBV DNA.

We did not evaluate HBV genotypes in all patients because of low levels of both HBV DNA and HBsAg, but all our patients were Japanese, and we presumed the most prevalent types would be genotype B or C.

Two billion people have been exposed to HBV worldwide, and our study indicates that one-third of patients with HCV infection were defined as showing prior HBV infection. Most countries perform universal vaccination to prevent HBV infection, but only high-risk groups such as health care workers and household contacts of HBV carriers are selected for HBV vaccination in Japan [23]. Vaccinated patients were easily distinguished from those with resolved HBV infection in this study. Rituximab has become the standard of care for patients with malignant lymphoma, and HBV reactivation has also been reported in lymphoma patients with prior HBV infection [17]. A low level of HBV is well recognized as persisting in the liver and peripheral blood mononuclear cells in patients with resolved HBV infection and a functioning immune system. Immunosuppressive agents or chemotherapy may block the immune functions that suppress HBV replication, thus accelerating HBV replication. HBV reactivation thus occurred in patients with prior HBV infection. The incidence of HBV reactivation in patients with chronic hepatitis C treated by DAAs among patients with prior HBV infection is not yet fully understood, but we speculate that DAAs lead to HBV reactivation in patients with resolved HBV infection. However, we failed to identify any cases representing HBV reactivation among patients with resolved HBV infection in this study. We have previously report a case of acute hepatitis B in a patient with HCV infection after DAA therapy [16]. However, the presence of HBcAb or HBsAb was not determined before DAA therapy, so prior HBV infection status was unclear. This case is speculated to represent HBV reactivation in a patient with previously resolved HBV induced by DAA therapy, based on virologic analysis and clinical status. Amino acid substitutions in the S region as immune escape mutants and minority patterns for HBV genotype and serological subtype were virologic features of HBV reactivation [24, 25]. DAAs were suspected to

http://dx.doi.org/10.5772/intechopen.70436

induce HBV reactivation, and effective strategies to prevent HBV reactivation are needed. However, data on the incidence of HBV reactivation with DAA therapy are limited. Larger studies are needed to establish whether the risk of HBV reactivation is increased during and after DAA therapy.

Several factors have been identified, including age, liver fibrosis, HCV genotype, HCV RNA levels, race, amino acid substitutions in the core and NS5A regions, and interleukin 28B polymorphisms have been reported as predictors of response to IFN therapy [26–31]. This study investigated whether HBV coinfection affects response to DAA therapy. However, HBV infection was not associated with SVR from DAA therapy. DAA could eradicate over 95% of HCV, and identification of predictors for SVR is difficult. The limitation of the present study was the small sample size, and larger prospective cohorts are needed to confirm our results.

In conclusion, although relatively few cases have been reported in the literature, we suggest caution regarding HBV reactivation in HCV and HBV coinfected patients undergoing treatment with DAA.

Acknowledgements

This study received a research grant from AMED. Hidemi Goto received research grants from Abbvie, AstraZeneca, Astellas Pharma, Bristol-Myers Squibb, Chugai Pharmaceutical Co, Daiichi Sankyo, Dainippon Sumitomo Pharma, Mitsubishi Tanabe Pharma, MSD, Otsuka Pharmaceutical Co, and Takeda Pharmaceutical Co.

Author details

Kazuhiko Hayashi[1], Masatoshi Ishigami[1]*, Yoji Ishizu[1], Teiji Kuzuya[1], Takashi Honda[1], Yoshihiko Tachi[2], Tetsuya Ishikawa[1], Yoshiaki Katano[3], Kentaro Yoshioka[4], Hidenori Toyoda[5], Takashi Kumada[5], Hidemi Goto[1] and Yoshiki Hirooka[1]

*Address all correspondence to: masaishi@med.nagoya-u.ac.jp

1 Department of Gastroenterology and Hepatology, Nagoya University Graduate School of Medicine, Nagoya, Japan

2 Department of Gastroenterology, Komaki City Hospital, Komaki, Japan

3 Department of Internal Medicine, Banbuntane Hotokukai Hospital, Fujita Health University, School of Medicine, Nagoya, Japan

4 Division of Liver and Biliary Diseases, Department of Internal Medicine, Fujita Health University, Toyoake, Japan

5 Department of Gastroenterology, Ogaki Municipal Hospital, Ogaki, Japan

References

[1] Seeff LB. Natural history of chronic hepatitis C. Hepatology. 2002;36:S35-S46. DOI: 10.1053/jhep.2002.36806

[2] Kumada H, Suzuki Y, Ikeda K, Toyota J, Karino Y, Chayama K, Kawakami Y, Ido A, Yamamoto K, Takaguchi K, Izumi N, Koike K, Takehara T, Kawada N, Sata M, Miyagoshi H, Eley T, McPhee F, Damokosh A, Ishikawa H, Hughes E. Daclatasvir plus asunaprevir for chronic HCV genotype 1b infection. Hepatology. 2014 Jun;59(6):2083-2091. DOI: 10.1002/hep.27113

[3] Mizokami M, Yokosuka O, Takehara T, Sakamoto N, Korenaga M, Mochizuki H, Nakane K, Enomoto H, Ikeda F, Yanase M, Toyoda H, Genda T, Umemura T, Yatsuhashi H, Ide T, Toda N, Nirei K, Ueno Y, Nishigaki Y, Betular J, Gao B, Ishizaki A, Omote M, Mo H, Garrison K, Pang PS, Knox SJ, Symonds WT, McHutchison JG, Izumi N, Omata M. Ledipasvir and sofosbuvir fixed-dose combination with and without ribavirin for 12 weeks in treatment-naive and previously treated Japanese patients with genotype 1 hepatitis C: An open-label, randomised, phase 3 trial. The Lancet Infectious Diseases. 2015 Jun;15(6):645-653. DOI: 10.1016/S1473-3099(15)70099-X

[4] Kumada H, Chayama K, Rodrigues L Jr, Suzuki F, Ikeda K, Toyoda H, Sato K, Karino Y, Matsuzaki Y, Kioka K, Setze C, Pilot-Matias T, Patwardhan M, Vilchez RA, Burroughs M, Redman R. Randomized phase 3 trial of ombitasvir/paritaprevir/ritonavir for hepatitis C virus genotype 1b-infected Japanese patients with or without cirrhosis. Hepatology. 2015 Oct;62(4):1037-1046. DOI: 10.1002/hep.27972

[5] Sulkowski M, Hezode C, Gerstoft J, Vierling JM, Mallolas J, Pol S, Kugelmas M, Murillo A, Weis N, Nahass R, Shibolet O, Serfaty L, Bourliere M, DeJesus E, Zuckerman E, Dutko F, Shaughnessy M, Hwang P, Howe AY, Wahl J, Robertson M, Barr E, Haber B. Efficacy and safety of 8 weeks versus 12 weeks of treatment with grazoprevir (MK-5172) and elbasvir (MK-8742) with or without ribavirin in patients with hepatitis C virus genotype 1 mono-infection and HIV/hepatitis C virus co-infection (C-WORTHY): A randomised, open-label phase 2 trial. Lancet. 2015 Mar 21;385(9973):1087-1097. DOI: 10.1016/S0140-6736(14)61793-1

[6] Forns X, Gordon SC, Zuckerman E, Lawitz E, Calleja JL, Hofer H, Gilbert C, Palcza J, Howe AY, DiNubile MJ, Robertson MN, Wahl J, Barr E, Buti M. Grazoprevir and elbasvir plus ribavirin for chronic HCV genotype-1 infection after failure of combination therapy containing a direct-acting antiviral agent. Journal of Hepatology. 2015 Sep;63(3):564-572. DOI: 10.1016/j.jhep.2015.04.009

[7] Roth D, Nelson DR, Bruchfeld A, Liapakis A, Silva M, Monsour H Jr, Martin P, Pol S, Londoño MC, Hassanein T, Zamor PJ, Zuckerman E, Wan S, Jackson B, Nguyen BY, Robertson M, Barr E, Wahl J, Greaves W. Grazoprevir plus elbasvir in treatment-naive and treatment-experienced patients with hepatitis C virus genotype 1 infection and stage 4-5 chronic kidney disease (the C-SURFER study): a combination phase 3 study. Lancet. 2015 Oct 17;386(10003):1537-1545. DOI: 10.1016/S0140-6736(15)00349-9

[8] Leroy V, Dumortier J, Coilly A, Sebagh M, Fougerou-Leurent C, Radenne S, Botta D, Durand F, Silvain C, Lebray P, Houssel-Debry P, Kamar N, D'Alteroche L, Petrov-Sanchez V, Diallo A, Pageaux GP, Duclos-Vallee JC, Agence Nationale de Recherches sur le SIDA et les Hépatites Virales CO23 Compassionate Use of Protease Inhibitors in Viral C in Liver Transplantation Study Group. Efficacy of Sofosbuvir and Daclatasvir in patients with Fibrosing Cholestatic hepatitis C after liver transplantation. Clinical Gastroenterology and Hepatology. 2015 Nov;13(11):1993-2001. DOI: 10.1016/j.cgh.2015.05.030

[9] Grebely J, Mauss S, Brown A, Bronowicki JP, Puoti M, Wyles D, Natha M, Zhu Y, Yang J, Kreter B, Brainard DM, Yun C, Carr V, Dore GJ. Efficacy and safety of Ledipasvir/Sofosbuvir with and without ribavirin in patients with chronic HCV genotype 1 infection receiving opioid substitution therapy: Analysis of phase 3 ION trials. Clinical Infectious Diseases. 2016 Dec 1;63(11):1405-1411. DOI: 10.1093/cid/ciw580

[10] Akuta N, Sezaki H, Suzuki F, Fujiyama S, Kawamura Y, Hosaka T, Kobayashi M, Kobayashi M, Saitoh S, Suzuki Y, Arase Y, Ikeda K, Kumada H. Retreatment efficacy and predictors of ledipasvir plus sofosbuvir to HCV genotype 1 in Japan. Journal of Medical Virology. 2017 Feb;89(2):284-290. DOI: 10.1002/jmv.24617

[11] Wands JR, Chura CM, Roll FJ, Maddrey WC. Serial studies of hepatitis associated antigen and antibody in patients receiving antitumor chemotherapy for myeloproliferative and lymphoproliferative disorders. Gastroenterology. 1975;68:105-112

[12] Hoofnagle JH, Dusheiko GM, Schafer DF, Jones EA, Micetich KC, Young RC, Costa J. Reactivation of chronic hepatitis B virus infection by cancer chemotherapy. Annals of Internal Medicine. 1982;96:447-449

[13] Collins JM, Raphael KL, Terry C, Cartwright EJ, Pillai A, Anania FA, Farley MM. Hepatitis B virus reactivation during successful treatment of hepatitis C virus with sofosbuvir and simeprevir. Clinical Infectious Diseases. 2015;61:1304-1306. DOI: 10.1093/cid/civ474

[14] Takayama H, Sato T, Ikeda F, Fujiki S. Reactivation of hepatitis B virus during interferon-free therapy with daclatasvir and asunaprevir in patient with hepatitis B virus/hepatitis C virus co-infection. Hepatology Research. 2016 Mar;46(5):489-491. DOI: 10.1111/hepr.12578

[15] De Monte A, Courjon J, Anty R, Cua E, Naqvi A, Mondain V, Cottalorda J, Ollier L, Giordanengo V. Direct-acting antiviral treatment in adults infected with hepatitis C virus: Reactivation of hepatitis B virus coinfection as a further challenge. Journal of Clinical Virology. 2016;78:27-30. DOI: 10.1016/j.jcv.2016.02.026

[16] Hayashi K, Ishigami M, Ishizu Y, Kuzuya T, Honda T, Nishimura D, Goto H, Hirooka Y. A case of acute hepatitis B in a chronic hepatitis C patient after daclatasvir and asunaprevir combination therapy: Hepatitis B virus reactivation or acute self-limited hepatitis? Clinical Journal of Gastroenterology. 2016 Aug;9(4):252-256. DOI: 10.1007/s12328-016-0657-4

[17] Dervite I, Hober D, Morel P. Acute hepatitis B in a patient with antibodies to hepatitis B surface antigen who was receiving rituximab. The New England Journal of Medicine. 2001;344:68-69. DOI: 10.1056/NEJM200101043440120

[18] Wang C, Ji D, Chen J, Shao Q, Li B, Liu J, Wu V, Wong A, Wang Y, Zhang X, Lu L, Wong C, Tsang S, Zhang Z, Sun J, Hou J, Chen G, Lau G. Hepatitis due to reactivation of hepatitis B virus in endemic areas among patients with hepatitis C treated with direct-acting antiviral agents. Clinical Gastroenterology and Hepatology. 2017 Jan;15(1):132-136. DOI: 10.1016/j.cgh.2016.06.023

[19] Sulkowski MS, Chuang WL, Kao JH, Yang JC, Gao B, Brainard DM, Han KH, Gane E. No evidence of reactivation of hepatitis B virus among patients treated with Ledipasvir-Sofosbuvir for hepatitis C virus infection. Clinical Infectious Diseases. 2016 Nov 1;63(9):1202-1204. DOI: 10.1093/cid/ciw507

[20] Yeo W, Chan PK, Zhong S, Ho WM, Steinberg JL, Tam JS, Hui P, Leung NW, Zee B, Johnson PJ. Frequency of hepatitis B virus reactivation in cancer patients undergoing cytotoxic chemotherapy: A prospective study of 626 patients with identification of risk factors. Journal of Medical Virology. 2000;62:299-307

[21] Lau GK, Leung YH, Fong DY, Au WY, Kwong YL, Lie A, Hou JL, Wen YM, Nanj A, Liang R. High hepatitis B virus (HBV) DNA viral load as the most important risk factor for HBV reactivation in patients positive for HBV surface antigen undergoing autologous hematopoietic cell transplantation. Blood. 2002;99(7):2324-2330

[22] Zhong S, Yeo W, Schroder C, Chan PK, Wong WL, Ho WM, Mo F, Zee B, Johnson PJ. High hepatitis B virus (HBV) DNA viral load is an important risk factor for HBV reactivation in breast cancer patients undergoing cytotoxic chemotherapy. Journal of Viral Hepatitis. 2004;11:55-59

[23] Zanetti AR, Van Damme P, Shouval D. The global impact of vaccination against hepatitis B: A historical overview. Vaccine. 2008;26:6266-6273. DOI: 10.1016/j.vaccine.2008.09.056

[24] Salpini R, Colagrossi L, Bellocchi MC, Surdo M, Becker C, Alteri C, Aragri M, Ricciardi A, Armenia D, Pollicita M, Di Santo F, Carioti L, Louzoun Y, Mastroianni CM, Lichtner M, Paoloni M, Esposito M, D'Amore C, Marrone A, Marignani M, Sarrecchia C, Sarmati L, Andreoni M, Angelico M, Verheyen J, Perno CF, Svicher V. Hepatitis B surface antigen genetic elements critical for immune escape correlate with hepatitis B virus reactivation upon immunosuppression. Hepatology. 2015;61:823-833. DOI: 10.1002/hep.27604

[25] Hayashi K, Ishigami M, Ishizu Y, Kuzuya T, Honda T, Tachi Y, Ishikawa T, Katano Y, Yoshioka K, Toyoda H, Kumada T, Goto H, Hirooka Y. Clinical characteristics and molecular analysis of hepatitis B virus reactivation in hepatitis B surface antigen-negative patients during or after immunosuppressive or cytotoxic chemotherapy. Journal of Gastroenterology. 2016 Nov;51(11):1081-1089. DOI: 10.1007/s00535-016-1187-z

[26] Berg T, Sarrazin C, Herrmann E, Hinrichsen H, Gerlach T, Zachoval R, Wiedenmann B, Hopf U, Zeuzem S. Prediction of treatment outcome in patients with chronic hepatitis C: Significance of baseline parameters and viral dynamics during therapy. Hepatology. 2003;37:600-609. DOI: 10.1053/jhep.2003.50106

[27] Conjeevaram HS, Kleiner DE, Everhart JE, Hoofnagle JH, Zacks S, Afdhal NH, Wahed AS, Virahep-C Study Group. Race, insulin resistance and hepatic steatosis in chronic hepatitis C. Hepatology. 2007 Jan;45(1):80-87. DOI: 10.1002/hep.21455

[28] Tanaka Y, Nishida N, Sugiyama M, Kurosaki M, Matsuura K, Sakamoto N, Nakagawa M, Korenaga M, Hino K, Hige S, Ito Y, Mita E, Tanaka E, Mochida S, Murawaki Y, Honda M, Sakai A, Hiasa Y, Nishiguchi S, Koike A, Sakaida I, Imamura M, Ito K, Yano K, Masaki N, Sugauchi F, Izumi N, Tokunaga K, Mizokami M. Genome-wide association of IL28B with response to pegylated interferon-alpha and ribavirin therapy for chronic hepatitis C. Nature Genetics. 2009;41:1105-1109. DOI: 10.1038/ng.449

[29] Akuta N, Suzuki F, Kawamura Y, Yatsuji H, Sezaki H, Suzuki Y, Hosaka T, Kobayashi M, Kobayashi M, Arase Y, Ikeda K, Kumada H. Predictive factors of early and sustained responses to peginterferon plus ribavirin combination therapy in Japanese patients infected with hepatitis C virus genotype 1b: Amino acid substitutions in the core region and low-density lipoprotein cholesterol levels. Journal of Hepatology. 2007;46:403-410. DOI: 10.1016/j.jhep.2006.09.019

[30] Honda T, Katano Y, Shimizu J, Ishizu Y, Doizaki M, Hayashi K, Ishigami M, Itoh A, Hirooka Y, Nakano I, Urano F, Yoshioka K, Toyoda H, Kumada T, Goto H. Efficacy of peginterferon-alpha-2b plus ribavirin in patients aged 65 years and older with chronic hepatitis C. Liver International. 2010;30:527-537. DOI: 10.1111/j.1478-3231.2009.02064.x

[31] Hayashi K, Katano Y, Honda T, Ishigami M, Itoh A, Hirooka Y, Ishikawa T, Nakano I, Yoshioka K, Toyoda H, Kumada T, Goto H. Association of interleukin 28B and mutations in the core and NS5A region of hepatitis C virus with response to peg-interferon and ribavirin therapy. Liver International. 2011 Oct;31(9):1359-1365. DOI: 10.1111/j.1478-3231.2011.02571.x

Chapter 5

Current Therapeutic Options for HCV-HIV Coinfection

Ljiljana Perić and Dario Sabadi

Additional information is available at the end of the chapter

http://dx.doi.org/10.5772/intechopen.70730

Abstract

Due to shared risk factors for transmission, coinfection with human immunodeficiency virus (HIV) and hepatitis C virus (HCV) is a very common event. The prevalence of HCV infection among HIV-positive patients averages about 35%. In HIV/HCV co-infected patients, liver-related morbidity and mortality is a prominent non-AIDS-defining complication: up to 90% of liver-related deaths in HIV-infected patients are attributable to HCV. The progression of liver fibrosis is accelerated in HIV/HCV-coinfected patients, particularly in individuals with low CD4 counts (≤350 cells/mm^3). Antiretroviral therapy may slow liver disease progression in HIV/HCV-coinfected patients and should, therefore, be considered for all coinfected patients regardless of CD4 cell count. Most patients with HIV/HCV coinfection are taking multi-drug antiretroviral therapy, which may pose a problem with drug–drug interactions when initiating therapy with HCV medications. Rapid advances in HCV drug development led to the discovery of new classes of direct-acting antiviral (DAA) agents that target the HCV replication cycle. Several studies demonstrated comparable rates of sustained virological response (SVR) in coinfected and monoinfected patients with new DAA-based therapy.

Keywords: HCV/HIV-coinfection, liver cirrhosis, CD4 T lymphocytes, antiretroviral therapy (ART), direct-acting antiviral (DAA) agents, drug–drug interaction

1. Introduction

By the Global AIDS Update: 2016, around 36.7 million people are living with human immunodeficiency virus (HIV) in the world today [1]. Five million of them are also infected with hepatitis C virus (HCV) [1]. HIV accelerate the progression of hepatitis C, inducing increased morbidity and mortality [2]. HIV-infected people are on average six times more likely than HIV-uninfected people to have HCV infection [3].

HIV and HCV share modes of transmission: often occurring by exposure to blood, sexual intercourse or by mother-to-child transmission.

2. Epidemiology

The prevalence of HCV antibodies varies widely among HIV transmission groups, ranging from 7–8% in men who have sex with men to 60–70% in hemophiliacs and 80–90% in intravenous drug users (IDUs), the most important group (**Figure 1**) [4].

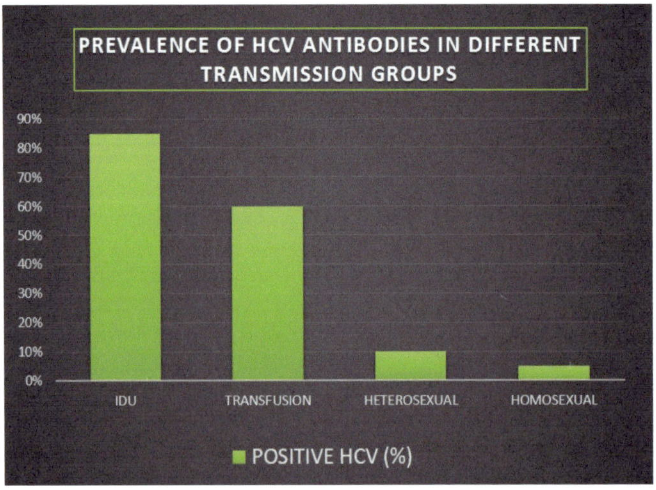

Figure 1. Prevalence of HCV antibodies in different transmission groups. IDU, intravenous drug users; HCV, hepatitis C virus. Inspired by Management of Hepatitis C and HIV coinfection, Clinical Protocol for the WHO European Region. Available at: http://www.euro.who.int/data/assets/pdf_file/0008/78146/E90840Chapter6.pdf, Version September 1th, 2015.

For HIV-infected patients with HCV coinfection, liver-related morbidity and mortality is a prominent non-AIDS-defining complication [5]. Up to 90% of liver-related deaths in HIV-infected patients are attributable to HCV [5].

Among patients with chronic HCV infection, approximately one-third progress to cirrhosis, at a median time of 20 years [6–8]. The risk of progression is even greater in HCV/HIV-coinfected patients with low CD4 T lymphocyte (CD4) cell counts (≤350 cells/mm^3) [6, 9, 10]. Cirrhosis has been observed to occur 12–16 years earlier in HIV/HCV-coinfected patients compared with those who have HCV monoinfection [11].

3. Antiretroviral therapy (ART) in HIV/HCV-coinfected patients

Antiretroviral therapy (ART) may slow liver disease progression in HIV/HCV-coinfected patients and should, therefore, be considered for all coinfected patients regardless of CD4

http://dx.doi.org/10.5772/intechopen.70730

NRTIs	NNRTIs	Protease inhibitors	Entry inhibitors	Integrase inhibitors
Abacavir	Efavirenz	Atazanavir, atazanavir/ritonavir	Enfuvirtide	Dolutegravir
Didanosine	Etravirine	Darunavir/ritonavir Darunavir/cobicistat	Maraviroc	Raltegravir
Emtricitabine	Nevirapine	Fosamprenavir		
Lamivudine	Rilpivirine	Lopinavir		
Stavudine		Saquinavir		
Tenofovir				
Zidovudine				

Table 1. Standard recommended treatments for naive patients with HIV-1 infection.

cell count [12]. This recommendation is supported by observational studies that suggest that antiretroviral therapy may reduce the risk of liver-related morbidity. The key issues in the clinical management of HIV/HCV-coinfected patients are which treatment for each condition and when to initiate it [12].

Classes of antiretroviral agents are nucleoside reverse transcriptase inhibitors (NRTIs), non-nucleoside reverse transcriptase inhibitors (NNRTIs), protease inhibitors (PIs), integrase inhibitors (INSTIs), entry/fusion inhibitors (FIs) and chemokine receptor antagonists (CCR5 antagonists).

Standard recommended treatments for naive patients with HIV-1 infection (**Table 1**) generally consist of two nucleoside reverse transcriptase inhibitors (NRTIs) in combination with a third active antiretroviral drug from one of three drug classes: an integrase strand transfer inhibitor (INSTI), a non-nucleoside reverse transcriptase inhibitor (NNRTI) or a protease inhibitor (PI) with a pharmacokinetic (PK) enhancer (booster) (cobicistat or ritonavir) [12].

Antiretroviral therapy (ART) associated with liver injury is more common in HIV/HCV-coinfected patients than in those with HIV monoinfection [6, 13]. Some older ART have been associated with higher rates of liver injury in patients with chronic HCV infection, but newer ART drugs currently in use appear to be less hepatotoxic [6, 13]. Patients with significant alanine aminotransferase (ALT) and/or aspartate aminotransferase (AST) elevation should be carefully evaluated for signs and symptoms of liver insufficiency and for alternative causes of liver injury (e.g., acute HAV or HBV infection, hepatobiliary disease, or alcoholic hepatitis) [6, 14]. Short-term interruption of the ART regimen or of the specific drug suspected of causing the liver injury may be required [6, 14].

4. Concurrent treatment of HIV and HCV by the Office of AIDS Research advisory council (OARAC 2016)

If the decision is made to treat HCV, the antiretroviral regimen may need to be modified before HCV treatment is initiated to reduce the potential drug–drug interactions and/or toxicities that may develop during the period of concurrent HIV and HCV treatment [6].

In patients with suppressed plasma HIV RNA and modified antiretroviral therapy, HIV RNA should be measured within 4–8 weeks after changing antiretroviral therapy to confirm the effectiveness of the new regimen [6]. After completion of HCV treatment, the modified ART regimen should be continued for at least 2 weeks before reinitiating the original regimen [6]. This is necessary because of the prolonged half-life of some HCV drugs and the potential risk of drug–drug interactions if a prior HIV regimen is resumed soon after HCV treatment is completed [6].

5. HCV therapy in HIV/HCV-coinfected patients by EASL recommendations on treatment of hepatitis C, 2016

With direct-acting antivirals (DAAs), HCV cure rates of both HCV mono and HIV/HCV-coinfected persons are greater than 95% [15]. Current treatment guidelines no longer separate these two groups. Indications for HCV treatment and choice of direct-acting antiviral (DAA) agents combination are now the same for all HCV patients. In HIV/HCV co-infection, drug interactions between HIV and HCV agents need be checked prior to starting HCV therapy [15]. The higher risk of hepatic decompensation in HIV/HCV-coinfected patients, including those receiving successful antiretroviral therapy, continues to make these patients a high priority group for receiving access to direct-acting antiviral (DAA) agents as combination therapy [15].

6. Key studies for treatment of HCV with HIV coinfection

Using DAA therapy, several studies demonstrated comparable rates of sustained virological response (SVR) in coinfected and monoinfected patients.

These trials, however, have primarily included individuals with CD4 counts >200 cells/mm^3, and most patients in these trials did not have cirrhosis.

6.1. Sofosbuvir for genotype 1–4 in HIV coinfection by Rodriguez-Torres et al.

In an open-label trial, 23 HCV/HIV-coinfected treatment-naive patients with genotype 1–4 received the 12-week triple therapy of peginterferon alfa-2a, ribavirin (weight-based) and sofosbuvir [16]. Mean CD4 count was 562 cells/mm^3, and all were on antiretroviral therapy (tenofovir-emtricitabine plus one of the following: efavirenz, atazanavir plus ritonavir, darunavir plus ritonavir, rilpivirine or raltegravir) [16]. The overall SVR12 rate was 91%; of the 19 patients with genotype 1, 89% achieved an SVR12 (**Figure 2**) [16].

6.2. TURQUOISE-I by Wyles et al.

This open-label study randomized treatment-naive and experienced patients with chronic HCV genotype 1 and HIV coinfection to receive a 12- or 24-week course of ombitasvir-paritaprevir-ritonavir and dasabuvir plus ribavirin [17]. Patients were required to have

http://dx.doi.org/10.5772/intechopen.70730

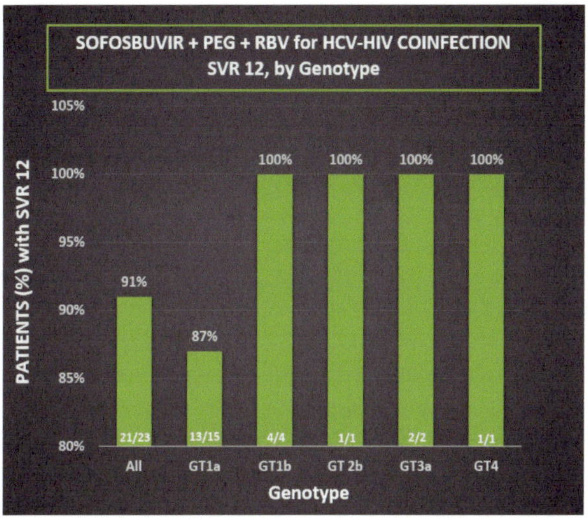

Figure 2. Sofosbuvir for genotype 1-4 in HIV coinfection. PEG, peginterferon alfa-2a; RBV, ribavirin; SVR12, sustained viral response 12 weeks after the end of treatment; GT, genotype. Inspired by http://slides.hcvonline.org/uploads/151/sofosbuvir_for_genotype_14_in_hiv_coinfection.pdf

a CD4 > 200 cells/mm^3 and an HIV RNA level < 40 copies while receiving an atazanavir- or raltegravir-based regimen [17]. The sustained virological response (SVR) 12 rates were 93.5% (29 of 31) in the 12-week group and 90.6% (29 of 32) in the 24-week group (**Figure 3**) [17].

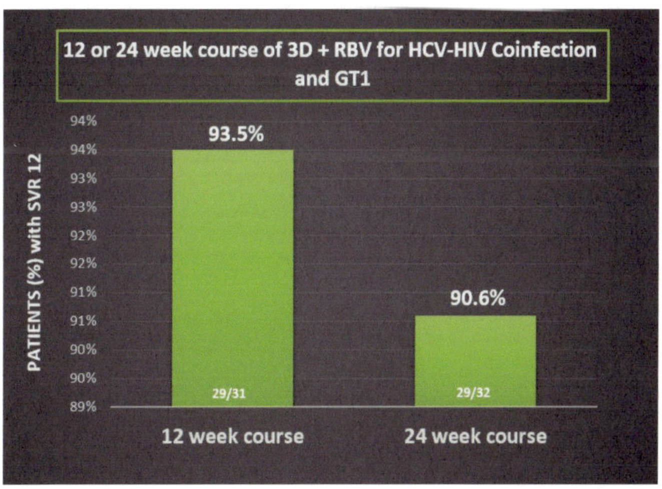

Figure 3. TURQUOISE-I. 3 D, Ombitasvir-Paritaprevir-Ritonavir and Dasabuvir; RBV, ribavirin; GT, genotype; SVR, sustained viral response. Inspired by https://depts.washington.edu/hepstudy/presentations/uploads/137/turquoise13d.pdf

6.3. ALLY-2 study (daclatasvir + sofosbuvir in HCV GT 1–4 and HIV coinfection) by Wyles et al.

Among HIV/HCV-coinfected patients who received 12 weeks of daclatasvir plus sofosbuvir, sustained virologic response across all genotypes was 97.0% (including black patients and those with cirrhosis) and 76.0% after 8 weeks [18].

6.4. ION-4 study (ledipasvir and sofosbuvir for HCV genotype 1 or 4 in patients coinfected with HIV-1) by Naggie et al.

In this multicenter, open-label, single-group study, 12 weeks of treatment with the once-daily, single-tablet regimen of ledipasvir-sofosbuvir resulted in a sustained virologic response in 96% of patients [19]. In exploratory subgroup analyses, rates of sustained virologic response 12 weeks after the end of therapy (the primary efficacy end point) were similar across all subgroups except that black patients, who made up 34% of the study population, had lower rates of sustained virologic response (**Figure 4**) [19].

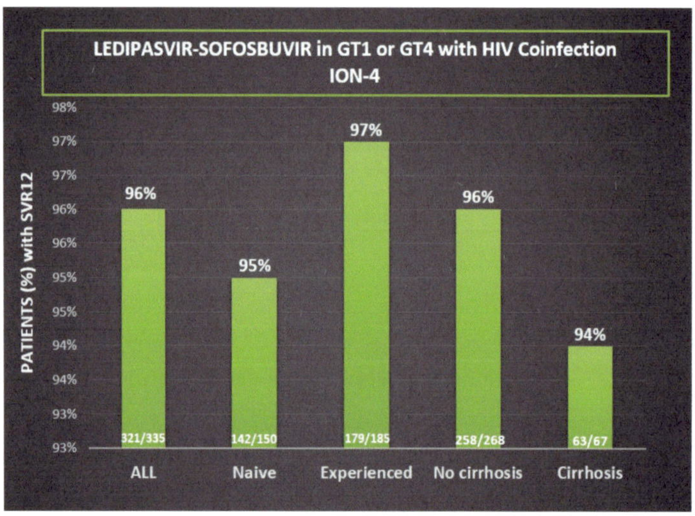

Figure 4. Ledipasvir and sofosbuvir for HCV genotype 1 or 4 in patients coinfected with HIV-1. GT 1 or 4, genotype 1 or 4; SVR 12, sustained viral response 12 weeks after the end of treatment. Inspired by http://slides.hcvonline.org/uploads/149/ion4_ls.pdf

7. Conclusions

Due to shared risk factors for transmission, HIV/HCV coinfection is a very common event, the prevalence averages about 35% in the United States and Europe [20, 21].

http://dx.doi.org/10.5772/intechopen.70730

The progression of liver fibrosis is accelerated in HIV/HCV-coinfected patients. HCV guidance recommends using the same HCV treatment approach for patients coinfected with HIV as those with HCV monoinfection.

DAAs and interferon-free combination therapy has changed the landscape of therapy for HIV/HCV-coinfected patients.

Multiple studies demonstrating comparable rates of SVR in coinfected and monoinfected patients.

Author details

Ljiljana Perić[1,2]* and Dario Sabadi[1,2]

*Address all correspondence to: ljiljana.peric@mefos.hr

1 Department of Infectious Diseases and Dermatology, Faculty of Medicine Osijek, University of Osijek, Osijek, Croatia

2 Clinic for Infectious Diseases, University Hospital Center Osijek, Osijek, Croatia

References

[1] Global AIDS Response Progress Reporting (GARPR) 2016. Geneva, Switzerland: UNAIDS 2016 Estimates; 2016

[2] Operskalski EA, Kovacs A. HIV/HCV co-infection: Pathogenesis, clinical complications, treatment, and new therapeutic technologies. Current HIV/AIDS Reports. 2011;**8**(1):12-22

[3] Platt L, Easterbrook P, Gower E, McDonald B, Sabin K, McGowan C, Yanny I, Razavi H, Vickerman P. Prevalence and burden of HCV co-infection in people living with HIV: A global systematic review and meta-analysis. 2016.

[4] Management of hepatitis C and HIV coinfection, Clinical Protocol for the WHO European Region, Chapter6.pdf, Version 1 September 2015. Available from: http://www.euro.who.int/data/assets/pdf_file/0008/78146/ E90840

[5] Spach DH, Nina Kim H. Treatment of Chronic Hepatitis C Infection Overview. Available from: http://www.hepatitisc.uw.edu/go/treatment-infection

[6] Guidelines for the Use of Antiretroviral Agents in HIV-1-Infected Adults and Adolescents, Developed by the DHHS Panel on Antiretroviral Guidelines for Adults and Adolescents – A Working Group of the Office of AIDS Research Advisory Council (OARAC), 8/25/2017. Available from: https://aidsinfo.nih.gov/contentfiles/lvguidelines/AdultandAdolescentGL.pdf

[7] Alter MJ, Margolis HS, Krawczynski K, et al. The natural history of community-acquired hepatitis C in the United States. The Sentinel Counties Chronic non-A, non-B Hepatitis

Study Team. The New England Journal of Medicine 1992;**327** (27):1899-1905. Available at: http://www.ncbi.nlm.nih.gov/entrez/query.fcgi?cmd=Retrieve&db=PubMed&dopt=Citation&list_uids=1280771

[8] Thomas DL, Astemborski J, Rai RM, et al. The natural history of hepatitis C virus infection: Host, viral, and environmental factors. Journal of the American Medical Association. 2000;**284**(4):450-456 Available from: http://www.ncbi.nlm.nih.gov/entrez/query.fcgi?cmd=Retrieve&db=PubMed&dopt=Citation&list_uids=10904508

[9] Considerations for Antiretroviral Use in Patients with Coinfections, Hepatitis C (HCV)/HIV Coinfection, Last Updated: July 14, 2016; Last Reviewed: July 14, 2016. Developed by the DHHS Panel on Antiretroviral Guidelines for Adults and Adolescents – A Working Group of the Office of AIDS Research Advisory Council (OARAC) , Available at: https://aidsinfo.nih.gov/guidelines/html/1/adult-and-adolescent-arv-guidelines/26/hcv-hiv

[10] Graham CS, Baden LR, Yu E, et al. Influence of human immunodeficiency virus infection on the course of hepatitis C virus infection: A meta-analysis. Clinical Infectious Diseases. 2001;**33**(4):562-569 Available from: http://www.ncbi.nlm.nih.gov/entrez/query.fcgi?cmd=Retrieve&db=PubMed&dopt=Citation&list_uids=11462196

[11] Benhamou Y, Bochet M, Di Martino V, Charlotte F, Azria F, Coutellier A, Vidaud M, Bricaire F, Opolon P, Katlama C, Poynard T. Liver fibrosis progression in human immunodeficiency virus and hepatitis C virus coinfected patients. Hepatology. 1999;**30**:1054-1058

[12] Considerations for Antiretroviral Use in Patients with Coinfections, Hepatitis C (HCV)/HIV Coinfection, Last Updated: 14 July 2016; Last Reviewed: 14 July 2016. Available from: https://aidsinfo.nih.gov/guidelines/html/1/adult-and-adolescent-arv-guidelines/26/hcv-hiv

[13] Aranzabal L, Casado JL, Moya J, et al. Influence of liver fibrosis on highly active antiretroviral therapy-associated hepatotoxicity in patients with HIV and hepatitis C virus coinfection. Clinical Infectious Diseases. 2005;**40**(4):588-593 Available from: http://www.ncbi.nlm.nih.gov/entrez/query.fcgi?cmd=Retrieve&db=PubMed&dopt=Citation&list_uids=15712082

[14] Sulkowski MS, Thomas DL. Hepatitis C in the HIV-infected patient. Clinics in Liver Disease. 2003;**7**(1):179-194 Available from: http://www.ncbi.nlm.nih.gov/entrez/query.fcgi?cmd=Retrieve&db=PubMed&dopt=Citation&list_uids=12691466

[15] Rockstroh JK, Hardy WD. Current treatment options for hepatitis C patients co-infected with HIV, Expert Rev Gastroenterol Hepatol. 2016;**10**:689-695. Available from: https://www.ncbi.nlm.nih.gov/pubmed/26799571

[16] Rodriguez-Torres M et al. Sofosbuvir for chronic hepatitis C virus infection genotype 1-4 in patients coinfected with HIV. Journal of Acquired Immune Deficiency Syndrome. 2015;**68**:543-549 Available from: https://www.ncbi.nlm.nih.gov/pubmed/25622055, http://slides.hcvonline.org/uploads/151/sofosbuvir_for_genotype_14_in_hiv_coinfection.pdf

[17] Wyles D et al. TURQUOISE-I Part 1b: Ombitasvir/Paritaprevir/Ritonavir and Dasabuvir with Ribavirin for Hepatitis C Virus Infection in HIV-1 Coinfected Patients on Darunavir. The Journal of Infectious Disease. 2017;**215**(4):599-605. doi: 10.1093/infdis/jiw597. Available from: https://www.ncbi.nlm.nih.gov/pubmed/28329334 and https://depts.washington.edu/hepstudy/presentations/uploads/137/turquoise13d.pdf

[18] Wyles DL et al. Daclatasvir in combination with sofosbuvir for HIV/HCV coinfection: ALLY-2 Study. The New England Journal of Medicine. 2015;**373**:714-725 Available from: http://slides.hcvonline.org/uploads/163/ally2_daclatasvir.pdf and http://www.nejm.org/doi/full/10.1056/NEJMoa1503153#t=article

[19] Naggie S et al. Ledipasvir and sofosbuvir for HCV in patients coinfected with HIV-1-ION-4 Study. The New England Journal of Medicine. 2015;**378**:705-713 Available at http://www.nejm.org/doi/full/10.1056/NEJMoa1501315?rss=searchAndBrowse#t=article and http://slides.hcvonline.org/uploads/149/ion4_ls.pdf

[20] Nina Kim H, Spach DH. Treatment of Hepatitis C in Patients with HIV Coinfection. Available from: http://www.hepatitisc.uw.edu/go/special-populations-situations/treatment-hiv-coinfection/core-concept/all#drug-drug-interactions-hiv-hcv-coinfection-treatment

[21] Verucchi G et al. Human immunodeficiency virus and hepatitis C virus coinfection: Epidemiology, natural history, therapeutic options and clinical management. Infection. 2004;**32**(1):33-46 Available from: https://www.ncbi.nlm.nih.gov/pubmed/15007741

Section 2

HCV Today's Challenges

Chapter 6

Hepatitis C Treatment in Elderly Patients

Takashi Honda, Masatoshi Ishigami,
Kazuhiko Hayashi, Teiji Kuzuya, Yoji Ishizu,
Yoshiki Hirooka and Hidemi Goto

Additional information is available at the end of the chapter

http://dx.doi.org/10.5772/intechopen.70437

Abstract

The patients with chronic hepatitis C (CHC) are getting older and the demands for treatment to those patients are increasing due to the high risk of development of hepatocellular carcinoma. Elderly patients were previously defined as 60 years and over, however definition of the elderly patients shifted to be older year to year. Interferon (IFN) and ribavirin combination therapy was significantly improved efficacy of treatment, however ribavirin induces anemia, resulted in lower efficacy due to reduction of ribavirin for the elderly patients. And efficacy of over 60 years old was comparable to the patients under 60 years. In the CHC patients with genotype 1, the efficacy of elderly patient was significantly lower than that of younger patients, especially in female. Direct-acting antivirals (DAAs) therapy makes treatment efficacy improved to over 90% and side effect of treatment was dramatically reduced compared to IFN-based therapy. The efficacy of dual oral therapy by using asunaprevir (ASV) and daclatasvir (DCA) for elderly patients with hepatitis C virus (HCV) genotype 1b has not been fully clarified. In this article we would like to show the efficacy of elderly patients with CHC, especially patients infected with genotype 1b, from the era of IFN monotherapy to the era of new DAAs.

Keywords: hepatitis C virus, peginterferon, ribavirin, direct-acting antivirals, elderly patient

1. Introduction

The first in the world, the demand for treatment to the elderly patients with chronic hepatitis C (CHC) has increased in Japan. The prevalence of anti-hepatitis C virus (HCV) shows the peak is in the older generation and the rate of anti-HCV increases with the increase in age in Japan. In other country, the peak of prevalence differs from country to country. These differences

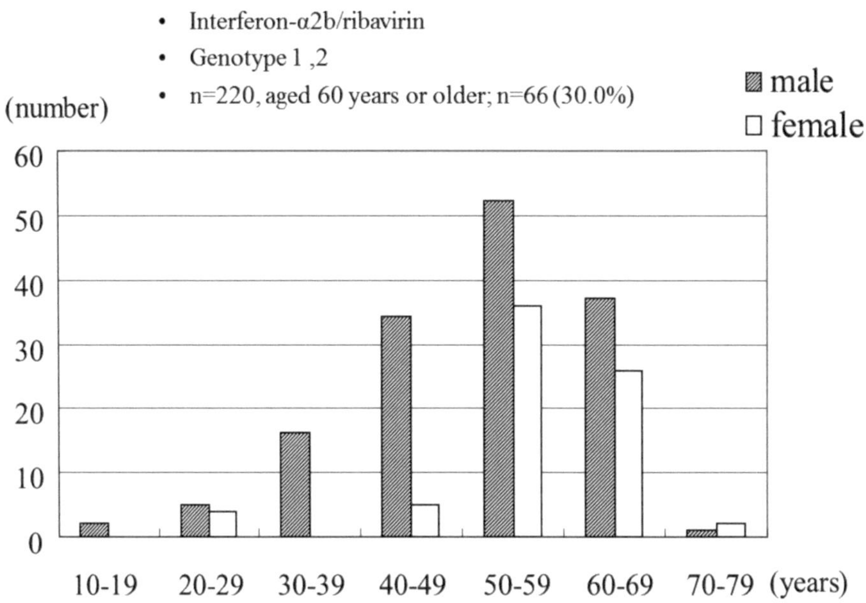

Figure 1. Patient age distribution by decade.

come from one of the reasons when the war was held in each country. During the war, HCV infection spread among drug users, blood donors and the wounded. Thereafter medical treatment with intravenous injection using contaminated needles and syringes during that time easily transmitted HCV. Therefore in Japan the peak of prevalence of anti-HCV was shifted to the older comparing to other country [1]. Previously, we compared SVR rate of ribavirin plus interferon (IFN)-α2b in CHC patients aged ≥60 years with patients aged <60 years [2]. Our study showed age distribution of the CHC patients treated by IFN-α plus ribavirin was peaked around 50 generation in 2002 (**Figure 1**). At that time we defined over 60 years as elderly patients.

2. Ribavirin and IFN-based treatment

The sustained virological response (SVR) rates of treatment in the patients with genotype 1 and a high viral load aged 60 years and older was below 10% by IFN monotherapy. However, SVR rate of IFN and ribavirin combination therapy was significantly improved by over 20%. And efficacy of over 60 years old was comparable to the patients under 60 years (**Figure 2**) [2]. In this study adding of ribavirin increased SVR rate, but ribavirin induces anemia, resulted in lower SVR rate due to reduction of ribavirin in the elderly patients. During combination of IFN-α2b plus ribavirin therapy, over 50 generation and 60 generation had high dose reduction and cessation of treatment (**Figure 3**) [2].

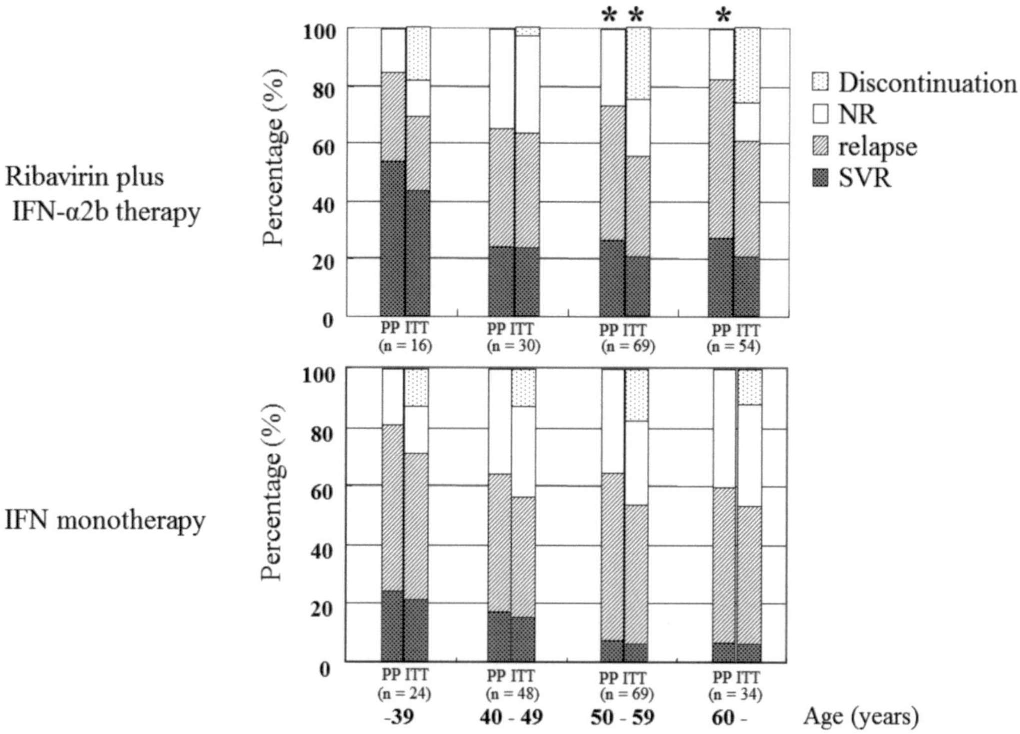

Figure 2. Virologic response to combination therapy and interferon monotherapy. * Indicate significant differences vs the respective IFN monotherapy (*P < 0.05).

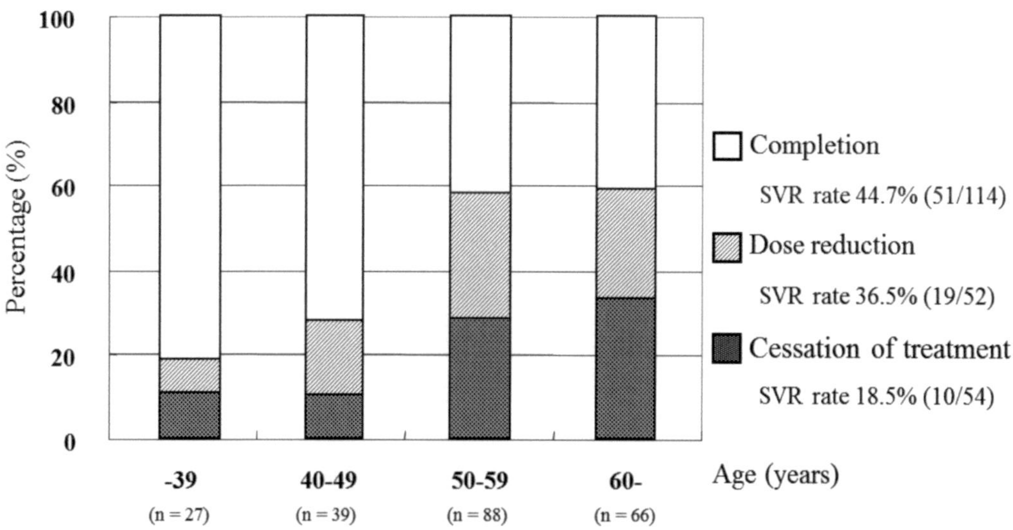

Figure 3. Ribavirin dose reduction and discontinuation rates according age of patients.

3. Ribavirin and PegIFN-based treatment

Peginterferon (PegIFN) plus ribavirin therapy improved the SVR rate of HCV treatment. We conducted the study of efficacy of PegIFN-α2b plus ribavirin and the number of the CHC patients in that study was 591. The distribution of elderly patients was around 20% in 2007. At that time elderly patients were defined as aged 65 years or older [3]. In the CHC patients with genotype 1, the SVR rate of elderly patient was significantly lower than that of younger patients, especially in female (**Figure 4**) [3]. On the other hand, patients with genotype 2 had comparable SVR rate of elderly patients to the younger patients (**Figure 5**) [3].

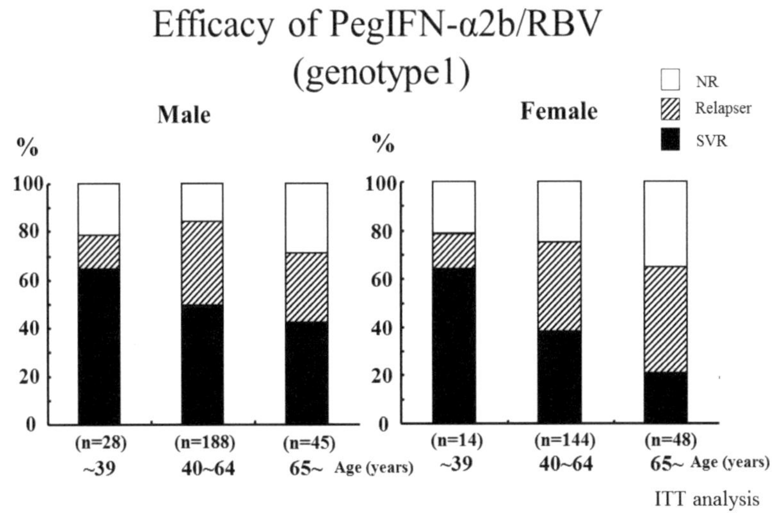

Figure 4. A virological response to combination therapy according to the age and gender of patients with genotype 1.

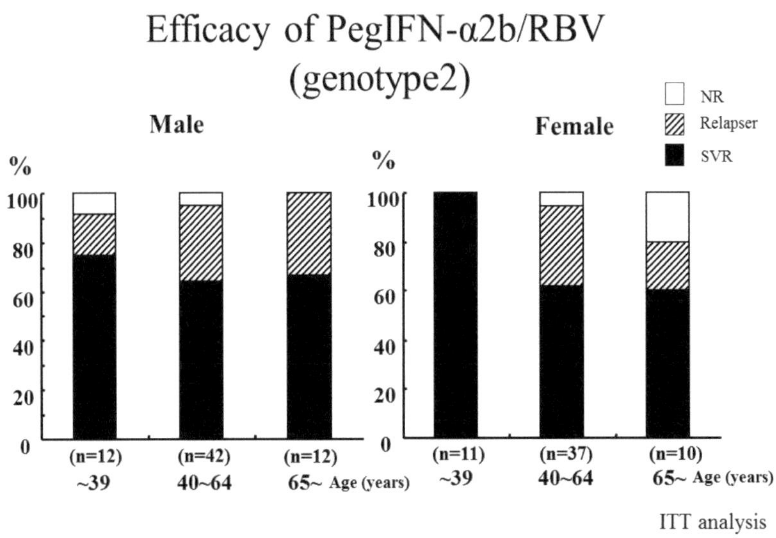

Figure 5. A virological response to combination therapy according to the age and gender of patients with genotype 2.

http://dx.doi.org/10.5772/intechopen.70437

4. DAA-based treatment

Emerge of direct-acting antiviral's (DAA's) therapy makes SVR rate improved to over 90% and side effect of treatment was dramatically reduced compared to IFN-based therapy. Ribavirin free regimen also has benefit for the elderly patients due to avoidance of ribavirin-induced anemia. Akuta et al. reported that high SVR rate was achieved by daclatasvir (NS5A replication complex inhibitor) (DCA) and asunaprevir (NS3 protease inhibitor) (ASV) even in the elderly patients infected with HCV genotype 1b aged 70 and older [4]. They showed predictive factors associated with SVR12 in elderly patients was NS5A-Y93H mutation under 20%, non-treated by triple therapy with simeprevir, lower level of viremia under 6 logIU/mL, hemoglobin under 13.0 g/dl.

We also conducted the study of efficacy of DAA's therapy for the genotype 1-infected patients with CHC. Here we show the results of the patients with DCA and ASV therapy, 287 patients were analyzed and the patient's background shows that patients were getting older and we defined elderly patients as aged 70 older. The study protocol was approved by the ethics committee of our hospital and affiliated hospital. The inclusion criteria included positive anti-HCV and positive HCV RNA and having findings of active hepatitis. Exclusion criteria included positive for serum hepatitis B surface antigen, alcohol abuse, autoimmune hepatitis, primary biliary cirrhosis, coexisting serious psychiatric or medical illness.

Elderly patients account for 57.8% (166/287) of total treated patients (**Table 1**). Baseline ALT, γ-glutamyl transpeptidase (GGT) hemoglobin and eGFR in elderly patients were significantly lower than that of younger patients. Renal function in elderly patients was worse comparing

	Total patients (n = 287)	Patients aged <70 years (n = 121)	Patients aged ≥70 years (n = 166)	P value
Sex ratio (male/female)	123/164	55/66	68/98	0.448
Age (years)	72.0 (65.0–77.0)	63.0 (58.0–66.0)	76.0 (73.0–79.0)	<0.001
AST (IU/L)	46.0 (35.0–68.0)	48.0 (35.0–75.0)	44.0 (34.0–60.3)	0.124
ALT (IU/L)	39.0 (27.0–63.0)	48.0 (30.5–74.0)	37.0 (23.8–52.3)	<0.001
GGT (IU/L)	32.0 (22.0–53.0)	35.0 (22.0–69.0)	29.5 (21.0–46.0)	0.021
Hemoglobin (g/dl)	13.2 (12.0–14.2)	13.5 (12.3–14.4)	13.0 (11.8–14.0)	0.010
Platelets (×10⁴/μL)	12.8 (8.8–17.1)	13.6 (9.2–18.1)	12.4 (8.5–16.8)	0.302
eGFR	71.7 (60.2–84.5)	80.6 (67.8–91.3)	68.2 (56.6–77.0)	<0.001
HCV RNA (KIU/mL)	6.1 (5.6–6.5)	6.1 (5.7–6.5)	6.1 (5.6–6.5)	0.556
Previous therapy (naive/ineligible/intolerant/NVR/relapse)	146/5/26/75/25	54/3/14/31/14	92/2/12/44/11	0.276
NS5A Y93H, n (%)	9 (3.1)	6 (5.0)	3 (1.8)	0.122
NS5A L31M, n (%)	4 (1.4)	3 (2.5)	1 (0.6)	0.230

ALT, alanine aminotransferase; GGT, γ-glutamyl transpeptidase; eGFR, estimated glomerular filtration rate; HCV RNA, hepatitis C virus RNA; KIU, kilo international units; NVR, null virological response.

Table 1. Baseline clinical characteristics of patients treated with DAA's therapy.

to the younger patients as expected. There was no patient with dose reduction due to renal insufficiency. The results of DAA's therapy showed that the SVR24 rate in elderly patients was high even in younger patients (92.2 vs. 85.1%). The factors associated with an SVR24 in DAA's therapy were determined by multivariate analysis. Gender [P = 0.014, odds ratio 0.301 (0.115–0.785)], GGT [P = 0.032, odds ratio 0.992 (0.985–0.999)] and absence of NS5A Y93H [P < 0.001, odds ratio 16.50 (3.801–71.66)] were significantly associated with an SVR24 while patient age did not affect SVR24. In elderly patients, the factors associated with an SVR24 in DAA's therapy were determined by multivariate analysis. Gender [P = 0.025, odds ratio 0.071(0.007–0.716)], GGT [P = 0.006, odds ratio 0.982 (0.970–0.995)] and absence of NS5A Y93H [P = 0.018, odds ratio 58.47 (2.024–1689.3)] were significantly associated with an SVR24.

5. Prevention of HCC

Aging is one of the factors associated with development of HCC in the CHC patients [5]. IFN therapy was reported to have reduction in development of HCC among virological or biochemical responders [6, 7]. We previously researched how benefit of reduction of HCC after eradication of HCV by PegIFN plus ribavirin. As shown in the **Figure 6** cumulative incidence of HCC in the elderly patients was higher than that in the younger patients [8]. However, if the elderly patients achieved a SVR, patients have marked reduction of cumulative incidence of HCC [8]. From the multivariate analysis in all patients age, advanced fibrosis, treatment efficacy and gender was associated with development of HCC. In elderly patients, GGT and treatment efficacy were factors associated with development of HCC. Receiver operating characteristic

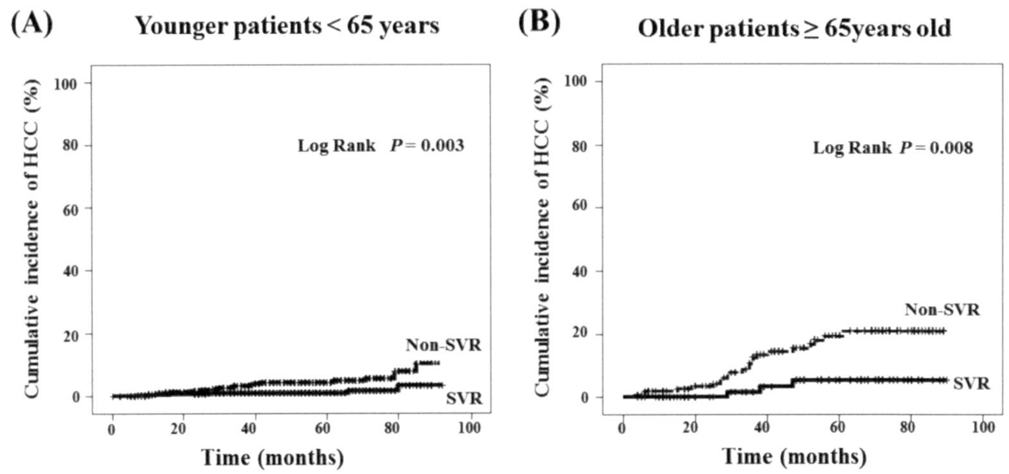

(A) Patients at risk

	0	20	40	60	80	HCC events
Non-SVR	422	354	278	190	76	19
SVR	604	462	308	186	62	6

(B) Patients at risk

	0	20	40	60	80	HCC events
Non-SVR	157	121	86	53	23	22
SVR	97	67	50	33	8	3

Figure 6. Cumulative incidence of HCC after peginterferon alfa-2b and ribavirin in patients who achieved SVR (solid line) or did not achieve SVR(dashed line) in younger patients < 65 years old (A) and older patients ≥ 65years old (B).

http://dx.doi.org/10.5772/intechopen.70437

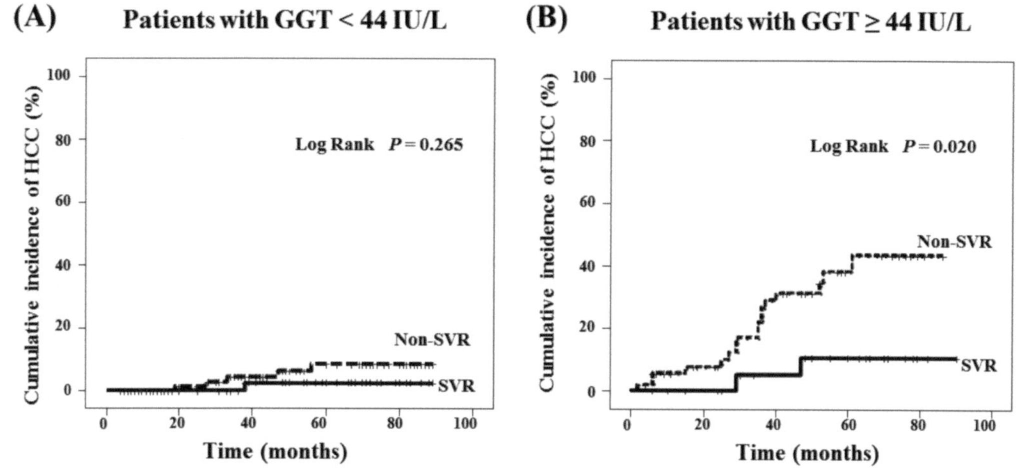

(A) Patients at risk

	0	20	40	60	80	HCC events
Non-SVR	95	76	54	40	20	5
SVR	67	45	34	21	6	1

(B) Patients at risk

	0	20	40	60	80	HCC events
Non-SVR	57	41	29	12	3	17
SVR	25	22	17	12	2	2

Figure 7. Cumulative incidence of HCC after peginterferon alfa-2b and ribavirin in older patients who achieved SVR (solid line) or did not achieve SVR(dashed line), among those with GGT < 44 IU/L (A) and GGT ≥ 44 IU/L (B). HCC, hepatocellular carcinoma; GGT, gamma-glutamyltranspeptidase; SVR,sustained virological response.

(ROC) curve indicated the cut off vale was 44 IU/L to predict for HCC. Among elderly patients with GGT < 44 IU/L, the cumulative incidence of HCC in patients with non-SVR was higher than patients with SVR, but this difference was not significant (**Figure 7A**). However, in elderly patients with SVR and GGT ≥ 44 IU/L, there was a marked reduction in the development of HCC compared with the elderly patients with SVR and GGT ≥ 44 IU/L (elderly patients with GGT < 44 IU/L, P = 0.265; elderly patients with GGT ≥ 44 IU/L, P = 0.020, log-rank test) (**Figure 7B**).

6. Discussion

Elderly patients with CHC are getting older and definition of elderly patients shifted from 60 to 70 years in our study during 13 years. In these days, the change of physical function according to age is seen 10 years older than that was seen in 10–20 years ago. Therefore, The Japan Geriatrics Society proposed elderly patients are defines as 75 years and over due to these rejuvenation phenomenon and the extension of the average life expectancy in 2017. If this phenomenon would be seen in all over the world, it will be globally accepted in the future.

DCV/ASV therapy for Japanese elderly patients with CHC had high SVR rate and is comparable to younger patients [4]. Our result indicated there is a possible to be higher SVR rate in elderly patients treated by DCV/ASV therapy than that in younger patients. For another type of DAA's therapy Ledipasvir/Sofosbuvir (LDV/SOF) therapy for the older CHC patients with genotype 1 from the Phase III had high SVR rate as well as younger patients [9]. They defined patients aged 65 years or older as elderly patients and those are still small population of CHC patients in the United States (12%). In other study CHC patients aged ≥65 years who were treated with different combinations of DAAs had high efficacy and took significantly more concomitant medications [10]. Therefore, they indicated assessment of concomitant medications and drug-drug interactions would be needed before DAAs therapy especially for the elderly patients. As well as PegIFN plus ribavirin therapy, DAA's therapy including ribavirin regimen needs close monitoring of anemia in the elderly patients. Elderly patients with GGT > 44 IU/L and advanced fibrosis have high risk of development of HCC when we treated older CHC patients by PegIFN plus ribavirin. These patients would be high priority to be treated with DAA, because patients who achieved SVR had a marked reduction in the development of HCC compared with elderly patients who did not achieve SVR. Compared to the RBV and IFN or PegIFN-based treatment, DAA-based treatment improved efficacy of treatment even in non-elderly patients. Therefore, indication for the elderly patients will expand. However, due to the high costs of current DAA's therapy at the moment, it is better to evaluate life expectancy. Higher age, HCV-related liver disease (advanced fibrosis, HCC) and other concomitant disease affect life expectancy. Elderly patients took many other medications, therefore evaluation of drug-drug interaction between DAA and other medication is necessary. If HCV-related liver diseases are likely to affect survival and quality of life (QOL) and there are no economic restrictions in country where patients will be treated, the patients are better to be treated. If HCV-related liver diseases are not likely to affect survival and QOL or there are economic restrictions in that country, the patients should be closely monitored and be regularly reevaluated. Therefore, physician needs more knowledge of interaction of other diseases and to have a long-term of view on the CHC patients.

Author details

Takashi Honda, Masatoshi Ishigami*, Kazuhiko Hayashi, Teiji Kuzuya, Yoji Ishizu, Yoshiki Hirooka and Hidemi Goto

*Address all correspondence to: masaishi@med.nagoya-u.ac.jp

Department of Gastroenterology and Hepatology, Nagoya University Graduate School of Medicine, Nagoya, Japan

References

[1] Yoshizawa H. Hepatocellular carcinoma associated with hepatitis C virus infection in Japan: Projection to other countries in the foreseeable future. Oncology. 2002;**62** Suppl 1: 8-17

[2] Honda T, Katano Y, Urano F, et al. Efficacy of ribavirin plus interferon-alpha in patients aged >or=60 years with chronic hepatitis C. Journal of Gastroenterology and Hepatology. 2007;**22**:989-995

[3] Honda T, Katano Y, Shimizu J, et al. Efficacy of peginterferon-alpha-2b plus ribavirin in patients aged 65 years and older with chronic hepatitis C. Liver International. 2010;**30**:527-537

[4] Akuta N, Sezaki H, Suzuki F, et al. Favorable efficacy of daclatasvir plus asunaprevir in treatment of elderly Japanese patients infected with HCV genotype 1b aged 70 and older. Journal of Medical Virology. 2017;**89**:91-98

[5] Asahina Y, Tsuchiya K, Tamaki N, et al. Effect of aging on risk for hepatocellular carcinoma in chronic hepatitis C virus infection. Hepatology. 2010;**52**:518-527

[6] Imai Y, Kawata S, Tamura S, et al. Relation of interferon therapy and hepatocellular carcinoma in patients with chronic hepatitis C. Osaka Hepatocellular Carcinoma Prevention Study Group. Annals of Internal Medicine. 1998;**129**:94-99

[7] Ikeda K, Saitoh S, Arase Y, et al. Effect of interferon therapy on hepatocellular carcinogenesis in patients with chronic hepatitis type C: A long-term observation study of 1,643 patients using statistical bias correction with proportional hazard analysis. Hepatology. 1999;**29**:1124-1130

[8] Honda T, Ishigami M, Masuda H, et al. Effect of peginterferon alfa-2b and ribavirin on hepatocellular carcinoma prevention in older patients with chronic hepatitis C. Journal of Gastroenterology and Hepatology. 2015;**30**:321-328

[9] Saab S, Park SH, Mizokami M, et al. Safety and efficacy of ledipasvir/sofosbuvir for the treatment of genotype 1 hepatitis C in subjects aged 65 years or older. Hepatology. 2016;**63**:1112-1119

[10] Vermehren J, Peiffer KH, Welsch C, et al. The efficacy and safety of direct acting antiviral treatment and clinical significance of drug-drug interactions in elderly patients with chronic hepatitis C virus infection. Alimentary Pharmacology & Therapeutics. 2016;**44**:856-865

Chapter 7

Direct-Acting Antivirals (DAAs): Drug-Drug Interactions (DDIs) in the Treatment of Hepatitis C Virus (HCV)

Sabina Steiner, Nikola Raguž-Lučić and Damir Erceg

Additional information is available at the end of the chapter

http://dx.doi.org/10.5772/intechopen.70788

Abstract

Hepatitis C virus (HCV)-infected patients often use multiple medications to treat infection, adverse events related to HCV therapy, or to manage other comorbidities. Drug-drug interactions (DDIs) associated with this polypharmacy are important in HCV pharmacotherapy, especially after introduction of direct-acting antivirals (DAAs). Knowledge about pharmacokinetics, metabolism, and disposition of drugs used in the treatment of HCV and comorbidities is crucial in the interpretation of these data and management of these interactions (e.g. dose adjustments, therapeutic drug monitoring, or safe alternatives). Web-based DDIs interactive tools like http://www.hep-druginteractions.org represent the most feasible and comprehensive way for an assessment of potential DDIs before, during, and after treatment. Additional helpful resources are data from clinical drug interaction studies as well as recent real-life data. This chapter is practical overview of DDIs in the treatment of HCV with the last update.

Keywords: hepatitis C virus, direct-acting antivirals, drug-drug interactions, cytochrome P450, antiviral therapy

1. Introduction

Hepatitis C virus (HCV) is one of the leading causes of liver disease in the world [1, 2]. HCV can cause acute and chronic infections. Acute infection is a non-life threatening disease and ranges from being asymptomatic to causing a self-limited hepatitis. Acute HCV infection is usually asymptomatic and is only very rarely associated with life-threatening disease. About 15–45% of acutely infected patients spontaneously clear HCV within several months after infection, but the remaining 55–85% of patients develop chronic infection [3, 4]. Currently, almost 180 million people in the world have chronic HCV infection [2, 3]. The risk of cirrhosis of the liver is between 15 and 30% within 20 years for patients with chronic HCV infection, and the risk of hepatocellular carcinoma increases (HCC) more than 20-fold within 20 years of infection. Approximately, 700,000 persons die each year from HCV-related complications, which include cirrhosis, hepatocellular carcinoma (HCC), and liver failure [4].

The goal of therapy is to cure HCV infection in order to prevent the complications of HCV-related liver and extrahepatic diseases, such as fibrosis, cirrhosis, decompensation of cirrhosis, HCC, severe extrahepatic manifestations, and death [4]. The gold standard of therapy for the treatment of chronic HCV infection for many years was pegylated interferon (Peg-INF) in combination with ribavirin (RBV). Over the past decade, the treatment of hepatitis C has dramatically improved. Limited efficacy in patients with HCV and side effects of indirect drugs, Peg-INF + RBV spurred the development of new therapeutic approaches. Almost 80 percent of patients receiving Peg-INF + RBV combination therapy for chronic HCV infection had side effects. The appropriate anticipation and prevention of side effects, proper response when they occur, as well as recognition of patients at increased risk for side effects have pivotal role in the care of patients with chronic HCV infection. Furthermore, the ability to achieve a sustained virologic response (SVR) to therapy depends in part upon the degree of compliance with therapy. Reduction of the dose of these agents as well as their discontinuation due to side effects could potentially compromise the outcome.

Peg-INF can cause in many cases bone marrow depression with decreased granulocytes, which can lead to opportunistic infections and decreased numbers of thrombocytes [5]. Neutropenia is one of the most common reasons for dose modification. Flu-like symptoms usually occur during the first week of treatment and include chills, headaches, myalgia, and fever. Severe fatigue, apathy, and irritability are neuropsychiatric side effects, which are great problem for patients and their families. They can even lead to suicide if they are not recognized on time [5]. A variety of autoimmune diseases can develop or be exacerbated during peginterferon-containing therapy, including psoriasis, vitiligo, rheumatoid arthritis, lichen planus, sarcoidosis, dermatitis herpetiformis, and type 1 diabetes mellitus [5]. Thus, peginterferon should be used with caution in patients with known autoimmune disease and is contraindicated in patients with known autoimmune hepatitis. The development of thyroid dysfunction is common in patients treated with peginterferon. On the other hand, most common side effect of RBV is hemolytic anemia. It may be necessary to lower the dose or even discontinue the therapy. In those cases, treatment with erythropoietin can reverse ribavirin-associated anemia and permit continuation of the RBV therapy [5]. The above-mentioned side effects, decreased adherence to therapy, prolonged treatment time as well as increased cost of HCV treatment are all hurdles to successful treatment.

2. Direct-acting antivirals (DAAs)

Before 2011, the gold standard of therapy was based on the combination of Peg-IFN and RBV that acts by mechanisms not completely known and exhibited low efficacy in most populations. In the recent years, thanks to basic research on HCV structure and replicative cycle, it has been possible to develop DAAs that have dramatically increased the viral clearance rates.

http://dx.doi.org/10.5772/intechopen.70788

Specifically, the advent of the combined therapy employing DAAs has dramatically increased the viral clearance rate from 40–50% with peginterferon + ribavirin to more than 95% with the current therapy [3, 6]. Initially, DAAs for treatments of chronic HCV were more efficacious, but had even more side effects at beginning due to combined therapy PEG INF + ribavirin + DAAs (protease inhibitor) (PI). Some of the side effects of combination Peg INF + RBV+ PI inhibitors appeared due to drug-drug interactions. The first generation of NS3/4APIs (boceprevir and telaprevir) was approved for clinical use in 2011. Since then, the new standard in the treatment of chronic HCV infection became triple therapy consisting PEG INF/ RBV and either boceprevir (BOC) or telaprevir (TVP). With the addition of boceprevir or telaprevir to PEG-IFN/RBV, cure rates for HCV genotype 1 increased to 60–70%. However, new protease inhibitors (PI)-containing triple therapy were also accompanied by new problems, including more complicated dosing regimens and increased adverse events, which were in some cases severe, particularly in patients with advanced liver disease. Furthermore, DDIs became additional challenges in HCV therapy. The first DAAs are metabolized by CYP3A4 and used transporter P-glycoprotein (P-gp) system. As a result, there is potential risk for DDIs with other drugs often used in the treatment of HCV patients. By 2013, the second generation of DAAs, including sofosbuvir, was introduced in the market.

Direct-acting antivirals target three of the main proteins involved in viral replication: the NS3/4A protease, the NS5B polymerase, and the NS5A [7].

2.1. NS3/4A protease inhibitors

NS3/4A protease inhibitors are inhibitors of the NS3/4A serine protease, an enzyme involved in post-translational processing and replication of HCV. Protease inhibitors disrupt HCV by blocking the NS3 catalytic site or the NS3/NS4A interaction. In addition to its role in viral processing, the NS3/NS4A protease blocks TRIF-mediated Toll-like receptor signaling and Cardif-mediated retinoic acid–inducible gene 1 (RIG-1) signaling, which result in impaired induction of interferons and blocking viral elimination. Thus, inhibition of the NS3/4A protease could contribute to antiviral activity through two mechanisms [7].

Following the introduction of other potent and better tolerated DAAs, the clinical importance of these agents diminished substantially because of their cumbersome administration, substantial adverse effects, drug-drug interactions, and low barrier to resistance. The subsequent wave of the first generation protease inhibitors (simeprevir, paritaprevir) as well as second generation (grazoprevir) offered several benefits over earlier protease inhibitors, including fewer drug-drug interactions, improved dosing schedules, and less frequent and less severe side effects. In addition, the newer protease inhibitors also appear to have increased efficacy against genotype 1 HCV and other genotypes. Grazoprevir, paritaprevir, and simeprevir are protease inhibitors available in the Europe and United States. Asunaprevir is a protease inhibitor used in Japan [7].

2.2. NS5A inhibitors

The NS5A protein plays a role in both viral replication and the assembly of the hepatitis C virus (HCV) [7]. However, the precise molecular mechanisms by which NS5A accomplishes these functions are unclear. NS5A inhibitors are generally quite potent and effective across all genotypes. However, they have a low barrier to resistance and have variable toxicity profiles (**Table 1**). They have been shown to significantly reduce HCV RNA levels and enhance SVR when given in conjunction with peginterferon and ribavirin [18]. They also result in very high SVR rates among patients with genotype 1 infection when given in combination with other DAAs with or without ribavirin [8].

Available NS5A inhibitors are ledipasvir, ombitasvir, velpatasvir, and elbasvir, each available in fixed-dose combinations with other direct-acting antivirals, and daclatasvir. Daclatasvir is a NS5A inhibitor that is used mainly in combination with sofosbuvir [7].

2.3. NS5B RNA-dependent RNA polymerase inhibitors

NS5B RNA-dependent RNA polymerase is an enzyme necessary for replication of HCV, involved in post-translational processing of HCV and has a catalytic site for nucleoside binding and at least four other sites at which a non-nucleoside compound can bind and cause allosteric alteration. The enzyme's structure is highly conserved across all HCV genotypes, giving agents that inhibit NS5B efficacy against all six genotypes [7]. There are two classes of polymerase inhibitors: non-nucleoside analogues (NNPIs) and nucleoside/nucleotide analogues (NPIs). The NNPIs act as allosteric inhibitors, whereas NPIs target the catalytic site of NS5B and result in chain termination during RNA replication of the viral genome.

Sofosbuvir was the first NS5B NPIs available in the Europe and United States and can be used in various combinations with other antivirals for different indications.

As a class, NNPIs are less potent, more genotype specific (optimized for genotype 1), have a low-to-moderate barriers to resistance and have variable toxicity profiles [7]. Consequently, this class of drug was developed primarily as an adjunct to more potent compounds with higher barriers to resistance. Dasabuvir is administered and packaged with ombitasvir-paritaprevir-ritonavir.

Also, "the second generation" PIs, simeprevir, resulted in similar SVR rates when added to PEG-IFN/RBV. By 2014, IFN-free regimens had essentially replaced interferon-based therapy. Sofosbuvir/ledipasvir and sofosbuvir/simeprevir/RBV resulted in genotype 1 SVR rates of 92–100%. Combination of ombitasvir, paritaprevir/ritonavir/dasabuvir with/without RBV achieved SVR rates as high as 100%. The next step in the clinical development of anti-HCV therapy was by 2016 with the availability of pangenotypic ultrarapid (4–8 weeks) single pill regimens such as grazoprevir/elbasvir. This review is focused on drug-drug interactions in the treatment of HCV infections in past several years.

3. Metabolic pathways of DAAs

Most of the interactions are linked to metabolism of cytochrome P450-3 A4 (CYP3A4) or hepatic and/or intestinal transporters such as organic anion-transporting polypeptide (OATP) and P-glycoprotein (P-gp) as shown in **Table 1** [8]. To a lesser extent, other pathways can be involved such as breast cancer resistance protein transporter (BCRP) or multi-drug resistance protein 2 (MDRP2).

http://dx.doi.org/10.5772/intechopen.70788

Direct antiviral agents (DAAs)	Metabolism	Transporter	Clinical DDI extent	Year of approval/ withdrawal	Drug in combination with	Brand name	Comment
Protease inhibitors-previrs							
Boceprevir	AKR, CYP3A4	P-gp BCRP	High	2011/2014	Not applicable	Victrelis	No longer available
Telaprevir	CYP3A4	P-gp, OATP1B1 OATP2B1	High	2011/2014	Not applicable	Incivo	No longer available
Simeprevir	CYP3A4	P-gp OATP1B1/3 OATP2B1	Moderate	2013	Sofosbuvir	Olysio	Approved as combination with sofosbuvir in 2014
Paritaprevir	CYP3A4	P-gp, BCRP OATP1B1/3	Height	2014 2015 2016	Ombitasvir, dasabuvir, ribavirin Ombitasvir, ribavirin Ombitasvir, dasabuvir, ribavirin	Viekira Pak (Technivie) Viekira XR	
Grazoprevir	CYP3A4	P-gp, MDRP2, OATP1B1	Low	2016	In combination with elbasvir	Zepatier	
NS5A inhibitors-buvirs							
Non-nucleoside inhibitors							
Sofosbuvir	Cathepsin A, esterases and kinases	P-gp and BCRP	Low	20132014	Ledipasvir	Sovaldi Harvoni	First treatment without interferon or ribavirin
Non-nucleoside inhibitors							
Dasabuvir			High	20142016	Ombitasvir, paritaprevir, and ribavirin	Viekira PakViekira XR	
NS5A inhibitors-asvirs							

Direct antiviral agents (DAAs)	Metabolism	Transporter	Clinical DDI extent	Year of approval/ withdrawal	Drug in combination with	Brand name	Comment
Ombitasvir	CYP 3A4	P-gp, BCRP	High	20142016	Paritaprevir, dasabuvir, and ribavirin	Viekira Pak Viekira XR	
Ledipasvir			Low	2014	Sofosbuvir	Harvoni	
Daclatasvir	CYP3A4	P-gp,BCRP, OATP1B1, OATP1B3	Low	2015		Daklinza	
Elbasvir	CYP3A4	P-gp and BCRP	Low	2016	Grazoprevir	Zepatier	To treat GT1–4 including compensated cirrhosis, or severe kidney disease and on dialysis
Velpatasvir	CYP3A4	Inhibits OATP1B1, OATP1B3, OATP2B1, P-gp, BCRP	Low	2016	Sofosbuvir	Epclusa	First therapy to treat all HCV GT 1–6

Adapted according to [8–10].

Table 1. DAAs, metabolism, transporters, potential for DDI, and some basics.

The good understanding of pharmacokinetic drug profiles is the key to interpret DDIs data. DDIs are more likely to occur with 3D regimen, followed by daclatasvir, simeprevir, and ledipasvir, as they are all both substrates and inhibitors of P-gp and/or CYP3A4, than with sofosbuvir [8–10]. Their concentrations may be influenced by CYP3A4 and P-gp inducers or inhibitors or they can increase concentrations of coadminstered drugs. Low dose or overdosage can be expected with potent inducers or inhibitors of drugs with narrow therapeutic range [8–10].

4. Drug-drug interactions with DAAs

Direct antiviral agents (DAAs) improved tolerability and efficacy for HCV-infected patients, but drug-drug interactions (DDIs) have the potential to cause harm due to liver dysfunction and multiple comorbidities. DDIs can be assessed based on information available at www.hep-druginteractions.org (http://www.hep-druginteractions.org/) [11]. This website was launched in 2010 by members of the Department of Pharmacology at the University of Liverpool to offer a resource for healthcare providers, researchers, and patients to be able to understand and manage drug-drug interactions. The fact sheets containing information on the pharmacokinetics, metabolism, and disposition of each drug are in PDF format. Data have been collected from company information, published literature, and are referenced at the end of each sheet. Since pharmacokinetic parameters are dependent on dose (and route of administration), data refer to the licensed dose unless otherwise stated.

According to the significance of interactions with DAA, DDIs were assigned to four risk categories as follows: classification not possible due to lack of information: category 0; no clinically significant interactions expected: category 1; significant interaction possible, may require dose adjustment/closer monitoring: category 2; and coadministration either not recommended or contraindicated: category 3. The regular comedication drugs were sorted into different groups according to the organ or system on which they act. When patient use more drugs with different risks for a DDI, the highest category was chosen to determine the risk for the patient with a respective treatment regimen. Also, the results are presented as a "Traffic Light" system (red, amber, and green) to indicate the recommendation. Last changes, made recently, include the new category, a yellow: potential interactions likely to be of weak intensity where additional action/monitoring or dosage adjustment is unlikely to be required [12].

DAAs may share metabolic pathways with drugs, such as antiretroviral drugs, cardiovascular drugs, lipid lowering drugs, immunosuppressive drugs, methadone, buprenorphine, herbal remedies, and commonly prescribed psychiatric medications, that are commonly used by populations with a high prevalence of hepatitis C. In the following text, we review drug interactions with some groups of drugs often used as comedications with DAAs in clinical practice.

4.1. Antiretroviral drugs

Coinfection with HIV and HCV is a serious problem resulting in many complications, including faster liver decompensation, cirrhosis, and hepatic carcinoma [4]. One-fourth of patients infected with HIV concomitantly have HCV infection [13]. After introducing highly active antiretroviral drugs in therapy, liver complications became the leading cause of morbidity and mortality in HIV-HCV coinfected population.

Optimal treatment is necessary to avoid such complications. It is very important to address drug-drug interactions between these two regimens to avoid adverse effects and a decrease in efficacy, thereby increasing adherence to therapy. Some of DAAs (e.g. simeprevir, following fixed combination VEL/SOF, 3D, and EBR/GZR) are not recommended for use with many HIV antiretroviral (ARV) drugs as well as efavirenz, etravirine, and nevirapine. Sofosbuvir and fixed combination LDV/SOF can be safely administered with many antiretroviral drugs used to treat coinfections (HCV and HIV) (**Table 2**).

The combination ledipasvir/sofosbuvir can be used with all ARVs. However, these combinations should be used with frequent renal monitoring when a pharmacokinetic enhancer (ritonavir or cobicistat) is present in an ARV regimen due to an increase in tenofovir concentrations. Also, tenofovir concentration is increased in efavirenz-containing regimens and renal monitoring is necessary.

Class	Drug	BOC	TLP	SOF	DCV	SIM	LDV/SOF	VEL/SOF	3D	EBR/GZR
NRTIs	Abacavir	Green	Amber	Green	Green	Green	Green	Green	Green	Green
	Emtricitabine	Green	Green	Green	Green	Green	Green	Green	Green	Green
	Lamivudine	Green	Green	Green	Green	Green	Green	Green	Green	Green
	Tenofovir	Green	Amber	Green	Green	Green	Amber	Amber	Green	Green
NNRTIs	Efavirenz	Green	Green	Green	Amber	Red	Amber	Red	Red	Red
	Etravirine	Amber	Green	Green	Amber	Red	Green	Red	Red	Red
	Neviparine	Amber	Amber	Green	Amber	Red	Green	Red	Red	Red
	Rilpivirine	Green	Green	Green	Green	Green	Green	Amber	Green	Green
PIs	A; A/r; A/C	Amber	Amber	Green	Amber	Red	Green	Amber	Red	Red
	D; D/C	Amber	Amber	Green	Red	Red	Green	Amber	Red	Red
	Lopinavir	Amber	Amber	Green	Red	Red	Green	Red	Red	Red
E/IIs	Doluteglavir	Amber	Amber	Green	Green	Green	Green	Green	Green	Green
	E/C/E/TDF	Amber	Green	Green	Amber	Red	Amber	Amber	Red	Red
	E/C/E/TAF	Red	Red	Green	Amber	Red	Green	Green	Red	Red
	Maraviroc	Amber	Amber	Green	Green	Green	Green	Green	Green	Green
	Raltegravir	Green	Green	Green	Green	Green	Green	Green	Green	Green

NRTIs, nucleoside analog reverse transcriptase inhibitors; NNRTIs, non-nucleoside reverse transcriptase inhibitors; PI, protease inhibitors; E/I i, entry and integrase inhibitors; A, atazanavir; A/r, atazanavir/ritonavir; A/C, atazanavir/cobicistat; D, darunavir; D/C, darunavir/cobicistat; E/C/E/TDF, elvitegravir/cobicistat/emtricitabine/tenofovir disoproxil fumarate; E/C/E/TA, elvitegravir/cobicistat/emtricitabine/tenofovir alafenamide; LDV/SOF-ledipasvir + sofosbuvir; VEL/SOF-velpatasvir + sofosbuvir; 3D, ritonavir boosted paritaprevir + ombitasvir + dasabuvir; EBR/GZR, elbasvir + grazoprevir.

Green-no clinically significant interaction expected. Red-contraindication. Amber-potential interaction; dose adjustment, altered timing of administration, or require monitoring.

Adapted according to www.hep-druginteractions.org (University of Liverpool).

Table 2. Drug-drug interactions between HCV DAAs and HIV antiretrovirals.

http://dx.doi.org/10.5772/intechopen.70788

4.2. Immunosuppressive agents (including steroids)

The most important drug interactions of DAAs are those with immunosuppressants, such as tacrolimus and cyclosporine [14]. These immunosuppressants are substrates of both CYP3A and P-gp, and inhibitory effects of boceprevir and telaprevir on CYP3A and P-gp increased plasma concentrations of the immunosuppressants. In particular, the interaction between tacrolimus and telaprevir had a magnitude that was unprecedented in clinical pharmacology: the AUC of tacrolimus is increased by 70.3-fold, and this combination would be lethal if doses were not adjusted [15]. From the start of combined treatment, therapeutic drug monitoring of immunosuppressants with dose adjustment can solve this problem (about 50% of observed differences in healthy volunteers) [16].

The combined therapy of telaprevir and boceprevir with systemically applied corticosteroids, such as methylprednisolone and prednisone, is not recommended due to risk of Cushing syndrome. These corticosteroids are CYP3A4 substrates and higher steroid levels can be expected. Similar situation is for locally applied corticosteroids by inhalation or intranasally such as fluticasone and budesonide. According to available data, beclomethasone can be used safely in patients on strong CYP3A inhibitors [16] and represents a corticosteroid of choice in patients with HCV therapy.

Also, sofosbuvir as DAAs in combination with daclatasvir or velpatasvir can be used when co-treatment is necessary with immunosuppressants or corticosteroids (**Table 3**).

Class	Drug	BOC	TLP	SOF	DCV	SIM	LDV/SOF	VEL/SOF	3D	EBR/GZR
Immunosuppressives	Azathioprine	Green	Green	Green	Green	Green	Green	Green	Green	Green
	Cyclosporine	Amber	Amber	Green	Green	Red	Green	Green	Amber	Red
	Everolimus	Green	Green	Green	Amber	Amber	Amber	Amber	Red	Amber
	Mycophenolate	Green	Green	Green	Green	Green	Green	Green	Amber	Green
	Sirolimus	Amber	Amber	Green	Green	Amber	Green	Green	Amber	Amber
	Tacrolimus	Amber	Amber	Green	Green	Amber	Green	Green	Amber	Amber
Corticosteroids.	Beclomethason	Green	Green	Green	Green	Green	Green	Green	Green	Green
	Dexamethasone	Amber	Amber	Green	Red	Red	Green	Green	Green	Green
	Momethasone	Amber	Amber	Green	Green	Green	Green	Green	Green	Green
	Prednisone	Amber	Amber	Green	Green	Amber	Green	Green	Green	Green
	Methylprednisolone	Amber	Amber	Green	Green	Amber	Green	Green	Green	Green
	Hydrocortsone top.	Green	Green	Green	Green	Amber	Green	Green	Green	Green

LDV/SOF, ledipasvir + sofosbuvir; VEL/SOF, velpatasvir + sofosbuvir; 3D, ritonavir boosted paritaprevir + ombitasvir + dasabuvir; EBR/GZR, elbasvir + grazoprevir; top, topical.

Green-no clinically significant interaction expected. Red-contraindication. Amber-potential interaction; dose adjustment, altered timing of administration, or require monitoring.

Adapted according to www.hep-drugineractions.org (University of Liverpool).

Table 3. DDIs between DAAs and immunosuppressive agents (including corticosteroids).

4.3. Psychoactive agents

The prevalence of mental disorders remains high among untreated HCV-infected patients [17, 18]. In one retrospective study, the authors reported that 86% of HCV-infected patients had at least one psychiatric-, drug-, or alcohol use-related disorder recorded in their patient data. The most common conditions were depressive disorders (50%) and psychosis (50%), followed by anxiety disorders (41%), post-traumatic stress disorders (34%), and bipolar disorders (16%) [19]. The majority of DAAs are extensively metabolized by liver enzymes and have the ability to influence cytochrome P450 (CYP) enzymes, as well as majority of psychoactive medications. However, remarkably little information is available on DDIs between psychoactive medications and DAAs. Smolders et al. made overview of the interaction mechanisms between DAAs and psychoactive agents [20]. In addition, they described evidenced-based interactions between DAAs and psychoactive drugs and identified safe options for the simultaneous treatment of mental illnesses and chronic HCV infection [20]. Boceprevir, telaprevir, and the combination paritaprevir/ritonavir plus ombitasvir with dasabuvir were most likely to cause drug interactions by inhibition of cytochrome P450 (CYP) 3A4 [11]. Escitalopram and citalopram have been studied in combination with most direct-acting antivirals (DAAs) and either of these drugs can be safely combined with hepatitis

Drug	Drug	BOC	TLP	SOF	DCV	SIM	LDV/SOF	VEL/SOF	3D	EBR/GZR
Anti-depressants	Amitriptyline	Green	Amber	Green	Green	Green	Green	Green	Amber	Green
	Citalopram	Amber	Amber	Green	Green	Green	Green	Green	Green	Green
	Duloxetine	Green	Green	Green	Green	Green	Green	Green	Green	Green
	Escitalopram	Amber	Amber	Green	Green	Green	Green	Green	Green	Green
	Fluoxetine	Green	Green	Green	Green	Green	Green	Green	Green	Green
	Paroxetine	Amber	Amber	Green	Green	Green	Green	Green	Green	Green
	Sertraline	Amber	Amber	Green	Green	Green	Green	Green	Amber	Green
	Trazodone	Amber	Amber	Green	Green	Amber	Green	Green	Amber	Green
	Trimipramine	Green	Green	Green	Green	Green	Green	Green	Green	Green
	Venlafaxine	Amber	Amber	Green	Green	Green	Green	Green	Amber	Green
Antipsychotics	Amisulpiride	Green	Green	Green	Green	Green	Green	Green	Green	Green
	Ariprazole	Amber	Amber	Green	Green	Amber	Green	Green	Amber	Amber
	Chlorpromazine	Amber	Amber	Green	Green	Green	Green	Green	Amber	Green
	Clozapine	Amber	Amber	Green	Green	Amber	Green	Green	Amber	Green
	Flupentixol	Amber	Amber	Green	Green	Green	Green	Green	Amber	Green
	Haloperidol	Amber	Amber	Green	Green	Amber	Green	Green	Amber	Green
	Olanzapine	Green	Green	Green	Green	Green	Green	Green	Amber	Green
	Paliperidone	Amber	Amber	Green	Amber	Amber	Amber	Green	Amber	Green
	Quetiapine	Red	Red	Green	Green	Amber	Green	Green	Red	Amber
	Risperidone	Amber	Amber	Green	Green	Amber	Green	Green	Amber	Green
	Zuclopentixol	Amber	Amber	Green	Green	Green	Green	Green	Amber	Green

LDV/SOF, ledipasvir + sofosbuvir; VEL/SOF, velpatasvir + sofosbuvir; 3D, ritonavir boosted paritaprevir + ombitasvir + dasabuvir; EBR/GZR, elbasvir + grazoprevir.

Green-no clinically significant interaction expected. Red-contraindication. Amber-potential interaction; dose adjustment, altered timing of administration, or require monitoring.

Adapted according to www.hep-druginteractions.org (University of Liverpool).

Table 4. DDI between DAAs and psychoactive agents.

http://dx.doi.org/10.5772/intechopen.70788

C virus (HCV) treatment besides boceprevir and telaprevir [11, 20]. No formal interaction studies between psychoactive agents and sofosbuvir or ledipasvir have been performed in humans. However, these DAAs are generally neither victims nor perpetrators of drug interactions and can, therefore, be safely used in combination with psychoactive drugs (**Table 4**) [11, 20].

Class	Drugs	BOC	TLP	SOF	DCV	SIM	LDV/SOF	VEL/SOF	3D	EBR/GZR
Antiarhytmyics	Amiodarone	Amber	Amber	Red	Red	Green	Red	Red	Red	Green
	Digoxine	Amber	Amber	Green	Amber	Amber	Amber	Amber	Amber	Green
	Flecainide	Amber	Amber	Green	Green	Amber	Green	Green	Amber	Green
	Vernakalant	Amber	Amber	Green	Green	Green	Green	Green	Amber	Green
Antiplatelets and anticaogulants	Clopidogrel	Amber	Amber	Green	Amber	Red	Green	Green	Amber	Red
	Dabigatran	Amber	Amber	Green	Amber	Red	Amber	Amber	Amber	Red
	Ticagretor	Amber	Amber	Green	Amber	Red	Amber	Amber	Red	Red
	Warfarin	Amber	Amber	Green	Green	Green	Green	Green	Green	Green
Beta blockers	Atenolol	Amber	Amber	Green	Green	Green	Green	Green	Green	Green
	Bisoprolol	Amber	Amber	Green	Green	Amber	Green	Green	Amber	Green
	Carvedilol	Amber	Amber	Amber	Amber	Amber	Amber	Amber	Amber	Green
	Propranolol	Amber	Amber	Green	Green	Green	Green	Green	Green	Green
Calcium channel blockers	Amlodipine	Amber	Amber	Green	Amber	Amber	Amber	Amber	Amber	Amber
	Diltiazem	Amber	Amber	Green	Amber	Amber	Amber	Amber	Amber	Green
	Nifedipine	Amber	Amber	Green	Amber	Amber	Green	Green	Amber	Green
HYpertension and heart failure agents	Aliskrein	Amber	Amber	Green	Amber	Amber	Amber	Amber	Red	Green
	Candesartan	Amber	Amber	Green	Green	Green	Green	Green	Amber	Amber
	Doxazosin	Amber	Amber	Green	Green	Amber	Green	Green	Amber	Green
	Enalapril	Amber	Amber	Green	Green	Green	Green	Green	Amber	Green
Statins	Atorvastatin	Amber	Red	Green	Amber	Amber	Amber	Amber	Red	Amber
	Fluvastatin	Amber	Amber	Green	Amber	Green	Amber	Amber	Amber	Amber
	Pivastatin	Green	Amber	Green	Amber	Amber	Amber	Amber	Amber	Green
	Pravastatin	Amber	Amber	Green	Amber	Amber	Amber	Amber	Amber	Green
	Rosuvastatin	Amber	Amber	Green	Amber	Amber	Red	Amber	Amber	Amber
	Simvastatin	Red	Red	Green	Amber	Amber	Amber	Amber	Red	Amber

LDV/SOF, ledipasvir + sofosbuvir; VEL/SOF, velpatasvir + sofosbuvir; 3D, ritonavir boosted paritaprevir + ombitasvir + dasabuvir; EBR/GZR, elbasvir + grazoprevir.

Green-no clinically significant interaction expected. Red-clinically significant interaction; contra-indication. Amber-clinically significant interaction; potential interaction-dose adjustment, altered timing of administration, or require monitoring.

Adopted according to www.hep-druginteractions.org (University of Liverpool).

Table 5. DDI between DAAs and cardiovascular drugs.

4.4. Cardiovascular drugs

Calcium channel blockers are CYP3A and partly P-gp substrates and, thus, increased exposure can be expected with CYP3A inhibitors. In that, sofosbuvir is drug of choice due to its metabolism by other metabolic pathways. Antiarrhythmics have a narrow therapeutic window, and some are CYP substrates (e.g. amiodarone). Amiodarone is contraindicated with many DAAs, except simeprevir and combination elbasvir/grazoprevir (**Table 5**). Digoxin has been tested with telaprevir as prototype of P-gp substrate. Levels of digoxin were increased by 85% with telaprevir, which is a moderate inhibitor [15]). Although, according to hep.interactions no clinically significant interactions between warfarin and DAAs, there is one case report in the available literature [21].

Many statins are both CYP3A substrates and inhibitors of telaprevir and boceprevir. DAAs are expected to increase statin levels and the associated risk of severe toxicity such as rhabdomyolysis [16]. Atorvastatin levels were elevated almost eight times with telaprevir, and this combination is contraindicated. Atorvastatin level were elevated 2.3 times with boceprevir, but this interaction can be manageable by staring with low dose of atorvastatin. In the case of pravastatin, levels were marginally increased when combined with boceprevir (1.5-fold), and it probably caused inhibition of OATP1B1. According to some clinicians, it is possible to temporarily stop the statins during relatively short treatment to avoid toxicity with DAAs.

4.5. Proton pump inhibitors (PPIs)

Depending on the DAA regimen, one of the most frequent drug classes involved in significant DDIs (category 2 or 3) is PPIs. Acid-reducing agents reduce the absorption of some DAAs (e.g. ledipasvir, velpatasvir) and, therefore, its serum concentrations. An observational study called Target has reported an association between the use of acid-reducing agents and decreased effectiveness of Harvoni (sofosbuvir-ledipasvir) [22]. In Target, participants who used PPIs had a cure rate of 93% vs. a cure rate of 98% in people who did not use PPIs. In that case, combination elbasvir/grazoprevir was a better choice (**Table 6**).

Class	Drug	BOC	TLP	DCL	SIM	SOF	LDV/SOF	VEL/SOF	3D	ELB/GRA
PPIs	Esomeprazole	Green	Green	Green	Green	Green	Amber	Red	Amber	Green
	Lansoprazole	Amber	Amber	Green	Green	Green	Amber	Red	Amber	Green
	Omeprazole	Green	Green	Green	Green	Green	Amber	Amber	Amber	Green
	Pantoprazole	Green	Green	Green	Green	Green	Amber	Red	Amber	Green
	Rabeprazole	Green	Green	Green	Green	Green	Amber	Red	Amber	Green

LDV/SOF, ledipasvir + sofosbuvir; VEL/SOF, velpatasvir + sofosbuvir; 3D, ritonavir boosted paritaprevir + ombitasvir + dasabuvir; EBR/GZR, elbasvir + grazoprevir.

Green-no clinically significant interaction expected. Red-contraindication. Amber-potential interaction; dose adjustment, altered timing of administration, or require monitoring.

Adopted according to www.hep-druginteractions.org (University of Liverpool).

Table 6. DDI between DAAs and PPIs.

http://dx.doi.org/10.5772/intechopen.70788

5. Real-life studies

The first real-life study with boceprevir and telaprevir was published in 2013 [23]. In this study, 101 patients were selected for treatment in one center. All changes to comedications before and during treatment were documented. Drugs were checked for DDIs with telaprevir and boceprevir using DDI website resources and categorized into groups according to traffic lights (red, amber, and green). Similar to the general population, HCV patients often suffered from various common comorbidities like hypertension, dyslipoproteinemia, or atrial arrhythmia. Furthermore, some comorbidities like diabetes and thyroid disorders may even be overrepresented in the HCV-infected population. There was no clinically significant risk in 62% drugs, whereas for 29% drugs, some DDI were suspected. However, dose modifications or careful monitoring were sufficient for management. Only 4% of drugs were contraindicated for co-administration with DAAs. However, 10% of patients took one of these contraindicated drugs. Fourthy nine of patients were suspected to be at risk for experiencing significant DDIs. Drug classes most often suspected to be involved in significant DDI were thyroid hormones, dihydropyridine derivatives, and herbal/alternative drugs. In 16% of the patients, at least one drug of the regular outpatient medication was stopped before DAA treatment. Overall, suspected DDIs were managed by dose adjustments and discontinuation of comedication before or during DAAs therapy in 75 and 21% of the patients.

After this study, the other real-life studies were published. They include monoinfected HCV group, coinfected HIV/HCV group, and elderly patients with different severity of liver disease [24–27]. In all studies, the potential for DDIs between DAAs and comedications was assessed using www.hep-druginteractions.org. In the real-word large cohort study, Ze Siederdissen et al. assessed significance of DDIs between DAAs therapies and regular medications. During the period between 2011 and 2014, 261 patients with HCV were selected for DAAs therapy and asked for their regular outpatient therapy. Twenty percent of patients did not use any comedications. The median number was two drugs (range 0–15). The highest risk to cause significant DDIs had ombitasvir/paritaprevir/ritonavir ± dasabuvir (66.3%), in contrast with sofosbuvir/ribavirin that possessed lowest risk (9.6%). Significant DDIs for sofosbuvir/ledipasvir would be expected in 40.2%, for sofosbuvir/daclatasvir in 36.8%, and for sofosbuvir/simeprevir in 31.4%. The most frequently used comedication drugs that possess risk of DDIs were proton pump inhibitors, thyroid hormones, and dihydropyridine derivatives.

Gussio et al. assessed the clinical significance of DDI with DAA in a real-world polycentric retrospective study involving five clinical unit of infectious diseases in south of Italy and Sardinia treating HCV monoinfected and coinfected subjects selected for DAA therapy [25]. Two hundred and fifteen (215) subjects were enrolled in the study. Of the total, 139 were HCV monoinfected and 76 HIV coinfected. One hundred and seventy patients (170 or 75%) were males; median age was 55 years with stage of fibrosis F4 in 70% of patients. At least one comorbidity was found in 146 patients (68 and 67%, respectively, within mono and HIV coinfected). HCV monoinfected and HIV coinfected subjects had medians of 2 and 1 comorbidities, respectively. Regarding DAA drug-drug interactions, sofosbuvir/daclatasvir had the lowest risk to cause a potentially significant DDI (20%). In contrast, for ombitasvir/paritaprevir/ritonavir ± dasabuvir, there was potentially significant DDIs (49.8%). Significant DDIs for sofosbuvir/simeprevir were expected in 30.8%, for sofosbuvir/ribavirin in 28.2%, and for sofosbuvir/ledipasvir in 39.8%. Proton pump inhibitors, diuretics, and some antihypertensive drugs were frequently used and presented a risk of interacting with the antiviral regimen. Antiretroviral regimens also showed a high risk of potential interactions, although 16% of patients had preventively modified this treatment.

Kondili et al. assessed the potential DDIs of DAAs in HCV-infected outpatients. They evaluated 449 patients in 25 clinical centers in one Italian prospective multicenter study [26]. Patients started a DAA regimen and received comedications between March 2015 and March 2016. From total number of patients, 86 had mild liver disease and 363 had moderate-to-severe disease. The utilization of more than three drugs was more frequent in the patients with moderate-to-severe disease, whereas the use of single drug as a comedication was more frequent in patients with mild liver disease. About 30% (26/86) of patients with mild liver disease used at least one drug with a potential DDI, whereas 44% (161/363) of patients with moderate-to-severe liver disease were at risk for one or more DDI. Twenty percent of drugs (27/142) used as comedications in 86 patients with mild disease may require dose adjustment or closer monitoring, whereas none was contraindicated. Twenty five percent (82/322) of comedicated drugs in 363 patients with moderate-to-severe liver disease were classified as potential DDOs that required monitoring and dose adjustments and 3% (10/322) were contraindicated in severe liver disease. Patients with moderate-to-severe liver disease require much more attention due to potential DDI during DAA therapy according to the data from this study.

Direct antiviral therapies for chronic hepatitis C virus (HCV) infection have expanded treatment options for neglected patient populations, including elderly patients who are ineligible/intolerant to receive interferon (IFN)-based therapy. Vermehren et al. followed 541 patients treated with different combinations of direct antiviral agents (DAAs: ledipasvir/sofosbuvir ±ribavirin; daclatasvir/sofosbuvir ±ribavirin; paritaprevir/ombitasvir ±dasabuvir ±ribavirin or simeprevir/sofosbuvir ±ribavirin or sofosbuvir/ribavirin in genotype) [27].

SVR rates were 91 and 98% in patients aged <65 years and ≥65 years, respectively. Elderly patients took significantly more concomitant drugs (79% vs. 51%). Patients over the age of 65 years with cirrhosis took the highest number of concomitant medications (three per patient-median; range, 0–10).

The number of patients who experienced treatment-associated adverse events was similar between the two age groups (63% vs. 65%). However, proportion of predicted clinically significant DDIs was significantly higher in elderly patients (54% vs. 28%). Elderly patients are at increased risk for significant DDIs when treated with DAAs for chronic HCV infection.

6. Conclusions

Based on these findings, a careful assessment of the regular outpatient medication (all drugs, including herbal products/alternative medicines and even illegal drugs e.g. HIV patients/intravenous users) and subsequent evaluation of potential DDIs with DAAs are absolutely crucial to ensure drug safety in all treated patients. Web-based DDI tools like www.hep-druginteractions.org represent the best way for an assessment of potential DDIs. However, although this web resource includes a huge number of drugs and regular update, some of the drugs are not probably covered.

Also, it is impossible to foresee each combination of drug used in the treatment, and data from real life are also useful source of information. Some DDIs may occur unexpectedly despite a careful evaluation before starting treatment, as demonstrated by the EMA and FDA warning against the concomitant use of amiodarone- and sofosbuvir-containing DAA therapy due to the occurrence of potentially life-threatening bradycardia.

In summary, thousands of patients are being treated with DAAs and a significant number of patients are at risk for DDIs. Although the use of strictly contraindicated comedications seems to be rare, a careful assessment of regular medications and a comprehensive evaluation of potential DDIs with each DAA used for therapy are essential to prevent adverse effects or unnecessary risks of treatment failure.

Author details

Sabina Steiner[1], Nikola Raguž-Lučić[1] and Damir Erceg[1,2,3]*

*Address all correspondence to: erceg@bolnica-srebrnjak.hr

1 Faculty of Medicine, Josip Juraj Strossmayer University of Osijek, Osijek, Croatia

2 Clinical Trials Unit, Children Hospital Srebrnjak, Zagreb, Croatia

3 Catholic University of Croatia, Zagreb, Croatia

References

[1] Lavanchy D. Evolving epidemiology of hepatitis C virus. Clinical Microbiology and Infection. 2011;**17**:107-115

[2] European Association for the Study of the Liver. EASL Recommendations on Treatment of Hepatitis C 2016. Journal of Hepatology. 2017;**66**(1):153-167

[3] Webster DP, Klenerman P, Dusheiko GM. Hepatitis C. Lancet 2015;**385**:1124-1135

[4] WHO. Guidelines for the screening care and treatment of persons with chronic hepatitis C infection. Updated version, April 2016. World Health Organisation. http://www.who.int/hepatitis/publications/hepatitis-c-guidelines-2016/en/ (Accessed on May 02, 2017)

[5] Kelleher TB. Management of the side effects of peginterferon and ribavirin used for treatment of chronic hepatitis C virus infection. Post TW, ed. UpToDate. Waltham, MA: UpToDate Inc http://www.uptodate.com (Accessed on February 02, 2017.)

[6] http://hepatitiscresearchandnewsupdates.blogspot.hr/2013/12/hcv-direct-acting-antiviral-agents-best.html

[7] Pockros PJ. Direct-Acting Antivirals for the Treatment of Hepatitis C Virus Infection. Post TW, ed. UpToDate. Waltham, MA: UpToDate Inc http://www.uptodate.com (Accessed on February 02, 2017.)

[8] Pons ST, Boyer A, Lamblin G, Chennell P, et al. Managing drug–drug interactions with new direct-acting antiviral agents in chronic hepatitis C. British Journal of Clinical Pharmacology. 2017;**83**:269-293

[9] Soriano V, Labarga P, Barreiro P, et al. Drug interactions with new hepatitis C oral drugs. Expert Opinion on Drug Metabolism & Toxicology. 2015;**11**(3):333-341

[10] Hill L. Hepatitis C virus direct-acting antiviral drug interactions and use in renal and hepatic impairment. Topics in Antiviral Medicine. 2015;**23**(2):

[11] http://www.hep-druginteractions.org (Accessed on 01, February 2017)

[12] http://www.hep-druginteractions.org /site_updates/284 (Accessed on 1 March 2017)

[13] Kaur K, Gandhi MA, Slish J. Drug-drug interactions among hepatitis C virus (HCV) and human immunodeficiency virus (HIV) medications. Infectious Disease and Therapy. 2015;**4**:159-172. DOI: 10.1007/s40121-015-0061-2

[14] Charlton M. Telaprevir, boceprevir, cytochrome P450 and immunosuppressive agents-a potentially lethal cocktail. Hepatology. 2011;**54**:3-5

[15] Garg V, van Heeswijk R, Lee JE, Alves K, Nadkarni P, Luo X. Effect of telaprevir on the pharmacokinetics of cyclosporine and tacrolimus. Hepatology 2011;**54**:20-27

[16] Burger D, Back D, Buggisch P, et al. Clinical management of drug-drug interactions in HCV therapy: challenges and solutions. Journal of Hepatology. 2013;**58**(4):792-800. DOI: 10.1016/j.jhep.2012.10.027

[17] Udina M, Castellvi P, Moreno-Espana J, et al. Interferon-induced depression in chronic hepatitis C: A systematic review and meta-analysis. The Journal of Clinical Psychiatry. 2012;**73**(8):1128-1138. DOI: 10.4088/JCP.12r07694

[18] Schaefer M, Capuron L, Friebe A, et al. Hepatitis C infection, antiviral treatment and mental health: A European expert consensus statement. Journal of Hepatology. 2012;**57**(6):1379-1390. DOI: 10.1016/j.jhep.2012.07.037

[19] El–Serag HB, Kunik M, Richardson P, Rabeneck L. Psychiatric disorders among veterans with hepatitis C infection. Gastroenterology. 2002;**123**(2):476-482. DOI: 10.1053/gast.2002.34750

[20] Smolders EJ, de Kanter CTMM, de Knegt RJ, et al. Drug–drug interactions between direct-acting antivirals and psychoactive medications. Clinical Pharmacokinetics 2016;**55**:1471-1494. DOI: 10.1007/s40262-016-0407-2

[21] Puglisi GM, Smith SM, Jankovich RD, Ashby CR, Jodlowski TZ. Paritaprevir/ritonavir/ombitasvir+dasabuvir plus ribavirin therapy and inhibition of the anticoagulant effect of warfarin: A case report. Journal of Clinical Pharmacy and Therapeutics. 2017;**42**(1):115-118

[22] Harvoni. SPC. http://www.ema.europa.eu/docs/en_GB/document_library/EPAR_-_Product_Information/human/003850/WC500177995.pdf. (Accessed on February 01, 2017.)

[23] Maasoumy B, Port K, Calle Serrano B, et al. The clinical significance of drug-drug interactions in the era of direct-acting anti-viral agents against chronic hepatitis C. Alimentary Pharmacology & Therapeutics. 2013;**38**(11-12):1365-1372

[24] Höner Z, Siederdissen C, Maasoumy B, Marra F, et al. Drug–drug interactions with novel all-oral interferon-free antiviral agents in a large real-world cohort. Clinical Infectious Diseases. 2016;**62**:561-567. DOI: 10.1093/cid/clv973

[25] https://www.researchgate.net/publication/304628441_Drug-Drug_Interactions_DDIs_With_New_anti_HCV_Oral_Interferon-Free_drugs_DAA_in_a_polycentric_cohort_of_HCV (Available on 1 March 2017.)

[26] Kondili LA, Gaeta GB, Ieluzzi D, et al. Real-life data on potential drug-drug interactions in patients with chronic hepatitis C viral infection undergoing antiviral therapy with interferon-free DAAs in the PITER Cohort Study. PLoS One. 2017;**12**(2):e0172159. DOI: 10.1371/journal.pone.0172159

[27] Vermehren J, Peiffer KH, Welsch C, et al. The efficacy and safety of direct acting antiviral treatment and clinical aliment. Pharmacology & Therapeutics. 2016;**44**(8):856-865

Chapter 8

Resistance to Direct-Acting Antiviral Agents in Treatment of Hepatitis C Virus Infections

Mostafa K. El Awady and Reham M. Dawood

Additional information is available at the end of the chapter

http://dx.doi.org/10.5772/intechopen.70729

Abstract

Compounds targeting nonstructural (NS) proteins of hepatitis C virus (HCV) demonstrate clinical promise, suggesting that NS3/NS4a, NS5A, or NS5B inhibitors are potential components in direct-acting antiviral (DAA) combination therapies. In vitro studies revealed dramatic inhibition of viral replication or alteration in subcellular localization of NS proteins. DAAs bind either to catalytic sites (NS3 and NS5B) or to domain-1 of NS5A. Although >90% of the patients clear HCV RNA from their sera, a significant portion of cirrhotic patients suffer from resistance or virological relapse. Mutations in specific residues (Q80K) in NS3 (M28, A30, L31, and Y93 in genotypes 1a and 1b or L28, L30, M31, and Y93 in genotype 4) in NS5A and A282T in NS5B are associated with resistance to DAA [resistance-associated variants (RAVs)]. Current knowledge on the NS functions, mode of action of DAAs, and impacts of RAVs on treatment response are discussed. Not only mutations affecting the binding of DAAs to target proteins but also substitutions affecting the replication fitness of mutant quasispecies are major determinants of treatment failures. These resistance-associated substitutions (RASs) are now considered the major viral mutants that influence the virological outcome after DAA treatment.

Keywords: hepatitis C virus, direct-acting antiviral agents, resistance-associated variants, resistance-associated substitutions

1. Introduction

Hepatitis C virus (HCV) infection is a major etiological factor for liver cirrhosis, steatosis, and hepatocellular carcinoma and represents a primary reason for liver transplantation in patients with end-stage disease. It is estimated that around 350,000 deaths each year occur worldwide as a result of HCV-related liver diseases [1]. Chronic infection with HCV afflicts around 185 million people which represents 2.8% of the world's population [2]. Phylogenetically, HCV exists as seven distinct genotypes each comprises several subtypes and many quasispecies. It was reported that more than 10% of the Egyptian population is infected with HCV, where genotype 4 represents >93% of the chronic infections [3]. The development of direct-acting antiviral (DAA) agents has dramatically enhanced sustained virological response (SVR) rates in genotype 1-infected patients [4]. Although the approval of IFN-free DAA combination treatments has been associated with high cure rates, the emergence of resistant HCV variants has an important role in treatment failure with DAA therapies.

2. Replication cycle of HCV

Elucidation of intracellular HCV replication has fostered the efforts toward development of DAA agents, since in the principle, each step represents a potential target for development of new DAA. Viral particles enter the host cell by endocytosis. After the release of HCV RNA from the virion, the former has two alternative pathways: (a) translated as (+) RNA strand at the rough endoplasmic reticulum into the polyprotein precursor that is cleaved by host and viral proteases into mature proteins, where viral proteins, with the help of host cell factors, stimulate the formation of a membranous web (MW). In the alternative pathway, (b) the negative-sense strand (−) RNA serves as a template for the production of extra copies of positive-sense (+) RNA strands. Since the nascent viral RNA could be a subject to excessive nucleases in the cytoplasm, the MW sequesters both viral and host factors are required for viral genomic replication process. Viral assembly occurs in the MW close to the ER and lipid, where core protein and viral RNA accumulate. During the lipoprotein synthesis in ER membrane, the latter buds to form viral envelope, and the newly formed HCV particles are released by exocytosis [5].

2.1. Direct-acting antiviral agents

The development of DAAs has been progressed through the accumulative information on HCV life cycle, improved cell culture technology, and establishment of a robust in vitro viral propagation system.

So far, four classes of DAAs targeting three HCV proteins [NS3, NS5A, and NS5B] [nucleotide/nucleoside polymerase inhibitors (NPI) and non-nucleotide polymerase inhibitors (NNPI)] are approved for HCV treatment in several countries around the globe as shown in **Figure 1**. Multiple DAAs target specific HCV-encoded nonstructural proteins leading to arrest of viral replication [6], thus achieving higher rates of SVR even in cirrhotic and difficult-to-treat patients.

Inhibitors of HCV replication target the NS3/NS4A protease, the NS5A, or the viral polymerase (NS5B) [7]. The first generation of DAAs included NS3/NS4A protease inhibitors (PI), telaprevir (TPV), and boceprevir (BOC). These drugs when given in combination with IFN + RBV, more than 30% increase in SVR rates were achieved, as compared with IFN + RBV; however, 20–40% of the patients suffer from breakthroughs or relapses after the end of treatment. New

http://dx.doi.org/10.5772/intechopen.70729

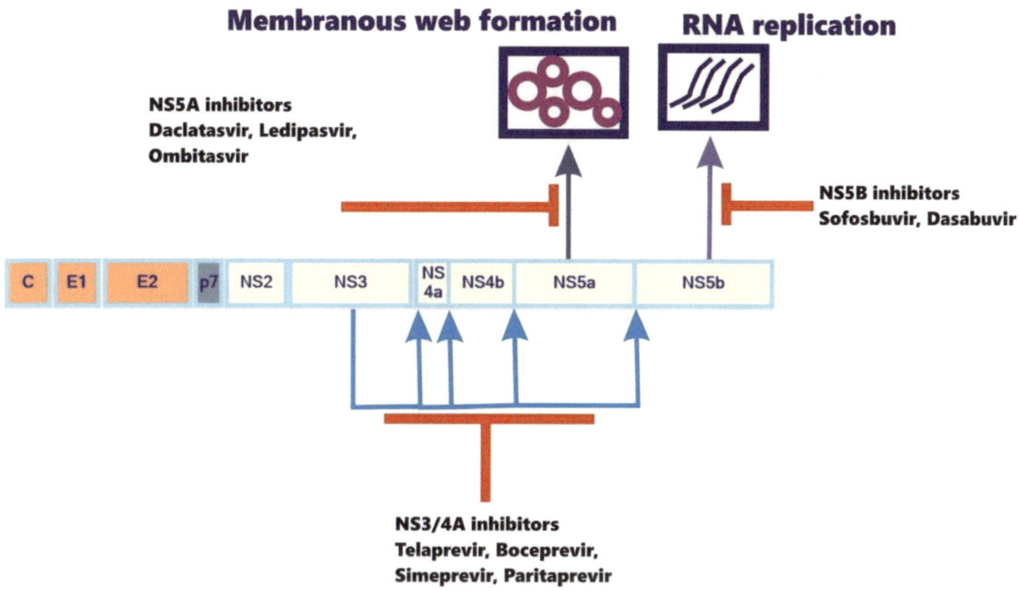

Figure 1. *HCV genome and potential drug discovery targets* shows the currently approved (particularly in Egypt) protease, polymerase, and NS5A inhibitors used as part of a multitargeted approach to HCV treatment.

DAAs were then approved such as simeprevir, an NS3/NS4A inhibitor; daclatasvir (DCV), an NS5A inhibitor; and sofosbuvir (SOF), an NS5B inhibitor as well as IFN-free combinations such as Harvoni [ledipasvir (LDV) + SOF] and paritaprevir/ritonavir + ombitasvir + dasabuvir (targeting NS3, NS5A, and NS5B, respectively). Rates of SVR were significantly increased (>90%) using these new combinations [8].

3. NS3/NS4A protease inhibitors

The viral protease NS3/NS4A is required to cleave the HCV polyprotein into individual viral proteins which are important for viral replication and assembly. It is formed by a heterodimer complex including NS3 and NS4A proteins. NS3 possesses the proteolytic site, while NS4 is a cofactor. This protease cleaves the HCV polyprotein at four sites to produce nonstructural viral proteins NS3, NS4A, NS4B, NS5A, and NS5B. The NS3 protease has a chymotrypsin-like fold consisted of two β-barrel subdomains separated by a groove containing the active site (comprising His57, Asp81, and Ser139) as in **Figure 2**. NS3/NS4A inhibitors block the NS3 catalytic site or inhibit NS3/NS4A interaction, thereby blocking HCV polyprotein cleavage [9]. In addition to this direct action, it is worth noting that NS3/NS4A protease has the ability to block interferon gene expression through the impairment of the retinoic acid-inducible gene I (RIG-I) and Toll-like receptor 3 (TLR3) pathways. Therefore, inhibition of NS3/NS4A protease restores the interferon expression and TLR3 production. Baseline sequencing analysis for NS3/NS4A region revealed the presence of resistance-associated variants (RAVs) in

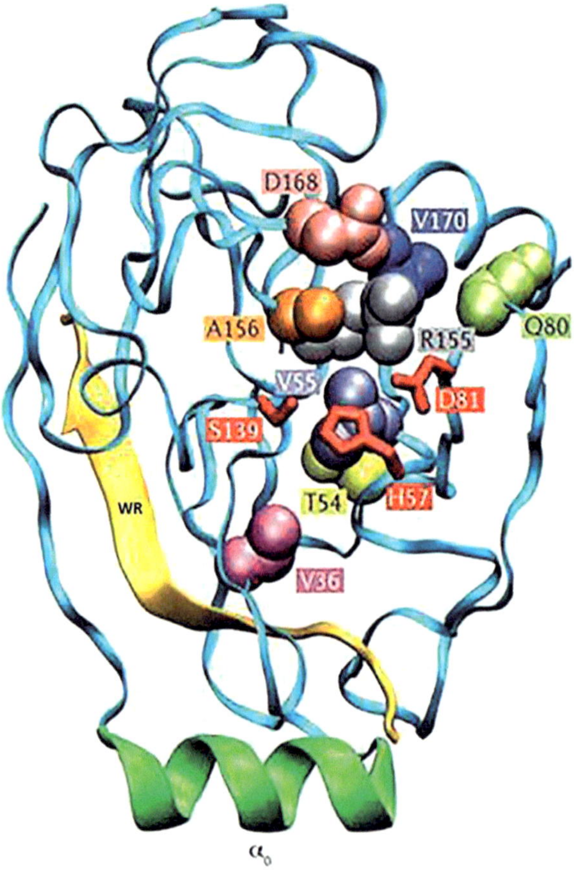

Figure 2. Membrane topology of NS3-4A and positions of mutations that confer resistance to NS3-4A inhibitors. A ribbon diagram of the NS3 protease domain with the central NS4A activation domain (wide ribbon, WR). The α_0 helix serves as an additional membrane anchor of NS3. The catalytic triad (His57, Asp81 and Ser139) is indicated as sticks (H 57, D81 and S139). Mutation of certain residues confers resistance to NS3-4A inhibitors, and the side chains of these residues are represented as van der Waals spheres. (cited with permission from Dr. *Ralf Bartenschlager* University of Heidelberg Department of Infectious Diseases, Molecular Virology, INF 345, 1st. Floor D-69120 Heidelberg Germany).

patients with HCV genotype 1. Although their presence did not have an impact on treatment success [10–12], the RAVs, however, have been detected during the breakthrough in the majority of non-SVR patients. Furthermore, sequence analysis for NS3/NS4A region in relapsers who received TPV-based regimen identified the following variants as RAV hotspots, as shown in **Figure 2**: V36A/V36M, T54A/T54S, R155K/R155T, A156S/A156T, and D168N [10]. These RAVs are situated close to the catalytic site in the NS3 protease domain, consistent with the mechanism of action of a protease inhibitor. Variants conferring low-level resistance had a 3–25-fold increase in IC50 from wild type, while those conferring the high level had >25-fold increase in IC50. The low genetic barrier for developing resistance in the second-generation protease inhibitors is still the major obstacle facing their activities. The sequence analysis for NS3 protease of genotype 1a in patients who received the simeprevir regimens detected a relevant polymorphism Q80K in 19–48% [13]. In vitro studies showed that this mutation decreases viral response to simeprevir by 10folds [13]. Less profound inhibition has been observed in other NS3 inhibitors including sovaprevir and asunaprevir. The presence of the baseline mutation Q80K in HCV genotype 1a-infected patients diminishes the viral response rate to simeprevir comparable to those without this mutation (58 vs. 84%). Therefore, it was recommended to test the presence of this mutation in HCV genotype 1a-infected patients and probably other genotypes to select the best treatment protocol [14].

4. NS5A inhibitors

Hepatitis C virus (NS5A) is a multifunctional phosphoprotein with an N-terminal amphipathic alpha-helix and is composed of 447 amino acids that are divided into 3 domains. It exists in two phosphorylated forms: basal (p56) and hyperphosphorylated (p58) NS5A. Phosphorylation is believed to regulate several NS5A functions, including RNA binding and self-interaction [15]. NS5A is a promiscuous protein which binds to viral (NS5B and RNA) and host factors including 13 different kinases, for example, PI4KIIIα as well as lipid membranes (ER). NS5A is composed of NH2-terminus domain I (amino acids 1–213), domain II (amino acids 250–342), and carboxy-terminus domain III (amino acids 356–447). Domains I and II play a major role in viral replication, while domain III is essential for virion assembly. Domain I is the highly conserved region among all HCV genotypes and contains the amphipathic membrane-anchoring helix and a Zn-binding motif that renders NS5A to exhibit high affinity for HCV RNA.

Nonstructural 5A protein has no enzymatic function, and its ultimate function is not fully understood. Daclatasvir, ledipasvir, and ombitasvir are among the currently available NS5A inhibitors. Daclatasvir (DCV) is believed to target the NH2-terminal region of NS5A, and it might stop the protein function through interfering with dimer formation, downregulating the NS5A phosphorylation which leads to unusual localization, prohibiting polyprotein processing, and eventually arresting viral replication. The mode of action of DCV contributes to blocking the formation of the MW. The latter is essential for replication, which does not occur at other sites in cytoplasm where exonucleases immediately destroy RNA. A description of NS5A inhibitors' mode of action is simplified in **Figure 3**. Targett-Adams et al. [16] suggested that NS5A inhibitors can change the subcellular localization of the NS5A in the infected cells from the endoplasmic reticulum to lipid droplets. Early proof of this mechanism was provided by Francis Chisari Laboratory [17], where amphipathic alpha-helical peptide mimicking the amino acid composition of the membrane anchor domain at the amino-terminal region of HCV NS5A could change the subcellular localization of NS5A that moved from the ER membrane to the lipid droplets.

The binding between the NS5A protein and its inhibitor changes the NS5A conformation and makes the NS5A unable to incorporate in the replication complex within the ER membrane; consequently, inhibited NS5A is no longer sequestered in the replication complex and is shuttled to the surface of the lipid droplets. It was demonstrated that the inhibited NS5A is localized at the lipid droplet surface where it remains nonfunctional and nonpermissive to

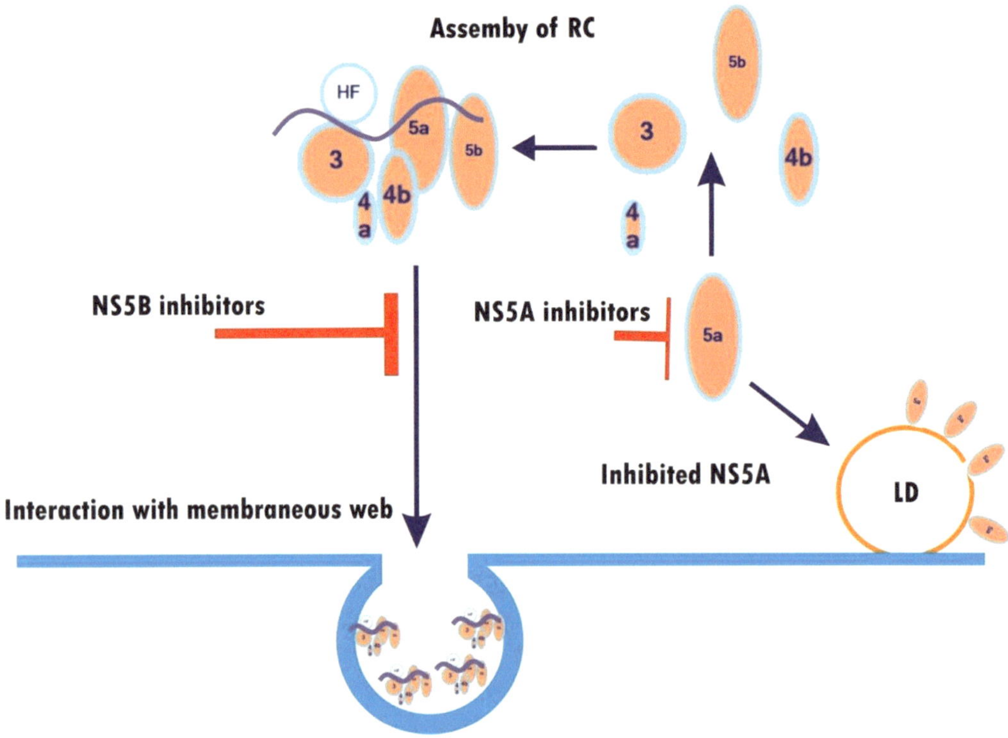

Figure 3. Intracellular trafficking of NS5A protein. Once cleaved out from the polyprotein precursor, NS5A mediates the formation of replication complex (RC) that contains host proteins, viral RNA, and nonstructural proteins of HCV. Host and viral components are sequestered in the membranous web to start genomic replication and viral assembly. Inhibitors of NS5A prevent it from migration to the MW, and alternatively NS5A is shuttled to the lipid droplets on the ER membrane. NS5A inhibitors therefore induce subcellular relocalization and cannot prevent replication of already formed RCs. In contrast NS5B inhibitors can arrest viral RNA replication from components within the RCs.

HCV genome synthesis (**Figure 3**) [16, 18]. An additional possible mechanism of inhibition is via inhibition of the hyperphosphorylation of the NS5A protein [19].

It was observed that the presence of single amino acid substitution in HCV genotype 1a is enough to lose response to DCV, while a couple of amino acid substitutions in HCV genotype 1b have led to minimal resistance such as Q54H-Y93H, whereas other double mutations such as L31V-Y93H in genotype 1b are associated with a high level of resistance [20]. The NS5A RAVs included M28, A30, L31, and Y93 in genotype 1a and L31 and Y93 for genotype 1b. The binding of DCV to NS5A dimer is blocked in NS5A RAVs, thus preventing the formation of MW at the ER membrane and the subsequent blocking of HCV replication. These sequels provide an explanation for the low susceptibility of HCV mutants to NS5A inhibitors in vitro. In phase III clinical trial, the use of combination therapy of NS5A inhibitor (DCV) with (NS3/NS4A inhibitor) asunaprevir revealed that the presence of double baseline NS5A mutations at amino acids L31 and Y93 was associated with low response to the combination therapy [21].

In HCV genotype 1a-infected patients, the baseline NS5A mutations conferred high-level resistance to NS5A inhibitors when treated for 24 weeks. These mutations included H58D, Y93H/

http://dx.doi.org/10.5772/intechopen.70729

Y93N/Y93F, or several RAV combinations [22]. A profound impact of RAVs was observed in cirrhotic patients treated for 24 weeks with SOF and LDV. However, SVR rates have not been changed in HCV genotype 1b-infected patients with or without baseline NS5A RAVs. The same study [22] concluded that IL28B-CC genotype is significantly associated with a higher prevalence of Y93H. This kind of association is not fully understood. One of the most relevant baseline mutations that were associated with alteration in clinical outcome is Y93H which was detected in 13 out of 148 genotype 3-infected patients treated with SOF and DCV, where SVR rates were significantly lower than the rest of patients in the same cohort [23].

There is a limited information on the RAVs' influence on efficacy of NS5A inhibitors in HCV genotype 4. In a study on HCV genotype 4d-infected patients treated with DCV [24], mutations associated with resistance after breakthrough at positions L28S, M31I, and Y93H were detected. Furthermore, in genotype 4-infected cirrhotic patients from Egypt, double or multiple baseline mutations were found associated with virological relapse after 24 weeks of treatment with SOF/DCV with or without RBV: L28M-L30S and L30R-M31C-A92T-Y93P [unpublished data]. An in vitro study revealed that replicons containing multiple NS5A mutations (L28S, M31I, and Y93H) conferred high resistance to DCV [24]. Hézode et al. [25] reported treatment failure to DCV in patients infected with genotype 4a mutants harboring double substitutions at positions 28 and 30. In a parallel in vitro study, double substitutions at L28M-R30H and L28M-L30S positions conferred >10,000-fold resistance against the NS5A inhibitors DCV and LDV [25]. The influence of baseline NS5A single or multiple mutations in genotype 4-infected patients was investigated in 186 patients receiving DCV. Interestingly, wild-type genotype 4 infection represented 44.1% of the baseline structure of NS5A, while L30R mutation represents ~43% of the polymorphisms in HCV genotype 4 infections regardless of the clinical outcome [26]. In an unpublished study from our laboratory, L30R mutation was detected in relapsers to SOF/DCV ± RBV. Mutations at L30 (L30R/L30H/L30I/L30S/L30A) were the most commonly detected substitutions among relapsers to DCV-based therapy in genotype 4 infections. In vitro testing of DCV and LDV efficacies on NS5A mutants created by cloning infusion in a 2a/4 hybrid replicon revealed that EC50 of both DCV and LDV was reduced >1 x 10^5 folds on the double mutants L30S-Y93H, L28M-L30H, L28M-L30S, and L30H-M31V as compared with wild-type hybrid. Although these polymorphisms confer high-level resistance in vitro, their presence in baseline samples prior to treatment was found not common, therefore reducing their impact on treatment response [26].

5. HCV population, replication fitness, and resistance to NS5A inhibitors

Hepatitis C virus exists in a mixture of related but genetically distinct viral populations known as viral quasispecies. The relative distribution of viral population depends on the replication capacity of each within a given environment. Emergence of quasispecies occurs as a result of polymorphism which either enhances or decreases the viral fitness of each quasispecies, thus leading to a change in the quasispecies distribution. Upon DAA treatment, viral polymorphisms may confer reduced susceptibility to DAAs. Such polymorphisms may be present in a fit viral population, thus leading to outgrowth of this mutant over the wild type that clinically leads to drug resistance either during DAA (breakthrough) or posttreatment (relapse). Alternatively, substitution may occur in a less fit population which might not be detectable during or after DAA treatment. Wild-type virus does not contain amino acids conferring resistance to DAAs, while one or more amino acid substitutions are associated with resistance to DAAs. The resistant variants may contain other substitutions that provide outgrowth over other variants during DAA treatment, that is, fitness-associated substitutions that eventually lead to viral breakthrough or relapse, that is, resistant fit variants. Alternatively, resistant variants remain relatively less fit to replicate under DAA treatment with higher possibility to achieve SVR.

Baseline sequencing of quasispecies population that represent low proportions requires deep sequencing which is not available in standard virology laboratories; however, resistant variants existing in low proportion (1–15%) of the total quasispecies population do not appear to significantly influence the virological response [27]. Using a cutoff of 15%, baseline resistance-associated substitutions (RASs) were detected in 13–16% of the naïve patients infected with genotype 1a and 16–20% of the patients infected with 1b [22]. All 1a infections who experienced a relapse had baseline RASs that confer in vitro reduced susceptibility to LDV >1000 folds [22].

6. NS5B inhibitors

The HCV NS5B protein is the key enzyme (RNA-dependent RNA polymerase) in the HCV replication cycle. It has the ability to initiate the de novo synthesis of viral RNA. Structurally, the NS5B protein appears as the right-hand shape and is divided into three domains, the palm domain which has the active catalytic site and surrounded by the thumb and finger domains [28]. The thumb domain contains the allosteric site which regulates the active site (**Figure 4**).

Inhibitors of this enzyme may bind either to the catalytic site, that is, nucleoside polymerase inhibitors (NPI), or to four allosteric sites responsible for the configuration of the protein, that is, non-nucleoside polymerase inhibitors (NNPI). Since the sequence of this protein retains genetic conservation across the viral genotypes, the rates of resistance to these inhibitors seem to be relatively rare [9].

6.1. Nucleoside/nucleotide analogue polymerase inhibitors (NPI)

Nucleoside analogue is administered in as a prodrug to facilitate its adsorption where it is activated in the hepatocytes. Several phosphorylation steps are required to convert the nucleoside into nucleoside triphosphate, and this step is mediated by the cellular kinases [29]. The insertion of the nucleoside analogue into RNA chain terminates its elongation. It was observed that the nucleoside inhibitors showed a high genetic barrier to resistance.

Any mutation occurring in the active site of polymerase confers resistance to NPI drugs and makes the mutant virus less fit compared to the wild type which renders the virus unable to replicate. A mutation at S282T has been detected in vitro and rarely in treatment failures to the first developed NPI, that is, sofosbuvir (SOF). Sofosbuvir is a uridine analogue and is highly tolerable compared to other polymerase inhibitors.

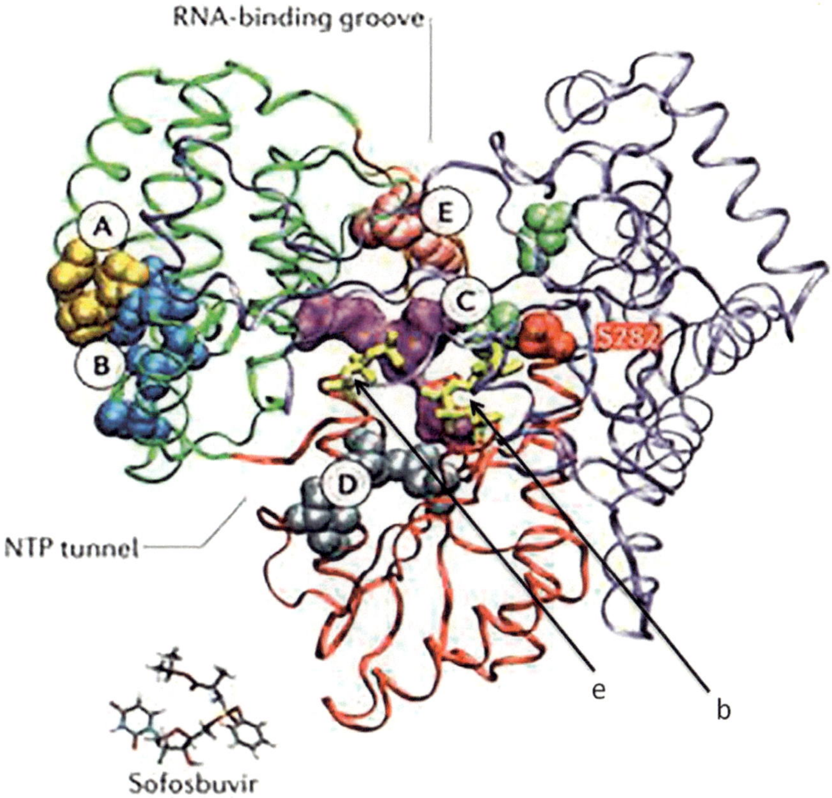

Figure 4. Ribbon diagram of full-length NS5B. Positions of the target regions of five distinct classes of non-nucleoside NS5B inhibitors (A–E) and of some side chains of amino acid residues involved in resistance to these drugs. The position of the major resistance mutation against nucleotide and nucleoside inhibitors (at Ser282) is also indicated. The C-terminal membrane anchor and the linker have been removed for clarity. The active site is indicated by two priming nucleotides (sticks, a,b). For a better comparison with already published structures, the orientation of the finger, palm and thumb subdomains has been rotated by 180° relative to parts. (cited with permission from Dr. *Ralf Bartenschlager* University of Heidelberg Department of Infectious Diseases, Molecular Virology, INF 345, 1st. Floor D-69120 Heidelberg Germany.)

Three mutations were detected through in vitro exposure to SOF, with little impact in patients, namely, S282T, L159F, and E341D. In replicon assays, the mutation S282T conferred resistance to SOF by genotypes 1a and b [30]. The presence of S282T combined with other mutations such as T179A, M289L, and I293L was found to be crucial for conferring resistance to SOF in genotype 2a.

In SOF monotherapy study, the S282T polymorphism was observed in HCV genotype 2-infected patient who relapsed at week 4 posttreatment [31]. In a phase III SOF clinical trials, the substitutions L159F and V321A have been detected in several HCV genotype 3-infected patients who did not achieve SVR. Treatment failure was experienced by six genotype 1b-infected patients and relapse in a genotype 1a-infected patient. Those patients were found to carry substitutions C316N/C316H/C316F in their baseline samples [29]. In another clinical trial at phases II and III where SOF was administered, the mutation S282T was not detected at baseline. An important phenomenon associated with the mutation S282T is that it confers low replication fitness and consequently virological failure that leads to uncommon emergence (1%).

6.2. Non-nucleoside polymerase inhibitors (NNPI)

The non-nucleosides target the allosteric site of the HCV polymerase. Non-nucleoside polymerase inhibitors bind to the non-catalytic site and change the conformational structure necessary for the HCV replication. The antiviral activities of these agents were determined and ranged from low to moderate, besides they have a low genetic barrier to resistance and inhibit HCV in a genotype-dependent manner. As a result of the low genetic barrier of NNPI to resistance, these agents have been studied in combination with other DAAs to target several regions of HCV genome and prevent the emergence of resistance-associated variants to an individual drug. At present, the approved NNPI is dasabuvir, which binds to palm 1 site of RNA polymerase, and beclabuvir, which binds to thumb 1 site [32].

Substitutions C316Y in genotypes 1a and b and Y448C/Y448H in genotype 1b induced resistance to dasabuvir >900 folds [33]. The 3D regimen is consists of dasabuvir in combination with ombitasvir (as an NS5A inhibitor), paritaprevir (as an NS3/NS4A inhibitor), and ritonavir (as a potent inhibitor of CYP3A4). The administration of the 3D regimen with ribavirin in HCV genotype 1-infected patients achieved 95–98% SVR [34, 35]. This provides evidence that a multitargeted approach can augment the rate of response. Substitutions in NS5A, NS3, and NS5B can emerge after exposure to ombitasvir, paritaprevir, and dasabuvir, respectively. In clinical trials, the common substitutions that were detected during treatment or at treatment failure in HCV genotype 1a-infected patients were D168V in NS3, M28A/M28T/M28V and Q30E/Q30K/Q30R in NS5A, and S556G/S556R in NS5B [35–38]. Whereas the observed substitutions in HCV genotype 1b-infected patients who did not achieve SVR were Y56H and D168V in NS3, L31 M and Y93H in NS5A and S556G in NS5B at the time of treatment failure [35].

7. Conclusion

The extensive use of the DAAs in the near future will end with the development of viral resistance and appearance of patients who failed to achieve SVR. The majority of available data on HCV infection susceptibility to the approved treatment regimens containing combined DAAs were derived from studies on genotypes 1a and 1b.

The HCV RNA-dependent RNA polymerase (NS5B) is characterized by the absence of proofreading activity which leads to production of a large number of viral variants. The persistence of these variants is dependent on its fitness (relative capacity of a viral variant to replicate normally). Prior to the DAA administration, most of the resistant variants are unfit to replicate, and the majority of viral variants are fit and sensitive to DAA drugs. After DAA administration, the antiviral activity of the DAAs will inhibit completely the sensitive fit wild-type variants and leads to positive selection for the resistant variants with low susceptibility to DAAs. The resistant variants may acquire substitutions rendering them fit and competently replicating. The emergence of the fitness-associated substitutions may be either preexisted naturally or acquired by replication in the presence of the drugs allowing the virus to be actively replicating during treatment (breakthrough) or after the end treatment (relapse). Luckily, S282T mutation is very rare, and if present it afflicts the replication capacity of HCV, thus rendering NS5B inhibitors specific for catalytic site binding, for example, SOF, the most effective NS5B inhibitor. Although S282T was the first described SOF-associated RAS [30], a couple of treatment emergent substitutions were identified such as L159F and V321A [39, 40]. Indeed, several factors determine the impact of RASs on SVR including susceptibility/fitness of a given viral population, patients' genetic identity, presence of liver cirrhosis, as well as treatment regimen and duration. In patients infected with genotype 1a, the efficacy of simeprevir + SOF treatment for 8 weeks has been significantly reduced to 73% SVR in the presence of NS3 Q80K substitution compared with 84% in the absence of this substitution [41]. The RAV test is then recommended and is in fact crucial to detect the prevalence of the common NS3 Q80K RAV that affects simeprevir efficacy in the HCV genotype 1a cirrhotic patients. In Japan, the protease inhibitor asunaprevir in combination with NS5A inhibitor DCV is approved for treatment with 84% SVR. The latter is reduced to 41% in NS5A baseline substitutions at L31 and Y93 [42].

Primary substitutions in NS5A sequences of genotype 1a that are associated with resistance to LDV involves residues K24, M28, Q30, L31, P32, H58, and Y93, while genotype 1b includes mainly L31, P58, A92, and Y93 [43, 44]. In genotype 4, mutations at residues L28 and L30 are associated with relapse after DCV-based treatment (unpublished data from our laboratory). Baseline substitutions at these two residues exist in more than 40% of the genotype 4 infections [26], while in genotypes 1a and b, substitutions Y93H and L31 M exist in 15 and 6.3%, respectively [45]. Besides, other substitutions exist in 0.3–3.5% of the population. The emergence of minor less fit variants in some patients rather than reinfection is believed to be associated with treatment failure in high-risk populations [46]. Well-tolerated variants persist >6 months posttreatment such as M28T, Q30R/Q30H, L31V, and Y93R [47]. Since most formulations contain NS5A inhibitors, these mutations represent a future challenge to the next-generation regimens.

Acknowledgements

The authors acknowledge Dr. Khaled Helmi El-Wakeel, for constructing **Figures 1** and **3**.

Author details

Mostafa K. El Awady* and Reham M. Dawood

*Address all correspondence to: mkawady49@yahoo.com

Department of Microbial Biotechnology, National Research Center (NRC), Giza, Egypt

References

[1] Mohd Hanafiah K, Groeger J, Flaxman AD, Wiersma ST. Global epidemiology of hepatitis C virus infection: New estimates of age-specific antibody to HCV seroprevalence. Hepatology. 2013 Apr;**57**(4):1333-1342. DOI: 10.1002/hep.26141

[2] Messina JP, Humphreys I, Flaxman A, Brown A, Cooke GS, Pybus OG, et al. Global distribution and prevalence of hepatitis C virus genotypes. Hepatology. 2015 Jan;**61**(1):77-87. DOI: 10.1002/hep.27259

[3] Kamal SM. Improving outcome in patients with hepatitis C virus genotype 4. The American Journal of Gastroenterology. 2007 Nov;**102**(11):2582-2588. DOI: 10.1111/j.1572-0241.2007.01538.x

[4] Liang TJ, Ghany MG. Current and future therapies for hepatitis C virus infection. The New England Journal of Medicine. 2013 May 16;**368**(20):1907-1917. DOI: 10.1056/NEJMra1213651

[5] Bartenschlager R, Lohmann V, Penin F. The molecular and structural basis of advanced antiviral therapy for hepatitis C virus infection. Nature Reviews. Microbiology. 2013 Jul;**11**(7):482-496. DOI: 10.1038/nrmicro3046

[6] Ahmed A, Felmlee DJ. Mechanisms of hepatitis C viral resistance to direct acting antivirals. Virus. 2015 Dec 18;**7**(12):6716-6729. DOI: 10.3390/v7122968

[7] Horner SM, Naggie S. Successes and challenges on the road to cure hepatitis C. PLoS Pathogens. 2015 Jun;**11**(6):e1004854. DOI: 10.1371/journal.ppat.1004854

[8] Pawlotsky JM. Hepatitis C treatment: The data flood goes on-an update from the liver meeting 2014. Gastroenterology. 2015 Mar;**148**(3):468-479. DOI: 10.1053/j.gastro.2015.01.002

[9] Pockros PJ. New direct-acting antivirals in the development for hepatitis C virus infection. Therapeutic Advances in Gastroenterology. 2010 May;**3**(3):191-202. DOI: 10.1177/1756283X10363055

[10] Kieffer TL, De Meyer S, Bartels DJ, Sullivan JC, Zhang EZ, Tigges A, et al. Hepatitis C viral evolution in genotype 1 treatment-naive and treatment-experienced patients receiving telaprevir-based therapy in clinical trials. PloS One. 2012;**7**(4):e34372. DOI: 10.1371/journal.pone.0034372

[11] Ogert RA, Howe JA, Vierling JM, Kwo PY, Lawitz EJ, McCone J, et al. Resistance-associated amino acid variants associated with boceprevir plus pegylated interferon-alpha 2b and ribavirin in patients with chronic hepatitis C in the SPRINT-1 trial. Antiviral Therapy. 2013;**18**(3):387-397. DOI: 10.3851/IMP2549

[12] Dierynck I, Ghys A, Witek J, Luo D, Janssen K, Daems B, et al. Incidence of virological failure and emergence of resistance with twice-daily vs every 8-h administration of telaprevir in the OPTIMIZE study. Journal of Viral Hepatitis. 2014 Dec;**21**(12):835-842. DOI: 10.1111/jvh.12347

[13] Bae A, Sun SC, Qi X, Chen X, Ku K, Worth A, et al. Susceptibility of treatment-naive hepatitis C virus (HCV) clinical isolates to HCV protease inhibitors. Antimicrobial Agents and Chemotherapy. 2010 Dec;**54**(12):5288-5297. DOI: 10.1128/AAC.00777-10

[14] Lawitz E, Poordad F, Brainard DM, Hyland RH, An D, Dvory-Sobol H, et al. Sofosbuvir with peginterferon-ribavirin for 12 weeks in previously treated patients with hepatitis C genotype 2 or 3 and cirrhosis. Hepatology. 2015 Mar;**61**(3):769-775. DOI: 10.1002/hep.27567

[15] Tellinghuisen TL, Marcotrigiano J, Gorbalenya AE, Rice CM. The NS5A protein of hepatitis C virus is a zinc metalloprotein. The Journal of Biological Chemistry. 2004 Nov 19;**279**(47):48576-48587. DOI: 10.1074/jbc.M407787200

[16] Targett-Adams P, Graham EJ, Middleton J, Palmer A, Shaw SM, Lavender H, et al. Small molecules targeting hepatitis C virus-encoded NS5A cause subcellular redistribution of their target: Insights into compound modes of action. Journal of Virology. 2011 Jul;**85**(13):6353-6368. DOI: 10.1128/JVI.00215-11

[17] Cheng G, Montero A, Gastaminza P, Whitten-Bauer C, Wieland SF, Isogawa M, et al. A virocidal amphipathic {alpha}-helical peptide that inhibits hepatitis C virus infection in vitro. Proceedings of the National Academy of Sciences of the United States of America. 2008 Feb 26;**105**(8):3088-3093. DOI: 10.1073/pnas.0712380105

[18] Pawlotsky JM. NS5A inhibitors in the treatment of hepatitis C. Journal of Hepatology. 2013 Aug;**59**(2):375-382. DOI: 10.1016/j.jhep.2013.03.030.

[19] Qiu D, Lemm JA, O'Boyle DR, 2nd, Sun JH, Nower PT, Nguyen V, et al. The effects of NS5A inhibitors on NS5A phosphorylation, polyprotein processing and localization. The Journal of General Virology 2011 Nov;**92**(Pt 11):2502-2511. doi: 10.1099/vir.0.034801-0

[20] Fridell RA, Wang C, Sun JH, O'Boyle DR 2nd, Nower P, Valera L, et al. Genotypic and phenotypic analysis of variants resistant to hepatitis C virus nonstructural protein 5A replication complex inhibitor BMS-790052 in humans: In vitro and in vivo correlations. Hepatology. 2011 Dec;**54**(6):1924-1935. DOI: 10.1002/hep.24594

[21] McPhee F, Hernandez D, Yu F, Ueland J, Monikowski A, Carifa A, et al. Resistance analysis of hepatitis C virus genotype 1 prior treatment null responders receiving daclatasvir and asunaprevir. Hepatology. 2013 Sep;**58**(3):902-911. DOI: 10.1002/hep.26388

[22] Zeuzem S, Mizokami M, Pianko S, Mangia A, Han K, Martin R., Svarovskaia E, Dvory-Sobol H, Doehle B, Pang P, et al. Prevalence of pre-treatment NS5A resistance associated variants in genotype 1 patients across different regions using deep sequencing and effect on treatment outcome with LDV/SOF. Hepatology. 2015;62:254A

[23] Nelson DR, Cooper JN, Lalezari JP, Lawitz E, Pockros PJ, Gitlin N, et al. All-oral 12-week treatment with daclatasvir plus sofosbuvir in patients with hepatitis C virus genotype 3 infection: ALLY-3 phase III study. Hepatology. 2015 Apr;**61**(4):1127-1135. DOI: 10.1002/hep.27726

[24] Bartolini B, Lionetti R, Giombini E, Sias C, Taibi C, Montalbano M, et al. Dynamics of HCV genotype 4 resistance-associated variants during virologic escape with pIFN/RBV + daclatasvir: A case study using ultra deep pyrosequencing. Journal of Clinical Virology. 2015 May;**66**:38-43. DOI: 10.1016/j.jcv.2015.02.001

[25] Hézode C, Hirschfield GM, Ghesquiere W, Sievert W, Rodriguez-Torres M, Shafran SD, et al. Daclatasvir plus peginterferon alfa and ribavirin for treatment-naive chronic hepatitis C genotype 1 or 4 infection: A randomised study. Gut. 2015 Jun;**64**(6):948-956. http://dx.doi.org/10.1136/gutjnl-2014-307498

[26] Zhou N, Hernandez D, Ueland J, Yang X, Yu F, Sims K, et al. NS5A sequence heterogeneity and mechanisms of daclatasvir resistance in hepatitis C virus genotype 4 infection. The Journal of Infectious Diseases. 2016 Jan 15;**213**(2):206-215. DOI: 10.1093/infdis/jiv379

[27] Pawlotsky JM. Hepatitis C virus resistance to direct-acting antiviral drugs in interferon-free regimens. Gastroenterology. 2016 Jul;**151**(1):70-86. DOI: 10.1053/j.gastro.2016.04.003

[28] Ranjith-Kumar CT, Kao CC. Biochemical activities of the HCV NS5B RNA-dependent RNA polymerase. Taylor & Francis; Wymondham, England: 2006. pp. 293-310

[29] Lontok E, Harrington P, Howe A, Kieffer T, Lennerstrand J, Lenz O, et al. Hepatitis C virus drug resistance-associated substitutions: State of the art summary. Hepatology. 2015 Nov;**62**(5):1623-1632. DOI: 10.1002/hep.27934

[30] Lam AM, Espiritu C, Bansal S, Micolochick Steuer HM, Niu C, Zennou V, et al. Genotype and subtype profiling of PSI-7977 as a nucleotide inhibitor of hepatitis C virus. Antimicrobial Agents and Chemotherapy. 2012 Jun;**56**(6):3359-3368. DOI: 10.1128/AAC.00054-12

[31] Gane EJ, Stedman CA, Hyland RH, Ding X, Svarovskaia E, Symonds WT, et al. Nucleotide polymerase inhibitor sofosbuvir plus ribavirin for hepatitis C. The New England Journal of Medicine. 2013 Jan 03;**368**(1):34-44. DOI: 10.1056/NEJMoa1208953

[32] Gerber L, Welzel TM, Zeuzem S. New therapeutic strategies in HCV: Polymerase inhibitors. Liver International. 2013 Feb;**33**(Suppl 1):85-92. DOI: 10.1111/liv.12068

[33] Kati W, Koev G, Irvin M, Beyer J, Liu Y, Krishnan P, et al. In vitro activity and resistance profile of dasabuvir, a nonnucleoside hepatitis C virus polymerase inhibitor. Antimicrobial Agents and Chemotherapy. 2015 Mar;**59**(3):1505-1511. DOI: 10.1128/AAC.04619-14

[34] Kowdley KV, Lawitz E, Poordad F, Cohen DE, Nelson DR, Zeuzem S, et al. Phase 2b trial of interferon-free therapy for hepatitis C virus genotype 1. The New England Journal of Medicine. 2014 Jan 16;**370**(3):222-232. DOI: 10.1056/NEJMoa1306227

[35] Feld JJ, Kowdley KV, Coakley E, Sigal S, Nelson DR, Crawford D, et al. Treatment of HCV with ABT-450/r-ombitasvir and dasabuvir with ribavirin. The New England Journal of Medicine. 2014 Apr 24;**370**(17):1594-1603. DOI: 10.1056/NEJMoa1315722

[36] Zeuzem S, Jacobson IM, Baykal T, Marinho RT, Poordad F, Bourliere M, et al. Retreatment of HCV with ABT-450/r-ombitasvir and dasabuvir with ribavirin. The New England Journal of Medicine. 2014 Apr 24;**370**(17):1604-1614. DOI: 10.1056/NEJMoa1401561

[37] Ferenci P, Bernstein D, Lalezari J, Cohen D, Luo Y, Cooper C, et al. ABT-450/r-ombitasvir and dasabuvir with or without ribavirin for HCV. The New England Journal of Medicine. 22 May 2014;**370**(21):1983-1992. DOI: 10.1056/NEJMoa1402338

[38] Andreone P, Colombo MG, Enejosa JV, Koksal I, Ferenci P, Maieron A, et al. ABT-450, ritonavir, ombitasvir, and dasabuvir achieves 97% and 100% sustained virologic response with or without ribavirin in treatment-experienced patients with HCV genotype 1b infection. Gastroenterology. 2014 Aug;**147**(2):359-365 e1. DOI: 10.1053/j.gastro.2014.04.045

[39] Svarovskaia ES, Dvory-Sobol H, Parkin N, Hebner C, Gontcharova V, Martin R, et al. Infrequent development of resistance in genotype 1-6 hepatitis C virus-infected subjects treated with sofosbuvir in phase 2 and 3 clinical trials. Clinical Infectious Diseases. 2014 Dec 15;**59**(12):1666-1674. DOI: 10.1093/cid/ciu697

[40] Svarovskaia ES, Gane E, Dvory-Sobol H, Martin R, Doehle B, Hedskog C, et al. L159F and V321A sofosbuvir-associated hepatitis C virus NS5B substitutions. The Journal of Infectious Diseases. 2016 Apr 15;**213**(8):1240-1247. DOI: 10.1093/infdis/jiv564

[41] Kwo P, Gitlin N, Nahass R, Bernstein D, Etzkorn K, Rojter S, et al. Simeprevir plus sofosbuvir (12 and 8 weeks) in hepatitis C virus genotype 1-infected patients without cirrhosis: OPTIMIST-1, a phase 3, randomized study. Hepatology. 2016 Aug;**64**(2):370-380. DOI: 10.1002/hep.28467

[42] Manns M, Pol S, Jacobson IM, Marcellin P, Gordon SC, Peng CY, et al. All-oral daclatasvir plus asunaprevir for hepatitis C virus genotype 1b: A multinational, phase 3, multicohort study. Lancet 2014 Nov 01;**384**(9954):1597-1605. DOI: http://dx.doi.org/10.1016/S0140-6736(14)61059-X

[43] Wong KA, Worth A, Martin R, Svarovskaia E, Brainard DM, Lawitz E, et al. Characterization of hepatitis C virus resistance from a multiple-dose clinical trial of the novel NS5A inhibitor GS-5885. Antimicrobial Agents and Chemotherapy. 2013 Dec;**57**(12):6333-6340. DOI: 10.1128/AAC.02193-12

[44] Cheng G, Tian Y, Doehle B, Peng B, Corsa A, Lee YJ, et al. In vitro antiviral activity and resistance profile characterization of the hepatitis C virus NS5A inhibitor ledipasvir. Antimicrobial Agents and Chemotherapy. 2016 Jan 11;**60**(3):1847-1853. DOI: 10.1128/AAC.02524-15

[45] Sarrazin C. The importance of resistance to direct antiviral drugs in HCV infection in clinical practice. Journal of Hepatology. 2016 Feb;**64**(2):486-504. DOI: 10.1016/j.jhep.2015.09.011

[46] Abdelrahman T, Hughes J, Main J, McLauchlan J, Thursz M, Thomson E. Next-generation sequencing sheds light on the natural history of hepatitis C infection in patients who fail treatment. Hepatology. 2015 Jan;**61**(1):88-97. DOI: 10.1002/hep.27192

[47] Wang C, Sun JH, O'Boyle DR, 2nd, Nower P, Valera L, Roberts S, et al. Persistence of resistant variants in hepatitis C virus-infected patients treated with the NS5A replication complex inhibitor daclatasvir. Antimicrobial Agents and Chemotherapy 2013 May;**57**(5):2054-2065. DOI: 10.1128/AAC.02494-12

Section 3

Many Faces of HCV Infection

Chapter 9

Extrahepatic Manifestations of Hepatitis C Virus Infection

Lucija Virović Jukić and Dominik Kralj

Additional information is available at the end of the chapter

http://dx.doi.org/10.5772/intechopen.70728

Abstract

Chronic hepatitis C virus (HCV) infection causes progressive liver fibrosis, cirrhosis, liver failure, and hepatocellular carcinoma. Additional to liver damage, HCV infection causes a variety of systemic disorders, some of which sometimes bear more severe morbidity than the liver disease itself. These extrahepatic manifestations represent a wide spectrum of disorders, ranging from the presence of a variety of clinically insignificant autoantibodies to diseases affecting a variety of organ systems. Mixed cryoglobulinemia is a common manifestation, and associated vasculitis can affect many organs (kidney, skin, and joints). The skin can also be affected by porphyria cutanea tarda and lichen planus. Other common extrahepatic manifestations include autoimmune disorders, lymphoproliferative disorders, and a number of neurological and neuropsychiatric disorders such as fatigue, depression, or cognitive impairment. Insulin resistance, diabetes mellitus, accelerated atherosclerosis, and increased cardiovascular disease morbidity and mortality have also been associated with chronic HCV infection. The existence and severity of extrahepatic manifestations do not correlate with the severity of liver disease, and the mainstay of treatment is HCV eradication. Patients with systemic manifestations of HCV infection should be prioritized for treatment, especially in the era of new interferon-free therapies with fewer side effects.

Keywords: chronic hepatitis C infection, extrahepatic manifestations, interferon therapy, direct-acting antiviral agents

1. Introduction

Hepatitis C virus (HCV) is a single-stranded RNA virus, a member of the *Flaviviridae* family. As a primarily hepatotropic virus, the main target of infection is hepatocytes, resulting in chronic inflammation in about 80% of cases of infection. It is well known that chronic hepatitis

C leads to cirrhosis, the terminal stage of liver disease, and hepatocellular carcinoma. It is, however, less known that chronic HCV infection leads to a series of systemic disorders and diseases that can often leave greater health consequences than the liver disease alone. These disorders are commonly called extrahepatic manifestations of chronic hepatitis C and encompass a wide spectrum of conditions, from a clinically insignificant presence of different autoantibodies to vasculitis, skin disease, kidney damage, lymphoproliferative disorders, diabetes, various neurological and neuropsychiatric changes, and even increased cardiovascular morbidity and mortality [1]. Extrahepatic manifestations in any form may appear in up to 74% of patients with chronic HCV infection and may long precede manifest hepatic disease presenting with various nonspecific health impairments including malaise, fatigue, nausea, weight loss, and musculoskeletal pain [2]. Specific extrahepatic manifestations of chronic hepatitis C can be divided according to the affected organ or organ system, pathological mechanism, or the strength of available evidence connecting them to chronic hepatitis C infection. Some of the extrahepatic manifestations according to organ system and proposed pathological mechanism are shown in **Tables 1** and **2**. The fact that the severity of these disorders does not necessarily correlate with the severity of hepatic disease is of great clinical significance because even in cases of mildly active chronic hepatitis, a considerable disruption of overall health and quality

Hematopoietic	Essential mixed cryoglobulinemia Monoclonal gammopathy B-cell non-Hodgkin lymphoma
Skin	Leukocytoclastic vasculitis Porphyria cutanea tarda Lichen planus
Kidneys	Membranoproliferative glomerulonephritis Membranous nephropathy Renal impairment
Immunological	Autoimmune antibodies: rheumatoid factor, antinuclear, antithyroid, anticardiolipin, anti-smooth muscle antibodies
Thyroid	Thyroiditis Hypothyroidism Hyperthyroidism
Endocrine and exocrine glands	Type 2 diabetes mellitus Sicca syndrome
Musculoskeletal	Arthralgia/myalgia
Neurological and neuropsychiatric disorders	Fatigue Depression Impaired cognitive function Sensory or sensorimotor polyneuropathy Mononeuritis multiplex
Cardiovascular	Accelerated atherosclerosis Increased rate of cardiovascular and neurovascular incident and peripheral artery disease Increased mortality from cardiovascular and neurovascular incidents

Table 1. The most common extrahepatic manifestations of chronic hepatitis C according to organ system involvement.

Autoimmune mechanism	Proliferative effect	Inflammatory/metabolic	Other mechanism
Autoantibodies	Essential mixed cryoglobulinemia	Insulin resistance and diabetes mellitus	Porphyria cutanea tarda
Thyroiditis	Monoclonal gammopathy	Fatigue/malaise	
Hepatitis	Non-Hodgkin lymphoma	Depression	
Sicca syndrome		Cognitive function damage	
Arthralgia/myalgia		Cardiovascular disease (coronary disease, stroke)	

Table 2. Proposed pathogenetic mechanism through which chronic HCV infection leads to extrahepatic manifestations.

of life can occur. On the other hand, numerous studies have shown that treatment of chronic HCV infection accomplishes the resolution of extrahepatic disease or greatly increases function of the affected organ and lowers accompanying morbidity and mortality risks. Because of this reason, it is accepted and highlighted in current European guidelines, as well as Croatian recommendations for treatment of chronic hepatitis C infection, that patients with extrahepatic manifestations should be prioritized for treatment, regardless of the activity/severity of their liver disease alone [3, 4].

2. Essential mixed cryoglobulinemia

Essential mixed cryoglobulinemia or type II cryoglobulinemia is classified into the group of lymphoproliferative disorders in which clonal B lymphocyte expansion leads to immunoglobulin production—polyclonal immunoglobulin (Ig) G class and monoclonal IgM as rheumatoid factor (RF)—leading to development of immune complexes that precipitate in the cold and are therefore called cryoglobulins. As a consequence of the precipitation of cryoglobulin complexes in small- and middle-sized blood vessels, the occurring complement activation leads to endothelial damage and cryoglobulinemic vasculitis [5]. The syndrome can affect blood vessels in different organs and manifest on the skin, large joints, peripheral nerves, or kidneys. Cryoglobulins are present in about 50% of patients with chronic hepatitis C infection, but do not always cause clinically manifest cryoglobulinemic vasculitis. On the other hand, over 90% of patients with essential mixed cryoglobulinemia have chronic hepatitis C infection. The skin is commonly affected in cryoglobulinemic syndrome manifesting as palpable purpura as a consequence of leukocytoclastic vasculitis [6]. Joint involvement manifests with arthralgias; perineural vasculitis is a cause of distal sensory or sensorimotor polyneuropathy, while kidney involvement most often leads to membranoproliferative glomerulonephritis with renal function impairment. Diagnosis is based on cryoglobulin presence, elevated RF, and immunofluorescence of complement fixing IgM in affected tissues. It is important to note that many studies have shown clinical manifestations of essential mixed cryoglobulinemia to withdraw after successful HCV infection treatment and that the presence of mixed cryoglobulinemia is associated with a reduced virological response rate [7]. Withdrawal of essential mixed cryoglobulinemia, with low recurrence levels, has been established earlier with interferon therapy, and recently some smaller scale studies showed a very good effect of combined direct-acting antiviral therapy (so-called "interferon-free" therapy) in cryoglobulin clearance, renal function improvement, and proteinuria reduction [8, 9]. The success rates seem to be lower than those observed in large registration studies, but the fact the treatment is new and that sample sizes were relatively small should be taken into account. It is important to highlight that, in some patients, interferon therapy can lead to the worsening of clinical manifestations and that in everyday practice optimal antiviral therapy with direct-acting antiviral drugs represents the standard of care for patients with clinically mild to moderate cryoglobulinemic vasculitis. In severe cases additional therapy modalities such as rituximab, corticosteroids, and plasmapheresis may be used before starting antiviral therapy. For refractory forms of cryoglobulinemia, cyclophosphamide and other immunosuppressants are sometimes used.

3. B-cell lymphoma and monoclonal gammopathies

Hepatitis C virus is primarily hepatotropic, but it has also been shown to be lymphotropic, and a connection between chronic HCV infection and B-cell non-Hodgkin lymphoma (NHL) has been established [10, 11]. It is assumed that chronic B lymphocyte stimulation by the HCV antigen leads to monoclonal B-cell expansion present in mixed cryoglobulinemia. This seems to predispose to NHL occurrence, with studies showing increased risk relative to the general population [12]. In a retrospective study comparing untreated HCV-infected patients to those treated with interferon, it has been shown that the rates of malignant lymphoma occurrence (diffuse large cell lymphoma and follicular lymphoma) were significantly higher in untreated patients, as well as in those who did not achieve sustained virologic response (SVR), compared to those who were cured [13]. The importance of chronic HCV infection in lymphoma development was additionally confirmed with reports of successful NHL remission after HCV eradication. Results with new interferon-free therapies are so far only available as case reports but point to lymphoma withdrawal after hepatitis C eradication. It can be expected that the wide use of new therapies will show results in larger cohorts of patients.

There are studies suggesting HCV to be a risk factor for monoclonal gammopathies, but the results are inconsistent, and a routine screening of patients with chronic hepatitis C for monoclonal gammopathies is not recommended. In patients with HCV infection, polyclonal or oligoclonal hypergammaglobulinemia (mostly IgG) is present. The gamma globulin level often correlates with disease severity on liver biopsy, and its decrease after successful HCV treatment has been noted.

4. Kidney impairment

Chronic hepatitis C infection is connected with glomerular disease which is most probably a consequence of immune complex deposition in glomerular capillaries. The most common form of kidney disease is membranoproliferative glomerulonephritis, typically connected with essential mixed cryoglobulinemia, while membranous nephropathy is less common [14, 15]. Other non-cryoglobulin-based renal diseases described in HCV-infected patients include IgA nephropathy, postinfectious glomerulonephritis, as well as focal and segmental glomerulosclerosis. Patients most often present with proteinuria and microhematuria with different degrees of renal impairment and with renal biopsy showing glomerular immune complex deposition. Acute nephrotic or nephritic syndrome with new onset of arterial hypertension is also possible. The Kidney Disease Improving Global Outcomes (KDIGO) guidelines thus recommend screening for renal impairment at the time of HCV infection diagnosis and then once a year by determining serum creatinine and performing urinalysis. All patients with chronic kidney disease should also be tested for HCV infection [16]. The existence of renal impairment, especially membranoproliferative glomerulonephritis, is an indication for HCV infection treatment. Until now the standard of treatment was combined interferon and ribavirin (with necessary precaution and kidney function-adjusted dosage), while rituximab, corticosteroids, or immunosuppressants are added in patients with severe cryoglobulinemic vasculitis. Data about the efficacy of new interferon-free therapies in this indication is only available from studies involving a relatively small number of patients, but it can be expected that it could significantly change the clinical presentation and improve treatment of this group of patients [8].

5. Skin manifestations

Porphyria cutanea tarda (PCT) is a disease caused by the reduced activity of the hepatic uroporphyrinogen decarboxylase (UROD) which leads to accumulation of uroporphyrinogen in the blood and urine and is the most common porphyria. PCT can be inherited (autosomal dominant) or acquired (sporadic), and exactly this form was connected with HCV infection in many studies. Meta-analysis that included 50 studies and a total of 2167 patients with PCT showed that the prevalence of HCV infection was around 50%, while the frequency of PCT in patients with chronic HCV infection is about 1–5% [17]. The exact mechanism by which HCV can cause or induce PTC is not known, but it is presumed to be mediated through changes in iron metabolism. Namely, increased iron saturation, estrogens, and alcohol consumption can provoke or induce PCT. Skin changes develop as a consequence of photosensitivity and skin friability and, upon sun exposure and/or minor trauma, manifest as erythema and bullae which may turn hemorrhagic [18, 19]. In later stages hyperpigmentation, hypopigmentation, hirsutism, and sclerodermic changes can appear. In the liver, a spectrum of histological changes can be found, including steatosis, mild to severe inflammation, fibrosis, and cirrhosis. Diagnosis of PCT is made on the basis of clinical suspicion and is confirmed by measuring increased levels of porphyrin in urine and, if available, direct measurement of the UROD enzyme activity. Treatment consists of avoiding precipitating factors (sun, alcohol, estrogens) and, if necessary, lowering iron overload (venipuncture) as well as treating HCV infection in affected patients. In general, treatment of chronic HCV infection leads to the normalization of UROD enzymatic activity, levels of liver aminotransferase and urine porphyrin, as well as disappearance of skin changes.

Lichen planus is a chronic inflammatory disease of the skin and mucosa which can affect hair and nails and is characterized by pruritic papulae. These most often appear on the skin of extremities, face, scalp, nails, and mucosa of the gastrointestinal and genitourinary tract. Lichen planus occurs in various chronic liver diseases, and anti-HCV antibodies can be found in 10–40% of patients with lichen planus [20]. It is assumed that the occurrence of lichen planus is immunologically mediated, but the exact mechanism is unknown. It is also considered a premalignant condition and is known to progress to squamous cell carcinoma. The treatment of HCV infection with interferon therapy did not result in regression of lichen planus in most studies; on the contrary, there are reports of appearance or exacerbation of lichen planus during interferon therapy. A recent case series involving seven patients with oral lichen planus treated with interferon-free protocols showed an improvement of symptoms without adverse events [21].

Leukocytoclastic vasculitis is associated with essential mixed cryoglobulinemia and is a consequence of blood vessel involvement. It is clinically characterized by palpable pruritic changes and petechiae which usually affect lower extremities and is treated as other manifestations of essential cryoglobulinemia.

Necrolytic acral erythema, a condition characterized by painful, pruritic, and erythematous skin lesions of extremities is reported to be strongly associated with chronic HCV infection. Zinc supplementation has been associated with improvement of the condition.

Some data supports a possible connection of chronic HCV infection with chronic pruritus, while sporadic reports also suggest an association of HCV infection with psoriasis, chronic urticaria, pyoderma gangrenosum, erythema nodosum, and erythema multiforme.

6. Ocular manifestations

Mooren's corneal ulcer represents a rare painful peripheral corneal ulceration, usually without accompanying scleritis. Some studies have made a connection between this rare form of corneal ulcer and chronic HCV infection, but the pathogenetic mechanism is not known [22]. Chronic HCV infection has been linked to other diseases of the eye such as sicca syndrome, keratitis, increased intraocular pressure, and episcleritis, while some disorders such as retinal bleeding, vision impairment, as well as rare cases of retinal artery or vein obstruction have been described as possible complications of interferon therapy.

7. Thyroid disorders

Thyroid disorders are relatively frequent in patients with chronic hepatitis C, especially in women. Antithyroid antibodies are, according to various reports, present in 5–17% (averaging at 10%) of patients with HCV infection, while thyroid diseases (mostly hypothyroidism) occur less often, in 2–13% of patients [23]. Thyroid function disorders appear even more often during interferon therapy, probably as a consequence of autoimmune activity precipitated by immunomodulatory therapy, but can persist even after treatment completion. There is some evidence of a possible HCV infection of thyroid tissue causing a local inflammatory response that might trigger the autoimmune process. In any case, determining thyroid hormones as well as

http://dx.doi.org/10.5772/intechopen.70728

anti-thyroglobulin and antithyroid peroxidase antibodies is necessary in all HCV-infected patients, especially before and periodically during interferon therapy. Substitution therapy with thyroid hormones is used in hypothyroidism treatment. In cases of mild hyperthyroidism, symptomatic therapy is used, while thyrostatic therapy is reserved for more severe cases. Interferon therapy should be stopped in cases of severe hyperthyroidism caused by the treatment. It will be interesting to see how the eradication of HCV infection with new drug combinations without interferon affects thyroid function disorders in patients with chronic hepatitis C.

8. Sicca syndrome

The sicca syndrome develops in most patients with Sjögren's syndrome. Lymphocytic sialadenitis resembling Sjögren's syndrome has been described in patients with chronic HCV infection who complain of mouth or eye dryness in 20–30% of cases [15]. There are, however, histological (milder, mostly pericapillary lymphocytic infiltration without ductal destruction in HCV infection as opposed to periductal infiltration with destruction of excretory ducts in classic Sjögren's syndrome) and clinical differences (less pronounced symptoms, later onset, increased levels of serum cryoglobulin and RF, lower complement levels, positive antinuclear, and negative Ro/La antibodies). Therefore, it seems that HCV does not cause Sjögren's syndrome but rather symptoms that imitate it [14]. Treatment of chronic HCV infection leads to symptom resolution in patients with the sicca syndrome.

9. Other autoimmune manifestations

Various autoantibodies are frequently found in patients with chronic HCV infection. Rheumatoid factor (around 60%) is most often present followed by antinuclear antibodies (ANA, around 40%), antithyroid (35%), anticardiolipin (15%), and anti-smooth muscle antibodies (ASMA, around 7%), respectively. These antibodies appear in about one-half of patients with chronic HCV infection (40–65% according to different studies) but are commonly present in low titer and, for the most part, do not seem to affect the clinical course of the disease [1]. Antibodies to liver and kidney microsomes (anti-LKM-1) and actin are an exception and can be of clinical significance in some HCV-infected patients. These antibodies are usually characteristic for autoimmune hepatitis, and it has been noticed that, although patients with hepatitis C and anti-LKM-1 antibodies mostly benefit from interferon therapy, in some cases an increase in liver function tests can be observed. Some of these patients respond well to standard therapy for autoimmune hepatitis which consists of azathioprine and corticosteroids. Determining the primary cause of hepatitis in patients with overlapping HCV infection and autoantibodies can be very challenging, even though it has been shown that anti-LKM-1 antibodies in these patients are directed against different epitopes of cytochrome P450 2D6 compared to patients with autoimmune hepatitis [24]. Even though there are no recommendations for routinely determining the presence of these antibodies, if they are known to be present, greater caution during interferon therapy is recommended. The role of direct-acting antiviral drugs in these patients is yet to be determined.

Numerous studies have shown a connection between HCV infection and immune thrombocytopenic purpura (ITP) and/or hemolytic anemia, whether as a consequence of the infection itself or of interferon therapy. According to the results of one of the largest studies, it seems that chronic HCV infection is associated with a higher frequency of ITP in both treated and untreated patients, while increased risk of autoimmune hemolytic anemia was only present in patients treated with interferon therapy.

10. Musculoskeletal system

Arthralgia is common and reported by 40–80% of patients with chronic hepatitis C [1]. The joints are usually symmetrically affected, mostly knees and hands. The afflicted joints are painful, without deformities. True arthritis is rare, presenting as rheumatoid like arthritis in two-thirds and oligoarthritis in one-third of patients. Rheumatoid factor is present in 70–80% of patients with mixed essential cryoglobulinemia, but its presence does not correlate with joint affection [15]. Likewise, cyclic citrulline antibodies characteristic for rheumatoid arthritis are usually not present. Myalgia is also a common complaint. According to epidemiological studies, chronic HCV infection is associated with reduced bone mineral density and increased risk of fractures. The mechanism is probably linked to chronic inflammation and liver disease. Hepatitis C-associated osteosclerosis, mostly reported in patients with a history of intravenous drug abuse, is an uncommon disorder characterized by an increase in bone mass during adulthood. The increased bone turnover in periosteal, endosteal, and trabecular bone leads to the thickening of the skeleton and may respond to bisphosphonate or calcitonin therapy.

11. Neurological manifestations

Neurological manifestations of HCV infection can vary from central nervous system (CNS) involvement to peripheral neuropathy including sensorimotor neuropathy and mononeuritis multiplex. Evidence of CNS involvement includes the demonstration of HCV RNA in brain tissue and cerebrospinal fluid suggesting active replication and as well as a possible association of HCV infection and small vessel cerebrovascular disease [25–27]. The most common form of nerve involvement is distal sensory or sensorimotor polyneuropathy, which clinically presents with painful, asymmetric paresthesia, while multiple mononeuropathy occurs rarely [15]. These changes are a consequence of vasculitis, sometimes associated with cryoglobulinemia, involving vasa nervorum.

In a recently published study, chronic HCV infection has been linked to Parkinson's disease [28].

12. Neuropsychiatric disorders

Neurocognitive damages can manifest with a wide array of neuropsychiatric conditions, such as tiredness, depression, and lack of concentration and working memory, of which patients with chronic HCV infection often complain. These disorders are often seen and intertwined with other associated additions, such as chronic liver disease, cirrhosis, the use of drugs, and others. Some studies have managed to show that these neurocognitive damages are a consequence of the HCV infection itself, regardless of comorbidities [29]. Functional imaging methods have shown metabolic changes in brains of chronic hepatitis C patients, with improvement of cognitive function and brain metabolism observed after treating the HCV infection [30]. Some of these disorders such as depression and fatigue are important because they can exacerbate under interferon therapy. This is why it is important to perform mental status evaluation at the beginning and during this therapy, so as to be able to timely act with suitable psychiatric support, antidepressants, and anxiolytics. Fatigue, depression, and cognitive damage significantly impair functional ability (at work and at home) and impact the quality of life of patients with chronic HCV infection, while the eradication of the virus positively correlates with an improvement in quality of life.

13. Metabolic manifestations: diabetes mellitus and insulin resistance

Disturbed glucose metabolism, onset of insulin resistance (IR), and type 2 diabetes mellitus (T2DM) are often associated with chronic HCV infection. A meta-analysis of 34 studies confirmed a positive correlation between HCV infection and risk of T2DM, which is 1.7 times greater than the general population and notably increased compared to chronic hepatitis B patients [31]. It appears that the risk of T2DM in patients with chronic HCV infection is increased in patients with risk factors such as older age, obesity, advanced liver fibrosis, and a family history of diabetes [32]. Likewise, results of multiple studies have shown that successful eradication of HCV infection decreases IR and that the risk of T2DM is decreased in patients who achieved SVR [33]. Multiple studies have confirmed an association between the HCV infection and IR development that can be present without manifest T2DM. Experimental studies have shown that HCV causes significant changes in the lipid and glucose metabolism and that it leads to IR in the liver and peripheral tissue through direct (immediate influence of HCV proteins on intracellular insulin signal pathways) and indirect (the influence of TNF-α and other cytokines on the development of peripheral IR) mechanisms. Insulin resistance causes a series of changes in lipid and lipoprotein metabolism and leads to the development of liver steatosis [34]. Clinical implications of HCV-induced IR, besides T2DM development, include a worse response to interferon therapy, accelerated fibrosis and development of cirrhosis, increased risk of hepatocellular carcinoma, as well as increased cardiovascular morbidity and mortality [35].

14. Cardiovascular disease

Chronic HCV infection has been associated with accelerated atherosclerosis [36]. Risk of early carotid artery atherosclerosis (determined by intima-media thickness measurement) was four times greater in HCV patients than noninfected patients [14, 37]. In several cohorts of HCV-positive patients, increased cardiovascular mortality (1.5–25 times) as well as a higher incidence of cerebrovascular and acute coronary syndromes was noted [38]. Besides coronary and cerebrovascular disease, an increased rate of peripheral arterial disease in patients with a chronic HCV infection has been described. Rates of acute coronary syndrome and ischemic stroke were significantly reduced in patients treated with peginterferon and ribavirin compared to untreated patients [39]. Although this association was found in studies originating from Far East countries, Western European and American studies, as well as a recent meta-analysis, have not established a clear correlation of HCV infection and increased cardiovascular and cerebrovascular risk [40, 41]. Likewise, the pathogenetic mechanism through which HCV leads to accelerated atherosclerosis has not been fully elucidated. There is evidence of HCV RNA presence in carotid plaques and endothelial cells in the brain, and it is possible that local infection leads to tissue damage, but atherosclerosis is more probably a consequence of the aforementioned IR, metabolism disturbance, and proinflammatory cytokine action. Many unsolved questions leave space for further research, and the arrival of new therapies opens new possibilities in treating patients with an expected decrease in cardiovascular morbidity and mortality.

15. Other HCV infection-associated diseases

Pulmonary fibrosis is a disease characterized by interstitial inflammation with focal fibroblast proliferation and collagen deposits leading to fibrosis, which clinically commonly manifests as dyspnea on exertion and nonproductive cough. The disease pathogenesis is unknown, and several studies have found a connection between pulmonary fibrosis and chronic HCV infection. A higher prevalence of pulmonary fibrosis was seen in HCV-infected patients than control groups, and vice versa, a group of patients with diagnosed idiopathic pulmonary fibrosis had an increased anti-HCV positivity rate (25%) [38].

Myasthenia gravis was associated with HCV infection in case reports only, and a clear link has not been established. Cases of this disease developing during interferon treatment have been described, but it is assumed that these cases were in fact exacerbations of subclinical disease precipitated by immunomodulatory therapy.

16. Conclusion

Chronic hepatitis C infection (HCV) is a systemic disease which, besides the liver as its primary target, affects a number of other organs and organ systems. So far more than 30 different conditions have been associated with chronic HCV infection. In general, the appearance of extrahepatic manifestations of HCV infection is unpredictable, that is, independent of the stage of the liver disease. A clear association with chronic hepatitis C has been established for many of these conditions, while, for some diseases, good-quality evidence linking them to HCV infection is still missing.

Considering the appearance of new direct-acting antiviral therapies that offer an excellent prospect for cure of infected patients, although at a relatively high expense, the practice in

Croatia, as well as in many economically limited countries, is to set treatment priorities, so as to sooner treat the patients that need it most. Taking this into regard, patients with established extrahepatic manifestations of HCV infection have priority in receiving treatment, regardless of the stage of their liver disease, as stated in the latest guidelines.

For example, patients with essential mixed cryoglobulinemia and its skin (leukocytoclastic vasculitis), kidney (membranoproliferative glomerulonephritis or membranous nephropathy, renal failure), or nerve (neuropathy) manifestations, as well as patients with non-Hodgkin lymphoma, porphyria cutanea tarda, and some other more rare autoimmune disease manifestations, will benefit from treatment not only by eradicating HCV but also in treating the extrahepatic manifestation and its sometimes very debilitating symptoms.

It can be expected, and recent studies show promising results, that new therapies without interferon which greatly improve therapeutic success with fewer adverse effects will prove especially beneficial in patients with immunologically mediated extrahepatic manifestations.

Author details

Lucija Virović Jukić[1]* and Dominik Kralj[2]

*Address all correspondence to: lucija.jukic@gmail.com

1 Division of Gastroenterology and Hepatology, Department of Internal Medicine, Sestre milosrdnice University Hospital Center, University of Zagreb School of Medicine, Zagreb, Croatia

2 Division of Gastroenterology and Hepatology, Department of Internal Medicine, Sestre milosrdnice University Hospital Center, Zagreb, Croatia

References

[1] Cacoub P, Renou C, Rosenthal E, et al. Extrahepatic manifestations associated with hepatitis C virus infection. A prospective multicenter study of 321 patients. The GERMIVIC. Groupe d'Etude et de Rescherche en Medecine interne et maladies Infectieuses sur le virus de l'Hepatite C Medicine. 2000;**79**:47-56

[2] Cacoub P, Poynard T, Ghillani P, et al. Extrahepatic manifestations of chronic hepatitis C. MULTIVIRC Group. Multidepartment Virus C. Arthritis Rheum. 1999;**42**:2204-2212

[3] European Association for the Study of the Liver. EASL recommendations on treatment of hepatitis C 2016. Journal of Hepatology. 2017;**66**:153-194

[4] Ministry of Health Referral Centre for Diagnosis and Treatment of Viral Hepatitis. Hepatitis C Treatment Recommendations. Available from: www.bfm.hr/page/hepatitis-c [Accessed: Sep 8, 2017]

[5] Lunel F, Musset L, Cacoub P, et al. Cryoglobulinemia in chronic liver diseases: Role of hepatitis C virus and liver damage. Gastroenterology. 1994;**106**:1291-1300

[6] Dedania B, Wu GY. Dermatologic Extrahepatic manifestations of hepatitis C. Journal of Clinical and Translational Hepatology. 2015;**3**:127-133

[7] Gragnani L, Fognani E, Piluso A, et al. Long-term effect of HCV eradication in patients with mixed cryoglobulinemia: A prospective, controlled, open-label, cohort study. Hepatology. 2015;**61**:1145-1153

[8] Saadoun D, Thibault V, Si Ahmed SN, et al. Sofosbuvir plus ribavirin for hepatitis C virus-associated cryoglobulinaemia vasculitis: VASCUVALDIC study. Annals of the Rheumatic Diseases. 2016;**75**:1777-1782

[9] Gragnani L, Visentini M, Fognani E, et al. Prospective study of guideline-tailored therapy with direct-acting antivirals for hepatitis C virus-associated mixed cryoglobulinemia. Hepatology. 2016;**64**:1473-1482

[10] Gisbert JP, Garcia-Buey L, Pajares JM, Moreno-Otero R. Prevalence of hepatitis C virus infection in B-cell non-Hodgkin's lymphoma: Systematic review and meta-analysis. Gastroenterology. 2003;**125**:1723-1732

[11] Giordano TP, Henderson L, Landgren O, et al. Risk of non-Hodgkin lymphoma and lymphoproliferative precursor diseases in US veterans with hepatitis C virus. Journal of the American Medical Association. 2007;**297**:2010-2017

[12] Marcucci F, Mele A. Hepatitis viruses and non-Hodgkin lymphoma: Epidemiology, mechanisms of tumorigenesis, and therapeutic opportunities. Blood. 2011;**117**:1792-1798

[13] Kawamura Y, Ikeda K, Arase Y, et al. Viral elimination reduces risk of lymphoma in patients with hepatitis C. The American Journal of Medicine. 2007;**120**:1034-1041

[14] Tang L, Marcell L, Kottilil S. Systemic manifestations of hepatitis C infection. Infectious Agents and Cancer. 2016;**11**:29

[15] Cacoub P, Comarmond C, Domont F, et al. Extrahepatic manifestation of chronic hepatitis C virus infection. Therapeutic Advances in Infectious Disease. 2016;**3**:3-14

[16] KDIGO (Kidney Disease: Improving Global Outcomes). KDIGO clinical practice guidelines for the prevention, diagnosis, evaluation, and treatment of hepatitis C in chronic kidney disease. Kidney Int Suppl. 2008;**109**:1-99

[17] Gisbert JP, Garcia-Buey L, Pajares JM, Moreno-Otero R. Prevalence of hepatitis C virus infection in porphyria cutanea tarda: Systematic review and meta-analysis. Journal of Hepatology. 2003;**39**:620-627

[18] Garcovich S, Garcovich M, Capizzi R, et al. Cutaneous manifestations of hepatitis C in the era of new antiviral agents. World Journal of Hepatology. 2015;**7**:2740-2748

[19] Dedania B, Wu GY. Dermatologic extrahepatic manifestations of hepatitis C. Journal of Clinical and Translational Hepatology. 2015;**3**:127-133

[20] Gumber SC, Chopra S. Hepatitis C: A multifaceted disease. Review of extrahepatic manifestations. Annals of Internal Medicine. 1995;**123**:615-620

[21] Nagao Y, Kimura K, Kawahigashi Y, et al. Successful treatment of hepatitis C virus-associated oral lichen planus by interferon-free therapy with direct-acting antivirals. Clinical and Translational Gastroenterology. 2016;**7**:e179

[22] Wilson SE, Lee WM, Murakami C, et al. Mooren's Corneal ulcers and hepatitis C virus infection. The New England Journal of Medicine. 1993;**329**:62

[23] Antonelli A, Ferri C, Pampana A, et al. Thyroid disorders in chronic hepatitis C. The American Journal of Medicine. 2004;**117**:10-13

[24] Muratori L, Lenzi M, Ma Y, et al. Heterogeneity of liver/kidney microsomal antibody type 1 in autoimmune hepatitis and hepatitis C virus related liver disease. Gut. 1995;**37**:406-412

[25] Weissenborn K, Krause J, Bokemeyer M, et al. Hepatitis C virus affects the brain-evidence from psychometric studies and magnetic resonance spectroscopy. Journal of Hepatology. 2004;**41**:845-851

[26] Laskus T, Radkowski M, Bednarska A, et al. Detection and analysis of hepatitis C virus sequences in cerebrospinal fluid. Journal of Virology. 2002;**76**:10064-10068

[27] Morgello S, Murray J, Van Der Elst S, et al. HCV, but not HIV, is a risk factor for cerebral small vessel disease. Neurology: Neuroimmunology & NeuroInflammation. 2014;**1**:27

[28] Tsai HH, Liou HH, Muo CH, et al. Hepatitis C virus infection as a risk factor for Parkinson disease: A nationwide cohort study. Neurology. 2016;**86**:840-846

[29] Monaco S, Mariotto S, Ferrari S, et al. Hepatitis C virus-associated neurocognitive and neuropsychiatric disorders: Advances in 2015. World Journal of Gastroenterology. 2015;**21**:11974-11983

[30] Byrnes V, Miller A, Lowry D, et al. Effects of anti-viral therapy and HCV clearance on cerebral metabolism and cognition. Journal of Hepatology. 2012;**56**:549-556

[31] White DL, Ratziu V, El-Serag HB. Hepatitis C infection and risk of diabetes: A systematic review and meta-analysis. Journal of Hepatology. 2008;**49**:831-844

[32] Petit JM, Bour JB, Galland-Jos C, et al. Risk factors for diabetes mellitus and early insulin resistance in chronic hepatitis C. Journal of Hepatology. 2011;**35**:279-283

[33] Aghemo A, Prati G, Rumi M, et al. Sustained virological response prevents the development of insulin resistance in patients with chronic hepatitis C. Hepatology. 2012;**56**:1681-1687

[34] Kralj D, Virović Jukić L, Stojsavljević S, et al. Hepatitis C virus, insulin resistance, and steatosis. Journal of Clinical and Translational Hepatology. 2016;**4**:66-75

[35] Adinolfi LE, Restivo L, Zampino R, et al. Chronic HCV infection is a risk of atherosclerosis. Role of HCV and HCV-related steatosis. Atherosclerosis. 2012;**221**:496-502

[36] Fukui M, Kitagawa Y, Nakamura N, Yoshikawa T, Hepatitis C. Virus and atherosclerosis in patients with type 2 diabetes. Journal of the American Medical Association. 2003;**289**:1245-1246

[37] Domont F, Cacoub P. Chronic hepatitis C virus infection, a new cardiovascular risk factor? Liver International. 2016;**36**:621

[38] Gill K, Ghazinian H, Manch R, Gish R. Hepatitis C virus as a systemic disease: Reaching beyond the liver. Hepatology International. 2016;**10**:415-423

[39] Adinolfi LE, Zampino R, Restivo L, et al. Chronic hepatitis C virus infection and atherosclerosis: Clinical impact and mechanisms. World Journal of Gastroenterology. 2014;**20**:3410-3417

[40] Hsu YC, Ho HJ, Huang YT, et al. Association between antiviral treatment and extrahepatic outcomes in patients with hepatitis C virus infection. Gut. 2015;**64**:495-503

[41] Wong RJ, Kanwal F, Younossi ZM, et al. Hepatitis C virus infection and coronary artery disease risk: A systematic review of the literature. Digestive Diseases and Sciences. 2014;**59**:1586-1593

Chapter 10

Hepatitis C–Associated Diabetes Mellitus

Ines Bilić-Ćurčić, Hrvoje Roguljić, Marul Ivandić, Aleksandar Včev, Robert Smolić and Martina Smolić

Additional information is available at the end of the chapter

http://dx.doi.org/10.5772/intechopen.70721

Abstract

Diabetes type 2 mellitus (T2DM) is the most common extrahepatic association of hepatitis C virus (HCV) infection. Substantial research has suggested that insulin resistance (IR) has crucial importance in development of type 2 diabetes in HCV-infected patients. Several pathophysiological mechanisms are proposed, such as direct effect of HCV proteins on inhibition of the insulin-signaling pathway inducing central insulin resistance (IR), while overproduction of inflammatory cytokines and increased lipolysis promote peripheral IR. IR in HCV-infected patients is associated with impaired sustained virologic response (SVR) and higher incidence of hepatocellular carcinoma (HCC). Some, but not all, studies have shown improvements in achieving SVR in patients with interferon/ribavirin (RBV) therapy co-treated with metformin or pioglitazone as well as beneficiary effect on the incidence of hepatocellular carcinoma. Recent studies indicate that response to the new direct-acting antiviral (DAA) treatments is unaffected by insulin resistance thus diminishing importance of IR in the new era of DAA. Additionally, viral eradication by DAAs has been shown to ameliorate insulin resistance, attenuating the risk of new-onset diabetes type 2. However, those metabolic improvements are sustainable long after the treatment remains unclear.

Keywords: hepatitis C infection, diabetes type 2, insulin resistance, insulin signaling, antiviral agents, antidiabetic agents

1. Introduction

Diabetes is a group of metabolic diseases characterized by hyperglycemia, which in vast majority of cases fall into two broad etiopathogenetic categories: type 1 (T1DM) and type 2 diabetes mellitus (T2DM) [1, 2]. Frequency of type 1 is relatively low in comparison with type 2, which accounts for over 90% of cases globally [3]. For development of type 2 diabetes mellitus, several pathophysiologic mechanisms are responsible such as insulin resistance

(IR), impairment of insulin secretion, and increased hepatic glucose production [4]. Chronic and uncontrolled diabetes results in serious comorbidities such as retinopathy, neuropathy, nephropathy, and cardiovascular diseases a leading cause of mortality [5].

So far, numerous studies indicate that diabetes mellitus could be the most common extrahepatic manifestation of chronic hepatitis C virus (HCV) [6]. A meta-analysis of 34 studies confirmed a positive correlation between HCV infection and increased prevalence of diabetes mellitus type 2 in comparison with general population [7]. Additionally, many epidemiological studies indicate that HCV-infected patients have higher prevalence of diabetes in comparison with hepatitis B virus (HBV)-infected patients [8].

2. Diabetes type 2 and chronic hepatitis C infection

Although HCV infection is primarily affecting liver, there are other well-known extrahepatic manifestations of chronic hepatitis C [9, 10]. Mechanisms of those disorders are related to extrahepatic tropism of the HCV or by immunological process in which chronic infection leads to the development of autoimmune-mediated disease [11].

Since the discovery of HCV in 1989, great attention is paid to the development of type 2 diabetes mellitus during chronic hepatitis C virus infection [12]. Already in 1994, Allison et al. showed that 50% of HCV-related cirrhosis have diabetes mellitus compared to 9% with cirrhosis related to other causes [13]. For a long time, a loss of liver endocrine function due to progression of fibrosis in chronic hepatitis was considered to be responsible for the development of insulin resistance [14]. To examine the effect of HCV infection without concomitant cirrhosis on development of diabetes mellitus, Knobler et al. performed an oral glucose tolerance test in patients with chronic hepatitis B and C without cirrhosis [15]. Study showed that 33% of HCV patients had type 2 diabetes, whereas only 12% of patients with chronic hepatitis B (HBV) infection and 6% of healthy volunteers had glucose metabolism impairment, indicating that diabetes occurs in the early stages of the HCV-induced liver disease. Also, liver biopsies from HCV-infected patients with diabetes had significantly higher fibrosis grade, inflammatory activity, and steatosis compared to HCV patients without diabetes.

The correlation between genotype of HCV and the level of insulin resistance has also been recognized. In a study of Hui, significantly lower insulin resistance index (HOMA-IR) was registered in patients with genotype 3 HCV in comparison with other genotypes [16]. Another study showed significantly higher median HOMA-IR in patients with hepatic steatosis infected with genotype 1 HCV than in patients with genotype 3 [17]. On the other hand, patients with genotype 3 had a higher probability of having moderate-to-severe steatosis, compared to those with non-3 genotypes [18]. Moreover, in type 1 genotype fatty liver disease occurred if there are other risk factors present at time like diabetes, adiposity, and insulin resistance implicating specific viral sequences responsible for fat accumulation independently of other risk factors. To clarify, there are two distinct disorders, viral, and metabolic steatosis [19]. This is important since whatever the mechanism, viral steatosis does not seem to impact liver fibrosis progression rate, although HCV genotype 3 is independently associated with increased fibrosis progression. Also, viral steatosis does not impair response to interferon-a (IFN-a). Alternatively, steatosis due to the metabolic syndrome and IR is associated with both accelerated fibrosis progression and poor response to IFN-a-based therapy.

2.1. Hepatitis C–induced insulin resistance

Substantial research has suggested that insulin resistance has crucial importance in development of type 2 diabetes in HCV-infected patients [17]. A study of Hui et al. showed higher levels of insulin, C peptide, and HOMA-IR in 121 hepatitis C virus patients with stage 0 or 1 hepatic fibrosis compared with healthy controls proposing that HCV may induce IR irrespective to stage of liver fibrosis [16], although higher levels of liver fibrosis were associated with increased stage of insulin resistance. These findings were confirmed with other studies, and dependence of insulin resistance is determined with severity of liver fibrosis [6].

HCV-infected patients also develop insulin resistance in hepatic and peripheral tissues while pathogenetic mechanism is not clear [20]. Although HCV is hepatotropic virus, its genome has been detected in numerous extrahepatic tissues including pancreatic acinar cells and epithelial cells of pancreatic duct [21, 22]. Several studies demonstrated direct effect of the HCV proteins on inhibition of the insulin-signaling pathway. Key mediators of insulin-signaling cascade are insulin receptor substrate (IRS) 1 and 2. Disruption of IRS1 results in insulin resistance, while for development of diabetes mellitus, disruption of IRS2 is needed [23, 24]. In HCV, core-transgenic mice as well core-transfected human hepatoma cells downregulation of IRS1 and IRS2 were observed [25]. A proposed mechanism was that HCV core protein induced upregulation of suppressor of cytokine signaling (SOCS) 3 resulting in proteasomal degradation of IRS1 and IRS2 through ubiquitination. Furthermore, Alberstein et al. reported several impairments in the insulin-signaling cascade linked to a proteasome degradation of IRS1 protein in cell lines transfected with HCV core protein [26]. HCV infection increased gluconeogenesis by promoting the expression of gluconeogenic genes, such as glucose 6 phosphatase (G6P) and phosphoenolpyruvate carboxyl kinase 2 (PCK2), which had adverse effect on insulin resistance [19]. On the other hand, HCV downregulated the expression of glucose transporter GLUT 4, which resulted in decreased glucose uptake and increased level of glucose in plasma leading to impairment of glucose metabolism [27].

Also, HCV core protein of genotype 3 downregulated peroxisome proliferator activating receptor (PPARγ) and upregulated SOCS 7 [28]. Beside its effect on insulin-signaling cascade, it is suggested that HCV has the ability to cause dysfunctions of cell organelles such as mitochondria and endoplasmatic reticulum which leads to further impairment of insulin-signaling pathway [29].

In studies where euglycemic insulin clamp was used, insulin resistance was determined mainly in peripheral tissues such as skeletal muscle rather than in liver [30]. Clearly, the effect of cytokines was necessary for the development of peripheral insulin resistance due to the tropism of HCV for hepatic tissue. Several studies emphasized the role of the overproduced tumor necrosis factor alpha (TNF-α) in HCV-induced insulin resistance [31–33]. Inhibitory role of TNF-α is achieved through activation of serine/threonine kinases, which resulted in uncoupling of insulin receptor substrate protein from downstream effectors [34]. Furthermore, the importance of the TNF-α in HCV-induced IR was confirmed by the study of Shintani et al., which used transgenic mice with characteristic expression of HCV core protein in the liver. Insulin resistance and impaired glucose metabolism were observed in this transgenic model, while administration of an antitumor necrosis factor-alpha antibody restored insulin sensitivity [35]. TNFα-induced insulin resistance was also achieved through indirect mechanisms such as increased lipolysis resulting in regulation of expression of several adipocyte genes that modulate insulin sensitivity [36]. Dysfunction of lipid metabolism triggers lipotoxicity through increased production of free fatty acids, which promotes insulin resistance [37]. Along TNF-α, it is proposed that some other cytokines such as IL-6 and numerous adipokines have a role in pathogenesis of HCV-induced IR as well in steatosis of nonalcoholic fatty liver disease [38, 39]. Possible pathophysiological mechanisms of HCV-induced IR are shown in **Figure 1**.

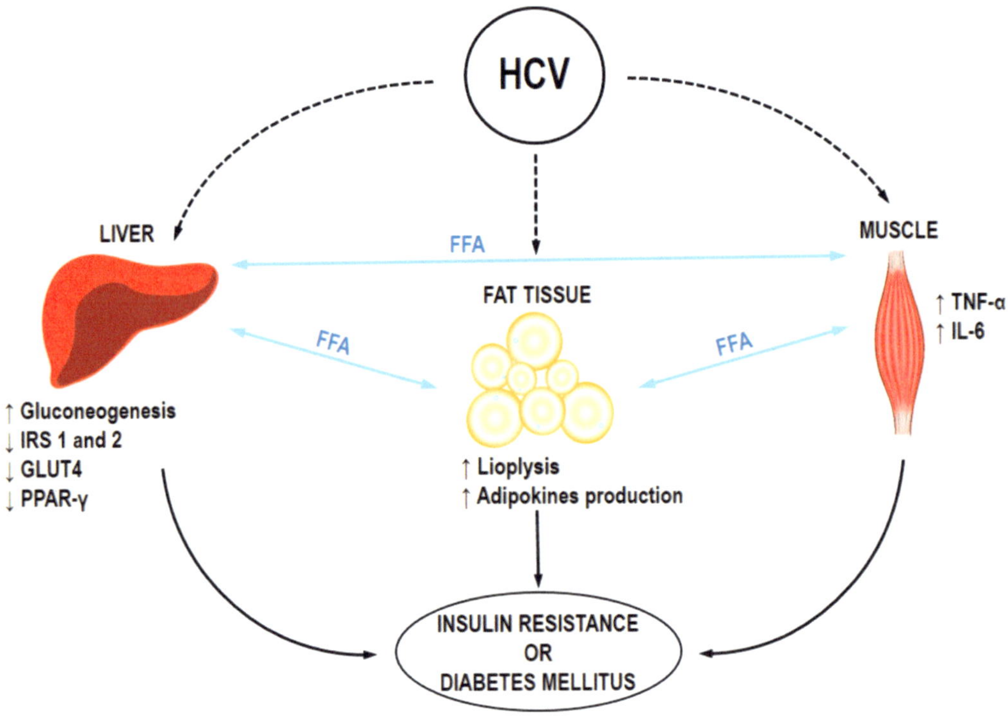

Figure 1. Proposed mechanisms involved in pathogenesis of HCV-induced insulin resistance and diabetes type 2.

3. Treatment of insulin resistance and diabetes with the eradication of viral infection

If HCV is one of the causal factors of insulin resistance, then clearance of viremia might be a way to reduce IR [40]. Additionally, viral eradication has been shown to ameliorate insulin resistance, attenuating the risk of new-onset T2DM [41].

Several observational studies indicated that eradication of HCV with interferon (IFN) and ribavirin (RBV) is associated with improved insulin sensitivity [42–44]. There are case reports that describe improvements in glycemic control with both IFN/RBV and IFN/RBV/telaprevir treatment. However, those improvements were observed only during the treatment phase, with the recurrence of diabetes when antiviral therapy ended [45, 46]. Case report by Doyle et al. was first to demonstrate complete remission of diabetes with viral clearance beyond the treatment phase, which may be due to the differences in antiviral treatment response [47]. In addition, several studies reported decreasing number of patients with IR treated with interferon IFN/RBV therapies after achievement of sustained virologic response (SVR) [40, 48–50]. Viral clearance is the most possible mechanism through which antiviral therapy ameliorates IR rather than a direct pharmacological effect of IFN/RBV.

A few studies [42, 43, 50] reported reduced incidence of T2DM among patients who achieved SVR. Although T2DM occurrence is associated with a genetic predisposition, it is also influenced by lifestyle-related aspects. For instance, one study showed that viral eradication induced a two-third reduction in the risk of T2DM incidence, but the authors did not report data regarding family history, smoking habit, and physical activity [42]. Reduced incidence of IR and T2DM in chronic hepatitis C (CHC) patients who achieved SVR after therapy, most likely depended on the genetic, demographic, clinical, histological, and lifestyle characteristics of the patients. For this reason, counseling on diet and physical activity should not be excluded by the eradication of HCV in patients with predisposing factors for T2DM.

The clinical impact of successful antiviral therapy on the long-term outcome of T2DM in diabetics with CHC is still unknown, mainly because of the lack in proper prospective studies although data from population-based research in Taiwan reported improved renal and cardiovascular outcomes in diabetic patients treated with antiviral HCV treatment [41].

High therapeutic efficacy of direct-acting antivirals (DAAs) will ensure viral eradication in a large number of diabetic cirrhotic patients, which will enable better understanding of the impact of the virus on T2DM outcome. One retrospective study reported a significant decrease in glycated hemoglobin (HbA1C) 6 months after HCV eradication with sofosbuvir, although the mechanism responsible for this improvement remains unknown [51]. In addition, other studies demonstrated the efficacy of DAAs (telaprevir and danoprevir) in improving IR and even restoring insulin sensitivity after achieving SVR, but only in genotype 1 patients [52, 53]. However, data for DAA effect on insulin resistance in other genotype HCV infected patients are lacking thus future studies are needed to conclude whether this effect is achievable in all genotypes.

4. Influence of insulin resistance and diabetes mellitus in treatment of hepatitis C infection

Since patients with chronic hepatitis C infection are twofold to threefold more likely to develop type 2 diabetes, which reduces their chances of achieving a sustained virologic response, the question is can we achieve better SVR by reducing insulin resistance. A meta-analysis of 17 studies has shown that insulin sensitivity was associated with a higher rate of SVR in comparison with insulin resistance. Elevated HOMA-IR was associated with a lower cure rate of patients with hepatitis C treated with Peg-IFN-α/ribavirin irrespective of genotype, and the more difficult-to-treat cohort, the better the HOMA-IR prediction [54]. In addition, IR was associated with a higher incidence of hepatocellular carcinoma (HCC) in patients with hepatitis C virus [55], thus improving IR and correcting hyperinsulinemia may improve the prognosis of HCV cirrhosis.

Therapy for the T2DM in patients with liver diseases is generally the same as that without liver disease. Only patients with evidence of liver cirrhosis have altered drug metabolism, and there is no evidence that patients with liver disease are predisposed to hepatotoxicity [56].

4.1. Biguanides

Metformin is considered as the drug of choice in HCV patients with IR or T2DM since it generally does not cause hepatotoxicity [57], although there are sporadic case reports of metformin induced acute liver injury [58]. Some, but not all studies, have shown improvements in achieving SVR in patients with interferon/ribavirin therapy co-treated with metformin

	Study population/design	Treatment	Outcome	Results
Yu et al. [59]	98 genotype 1 CHC patients with IR/ Prospective study	Metformin 500 TID vs. placebo	SVR	59.2 vs. 38.8% (p = 0.43)
Romero-Gomez et al. [60]	123 genotype 1 CHC with IR/ Prospective study	Metformin 850 mg TID vs. placebo	SVR	53 vs. 42%, p = NS
Sharifi et al. [61]	140 CHC patients/Prospective study	Metformin 500 mg TID vs. Placebo	SVR	75 vs. 79%, p = NS
Nkontchou et al. [62]	100 diabetic patients with HCV cirrhosis/Prospective study	Metformin, dose varied vs. therapy without metformin	Incidence of HCC	9.5 vs. 31.2% (p = .001)
Lee et al. [63]	800,000 health insurance beneficiaries/Prospective study	Metformin vs. no metformin in diabetic patients	HCC, colorectal, pancreatic cancer incidence	Reduced incidence to almost non-diabetic levels (HR, 0.12), p = significant
Chen et al. [64]	53 diabetic and 82 nondiabetic patients with HCC undergoing RFA/ Retrospective study	Metformin in diabetic patients (varied dose) vs. therapy without metformin	Survival probability	1 year, 95 vs. 74.5% 5 years, 60.5 vs. 26.2%
Donadon et al. [65]	465 HCC, 618 liver cirrhosis, 490 control patients/Retrospective study	Metformin in diabetic control and LC patients vs. SU and insulin	Risk of HCC	>80% risk reduction, p = significant

Table 1. Summary of trials evaluating metformin use in patients with chronic HCV and T2DM or IR.

[59–61] (**Table 1**). Increasing evidence points out that metformin is independently associated with reduced risk for HCC and liver-related death/transplantation [62–65] (**Table 1**). Metformin is frequently discontinued once cirrhosis is diagnosed because of concerns about an increased risk of adverse effects in patients with liver impairment. However, the study from Zhang et al. on 250 diabetic patients who developed cirrhosis showed that patients who continued metformin had a significantly longer median survival than those who discontinued metformin. In other words, metformin was found to be an independent predictor of better survival [66]. It is reasonable to conclude that metformin should remain a first-line option for patients with T2DM and chronic compensated HCV; however, more prospective, randomized controlled trials are needed to confirm safety and efficacy of metformin.

4.2. Thiazolidinediones

Thiazolidinediones (TZDs) are the only real insulin sensitizers available as they act primarily through stimulation peroxisome proliferator-activated receptor PPAR-Y decreasing insulin resistance in the liver and peripheral tissues. However, only few studies showed that pioglitazone improved virologic response to peginterferon alpha-2b/ribavirin combination therapy in overweight hepatitis C genotype 4 patients, while there was no effect in other genotypes [67–70] (**Table 2**). Also, recent data suggested that pioglitazone could decrease a risk of HCC recurrence in the group of patients with a BMI ≥24 [71] (**Table 2**).

	Study population/design	Treatment	Outcome	Results
Khattab et al. [68]	Ninety-seven previously untreated patients with CHC and IR/Prospective study	Pioglitazone vs. no pioglitazone + standard care PegIFN/RBV	SVR	SVR was significantly higher with pioglitazone (p = 0.04)
Harrison et al. [69]	150 treatment-naive HCV genotype 1 patients/Prospective study	Pioglitazone vs. no pioglitazone + standard care PegIFN/RBV	SVR	No significant difference between groups
Marks et al. [70]	19 previous non responders to PegIFN-RBV/Pilot study	Pioglitazone vs. no pioglitazone during 24 week before PegIFN/RBV/PIO	SVR	15% achieved SVR, no significant difference
Sumie et al. [71]	85 HCV-infected HCC patients/Prospective study	Pioglitazone vs. no pioglitazone in therapy	Recurrence-free survival	No significant difference, except in a group with BMI >24 kg/m2

Table 2. Summary of trials evaluating pioglitazone use in patients with chronic HCV and T2DM or IR.

TZD use is not recommended in advanced liver cirrhosis because of the reported cases of acute cholestatic hepatitis [72]. Current recommendation is that serum ALT levels are evaluated before the initiation of rosiglitazone and pioglitazone therapy and that therapy should not be initiated if there is evidence of active liver disease.

4.3. Incretin mimetics

Incretins are gut-derived hormones, mainly glucagon-like peptide 1 (GLP-1) and glucose-dependent insulinotropic peptide (GIP), that are secreted at low basal levels in the fasting state. Circulating levels increase rapidly and transiently following food ingestion. GLP-1R agonists control blood glucose through regulation of islet function, principally through activation of insulin-secreting beta cell in pancreas, and inhibition of glucagon secretion. In short term, it enhances glucose-induced insulin secretion, but continuous GLP-1 receptor activation also increases insulin synthesis, and beta cell proliferation and neogenesis. Dipeptidyl peptidase (DPP)-4 inactivates incretin hormones including GLP-1. Therefore, GLP-1 agonists as well as (DPP)-4 inhibitors are used as antidiabetic agents [73, 74].

Itou et al. found decreased serum GLP-1 levels and increased DPP-4 expression in the ileum, liver, and serum in HCV patients compared to control group and HBV group, thus concluding that altered expression of GLP-1 may play a role in the development of HCV-associated glucose intolerance [75]. Recent studies on GLP-1 have shown slowing of the progression of non-acoholic fatty liver disease (NAFLD) by direct effects on lipid metabolism in hepatocytes, and on inflammation in the liver [76]. A case–control study reported a reduction in HbA1C without side effects when treating HCV patients with DPP-4 inhibitors [77]. Nevertheless, further larger studies are needed to support the use of incretin mimetics in patients with advanced hepatic diseases.

4.3.1. Insulin

Insulin has been considered as the drug of choice in patients with diabetes and decompensated liver disease due to short half-life. However, one study in Japan found that exogenous insulin and a second-generation sulfonylurea were associated with a higher incidence of HCC in hepatitis C patients [78], whereas other studies showed reduced risk of HCC with the use of metformin, compared with SUs and insulin [79]. One meta-analysis of observational studies summarized the impact of antidiabetic medication on the risk of HCC: insulin and sulfonylurea (SU) increased the risk, metformin reduced it, and TDZs did not change it [80]. Insulin requirements may vary because patients with decompensated liver disease can have decreased requirements due to reduced capacity for gluconeogenesis or an increased need for insulin due to insulin resistance. Thus, there is need for careful glucose monitoring and frequent dose adjustments of insulin.

In conclusion, traditionally medications used to overcome IR are metformin and thiazolidinediones, but their effect on SVR and incidence of HCC remains an open question. However, new promising agents such as GLP-1 receptor agonists could further improve outcome and prognosis of HCV-infected patients with metabolic disturbances.

5. Conclusion

Without a doubt, IR in HCV-infected patients is associated with impaired SVR and higher incidence of hepatocellular carcinoma as well as higher incidence of diabetes type 2 accompanied

http://dx.doi.org/10.5772/intechopen.70721

by other metabolic disturbances. Evidence of beneficiary effect of metformin or pioglitazone co-treatment in patients with interferon/ribavirin therapy on achieving SVR or incidence of HCC in HCV patients are scarce and ambiguous, leaving more room for questions than offering potential solutions. However, recently published research suggests that response to the new direct-acting antiviral treatments is not dependent on insulin resistance thus diminishing importance of IR in the new era of DAA. Furthermore, if we postulate that HCV induces insulin resistance than achieving SVR could ameliorate it. Evidence supporting this hypothesis was recently published showing that insulin resistance disappeared after viral eradication by DAAs consequently decreasing a risk of diabetes type 2. In conclusion, further studies are needed to constitute how HCV induces insulin resistance, what effects different HCV therapies have on improving glycemic outcomes, and whether those metabolic improvements are permanent and still present after the treatment.

Author details

Ines Bilić-Ćurčić[1,2]*, Hrvoje Roguljić[1,2], Marul Ivandić[2], Aleksandar Včev[2,3], Robert Smolić[1,2] and Martina Smolić[1]

*Address all correspondence to: ibcurcic@mefos.hr

1 Department of Pharmacology, Faculty of Medicine, Josip Juraj Strossmayer University of Osijek, Osijek, Croatia

2 Clinic for Internal Medicine, University Hospital Center Osijek, Osijek, Croatia

3 Department of Internal Medicine, Faculty of Medicine, Josip Juraj Strossmayer University of Osijek, Osijek, Croatia

References

[1] Balakumar P, Maung-U K, Jagadeesh G. Prevalence and prevention of cardiovascular disease and diabetes mellitus. Pharmacological Research. 2016;**113**(Pt A):600-609

[2] Alberti KG, Zimmet PZ. Definition, diagnosis and classification of diabetes mellitus and its complications. Part 1: Diagnosis and classification of diabetes mellitus provisional report of a WHO consultation. Diabetic Medicine. 1998;**15**(7):539-553

[3] Zimmet P, Alberti KG, Shaw J. Global and societal implications of the diabetes epidemic. Nature. 2001;**414**(6865):782-787

[4] Defronzo RA. Banting Lecture. From the triumvirate to the ominous octet: A new paradigm for the treatment of type 2 diabetes mellitus. Diabetes. 2009;**58**(4):773-795

[5] Girach A, Manner D, Porta M. Diabetic microvascular complications: Can patients at risk be identified? A review. International Journal of Clinical Practice. 2006;**60**(11):1471-1483

[6] Knobler H, Malnick S. Hepatitis C and insulin action: An intimate relationship. World Journal of Hepatology. 2016;**8**(2):131-138

[7] White DL, Ratziu V, El-Serag HB. Hepatitis C infection and risk of diabetes: A systematic review and meta-analysis. Journal of Hepatology. 2008;**49**(5):831-844

[8] Bose SK, Ray R. Hepatitis C virus infection and insulin resistance. World Journal of Diabetes. 2014;**5**(1):52-58

[9] Cheng Z, Zhou B, Shi X, Zhang Y, Zhang L, Chen L, et al. Extrahepatic manifestations of chronic hepatitis C virus infection: 297 Cases from a tertiary medical center in Beijing, China. Chinese Medical Journal . 2014;**127**(7):1206-1210

[10] Tang L, Marcell L, Kottilil S. Systemic manifestations of hepatitis C infection. Infectious Agents and Cancer. 2016;**11**:29

[11] Gill K, Ghazinian H, Manch R, Gish R. Hepatitis C virus as a systemic disease: Reaching beyond the liver. Hepatology International. 2016;**10**(3):415-423

[12] Antonelli A, Ferrari SM, Giuggioli D, Di Domenicantonio A, Ruffilli I, Corrado A, et al. Hepatitis C virus infection and type 1 and type 2 diabetes mellitus. World Journal of Diabetes. 2014;**5**(5):586-600

[13] Allison ME, Wreghitt T, Palmer CR, Alexander GJ. Evidence for a link between hepatitis C virus infection and diabetes mellitus in a cirrhotic population. Journal of Hepatology. 1994;**21**(6):1135-1139

[14] Romero-Gómez M. Insulin resistance and hepatitis C. World Journal of Gastroenterology. 2006;**12**(44):7075-7080

[15] Knobler H, Schihmanter R, Zifroni A, Fenakel G, Schattner A. Increased risk of type 2 diabetes in noncirrhotic patients with chronic hepatitis C virus infection. Mayo Clinic Proceedings. 2000;**75**(4):355-359

[16] Hui JM, Sud A, Farrell GC, Bandara P, Byth K, Kench JG, et al. Insulin resistance is associated with chronic hepatitis C virus infection and fibrosis progression [corrected]. Gastroenterology. 2003;**125**(6):1695-1704

[17] Fartoux L, Poujol-Robert A, Guéchot J, Wendum D, Poupon R, Serfaty L. Insulin resistance is a cause of steatosis and fibrosis progression in chronic hepatitis C. Gut. 2005;**54**(7):1003-1008

[18] Rubbia-Brandt L, Fabris P, Paganin S, Leandro G, Male PJ, Giostra E, et al. Steatosis affects chronic hepatitis C progression in a genotype specific way. Gut. 2004;**53**(3):406-412

[19] Negro F. Facts and fictions of HCV and comorbidities: Steatosis, diabetes mellitus, and cardiovascular diseases. Journal of Hepatology. 2014 November;**61**(1 Suppl):S69-S78

[20] Kawaguchi Y, Mizuta T. Interaction between hepatitis C virus and metabolic factors. World Journal of Gastroenterology. 2014;**20**(11):2888-2901

[21] Gowans EJ, Jones KL, Bharadwaj M, Jackson DC. Prospects for dendritic cell vaccination in persistent infection with hepatitis C virus. Journal of Clinical Virology. 2004;**30**(4):283-290

[22] Masini M, Campani D, Boggi U, Menicagli M, Funel N, Pollera M, et al. Hepatitis C virus infection and human pancreatic beta-cell dysfunction. Diabetes Care. 2005;**28**(4):940-941

[23] Tamemoto H, Kadowaki T, Tobe K, Yagi T, Sakura H, Hayakawa T, et al. Insulin resistance and growth retardation in mice lacking insulin receptor substrate-1. Nature. 1994;**372**(6502):182-186

[24] Withers DJ, Gutierrez JS, Towery H, Burks DJ, Ren JM, Previs S, et al. Disruption of IRS-2 causes type 2 diabetes in mice. Nature. 1998;**391**(6670):900-904

[25] Kawaguchi T, Yoshida T, Harada M, Hisamoto T, Nagao Y, Ide T, et al. Hepatitis C virus down-regulates insulin receptor substrates 1 and 2 through up-regulation of suppressor of cytokine signaling 3. American Journal of Pathology. 2004;**165**(5):1499-1508

[26] Alberstein M, Zornitzki T, Zick Y, Knobler H. Hepatitis C core protein impairs insulin downstream signalling and regulatory role of IGFBP-1 expression. Journal of Viral Hepatitis. 2012;**19**(1):65-71

[27] Bose SK, Shrivastava S, Meyer K, Ray RB, Ray R. Hepatitis C virus activates the mTOR/S6K1 signaling pathway in inhibiting IRS-1 function for insulin resistance. Journal of Virology. 2012;**86**(11):6315-6322

[28] Bugianesi E, Salamone F, Negro F. The interaction of metabolic factors with HCV infection: Does it matter? Journal of Hepatology. 2012;**56**(Suppl 1):S56-S65

[29] Kralj D, Virović Jukić L, Stojsavljević S, Duvnjak M, Smolić M, Čurčić IB. Hepatitis C virus, insulin resistance, and steatosis. Journal of Clinical and Translational Hepatology. 2016;**4**(1):66-75

[30] Milner KL, van der Poorten D, Trenell M, Jenkins AB, Xu A, Smythe G, et al. Chronic hepatitis C is associated with peripheral rather than hepatic insulin resistance. Gastroenterology. 2010;**138**(3):932-941.e1-3

[31] Nelson DR, Lim HL, Marousis CG, Fang JW, Davis GL, Shen L, et al. Activation of tumor necrosis factor-alpha system in chronic hepatitis C virus infection. Digestive Diseases and Sciences. 1997;**42**(12):2487-2494

[32] Hotamisligil GS. The role of TNFalpha and TNF receptors in obesity and insulin resistance. Journal of Internal Medicine. 1999;**245**(6):621-625

[33] Zylberberg H, Rimaniol AC, Pol S, Masson A, De Groote D, Berthelot P, et al. Soluble tumor necrosis factor receptors in chronic hepatitis C: A correlation with histological fibrosis and activity. Journal of Hepatology. 1999;**30**(2):185-191

[34] Zick Y. Uncoupling insulin signalling by serine/threonine phosphorylation: A molecular basis for insulin resistance. Biochemical Society Transactions. 2004;**32**(Pt 5):812-816

[35] Shintani Y, Fujie H, Miyoshi H, Tsutsumi T, Tsukamoto K, Kimura S, et al. Hepatitis C virus infection and diabetes: Direct involvement of the virus in the development of insulin resistance. Gastroenterology. 2004;**126**(3):840-848

[36] Ruan H, Hacohen N, Golub TR, Van Parijs L, Lodish HF. Tumor necrosis factor-alpha suppresses adipocyte-specific genes and activates expression of preadipocyte genes in 3T3-L1 adipocytes: Nuclear factor-kappaB activation by TNF-alpha is obligatory. Diabetes. 2002;**51**(5):1319-1336

[37] Unger RH, Orci L. Lipotoxic diseases of nonadipose tissues in obesity. International Journal of Obesity and Related Metabolic Disorders. 2000;**24**(Suppl 4):S28-S32

[38] Cua IH, Hui JM, Bandara P, Kench JG, Farrell GC, McCaughan GW, et al. Insulin resistance and liver injury in hepatitis C is not associated with virus-specific changes in adipocytokines. Hepatology. 2007;**46**(1):66-73

[39] Stojsavljević S, Gomerčić Palčić M, Virović Jukić L, Smirčić Duvnjak L, Duvnjak M. Adipokines and proinflammatory cytokines, the key mediators in the pathogenesis of nonalcoholic fatty liver disease. World Journal of Gastroenterology. 2014;**20**(48): 18070-18091

[40] Delgado-Borrego A, Jordan SH, Negre B, Healey D, Lin W, Kamegaya Y, et al. Reduction of insulin resistance with effective clearance of hepatitis C infection: Results from the HALT-C trial. Clinical Gastroenterology and Hepatology. 2010;**8**(5):458-462

[41] Hsu YC, Lin JT, Ho HJ, Kao YH, Huang YT, Hsiao NW, et al. Antiviral treatment for hepatitis C virus infection is associated with improved renal and cardiovascular outcomes in diabetic patients. Hepatology. 2014;**59**(4):1293-1302

[42] Arase Y, Suzuki F, Suzuki Y, Akuta N, Kobayashi M, Kawamura Y, et al. Sustained virological response reduces incidence of onset of type 2 diabetes in chronic hepatitis C. Hepatology. 2009;**49**(3):739-744

[43] Simó R, Lecube A, Genescà J, Esteban JI, Hernández C. Sustained virological response correlates with reduction in the incidence of glucose abnormalities in patients with chronic hepatitis C virus infection. Diabetes Care. 2006;**29**(11):2462-2466

[44] Thompson AJ, Patel K, Chuang WL, Lawitz EJ, Rodriguez-Torres M, Rustgi VK, et al. Viral clearance is associated with improved insulin resistance in genotype 1 chronic hepatitis C but not genotype 2/3. Gut. 2012;**61**(1):128-134

[45] Tahrani A, Bowler L, Singh P, Coates P. Resolution of diabetes in type 2 diabetic patient treated with IFN-alpha and ribavirin for hepatitis C. European Journal of Gastroenterology and Hepatology. 2006;**18**(3):291-293

[46] Tallón de Lara P, Himschoot T, Frossard JL, Negro F. Does telaprevir possess a direct antidiabetic effect? Liver International. 2014;**34**(6):967-969

[47] Doyle MA, Cooper C. Successful hepatitis C antiviral therapy induces remission of type 2 diabetes: A case report. The American Journal of Case Reports. 2015;**16**:745-750

[48] Kawaguchi T, Ide T, Taniguchi E, Hirano E, Itou M, Sumie S, et al. Clearance of HCV improves insulin resistance, beta-cell function, and hepatic expression of insulin receptor substrate 1 and 2. American Journal of Gastroenterology. 2007;**102**(3):570-576

[49] Kawaguchi Y, Mizuta T, Oza N, Takahashi H, Ario K, Yoshimura T, et al. Eradication of hepatitis C virus by interferon improves whole-body insulin resistance and hyperinsulinaemia in patients with chronic hepatitis C. Liver International. 2009;**29**(6):871-877

[50] Romero-Gómez M, Fernández-Rodríguez CM, Andrade RJ, Diago M, Alonso S, Planas R, et al. Effect of sustained virological response to treatment on the incidence of abnormal glucose values in chronic hepatitis C. Journal of Hepatology. 2008;**48**(5):721-727

[51] Morales AL, Junga Z, Singla MB, Sjogren M, Torres D. Hepatitis C eradication with sofosbuvir leads to significant metabolic changes. World Journal of Hepatology. 2016;**8**(35):1557-1563

[52] Moucari R, Forestier N, Larrey D, Guyader D, Couzigou P, Benhamou Y, Voitot H, Vidaud M, Seiwert S, Bradford B, Zeuzem S, Marcellin P. Danoprevir, an HCV NS3/4A protease inhibitor, improves insulin sensitivity in patients with genotype 1 chronic hepatitis C. Gut. 2010;**59**(12):1694-1698

[53] Serfaty L, Forns X, Goeser T, Ferenci P, Nevens F, Carosi G, Drenth JP, Lonjon-Domanec I, DeMasi R, Picchio G, Beumont M, Marcellin P. Insulin resistance and response to telaprevir plus peginterferon α and ribavirin in treatment-naive patients infected with HCV genotype 1. Gut. 2012 October;**61**(10):1473-1480

[54] Eslam M, Aparcero R, Kawaguchi T, Del Campo JA, Sata M, Khattab MA, Romero-Gomez M. Meta-analysis: Insulin resistance and sustained virological response in hepatitis C. Alimentary Pharmacology and Therapeutics. 2011 August;**34**(3):297-305

[55] Khattab MA, Eslam M, Mousa YI, Ela-adawy N, Fathy S, Shatat M, Abd-Aalhalim H, Kamal A, Sharawe MA. Association between metabolic abnormalities and hepatitis C-related hepatocellular carcinoma. Annals of Hepatology. 2012 July-August;**11**(4):487-494

[56] Tolman KG, Fonseca V, Dalpiaz A, Tan MH. Spectrum of liver disease in type 2 diabetes and management of patients with diabetes and liver disease. Diabetes Care. 2007;**30**(3):734-743

[57] Hammerstad SS, Grock SF, Lee HJ, Hasham A, Sundaram N, Tomer Y. Diabetes and hepatitis C: A two-way association. Front Endocrinol (Lausanne). 2015;**6**:134

[58] Miralles-Linares F, Puerta-Fernandez S, Bernal-Lopez MR, Tinahones FJ, Andrade RJ, Gomez-Huelgas R. Metformin-induced hepatotoxicity. Diabetes Care. 2012;**35**(3):e21

[59] Yu JW, Sun LJ, Zhao YH, Kang P, Yan BZ. The effect of metformin on the efficacy of antiviral therapy in patients with genotype 1 chronic hepatitis C and insulin resistance. International Journal of Infectious Diseases. 2012;**16**(6):e436-e441

[60] Romero-Gómez M, Diago M, Andrade RJ, Calleja JL, Salmerón J, Fernández-Rodríguez CM, et al. Treatment of insulin resistance with metformin in naïve genotype 1 chronic hepatitis C patients receiving peginterferon alfa-2a plus ribavirin. Hepatology. 2009;**50**(6):1702-1708

[61] Sharifi AH, Mohammadi M, Fakharzadeh E, Zamini H, Zaer-Rezaee H, Jabbari H, et al. Efficacy of adding metformin to pegylated interferon and ribavirin in treatment naïve patients with chronic hepatitis C: A randomized double-blind controlled trial. Middle East Journal of Digestive Diseases. 2014;**6**(1):13-17

[62] Nkontchou G, Cosson E, Aout M, Mahmoudi A, Bourcier V, Charif I, et al. Impact of metformin on the prognosis of cirrhosis induced by viral hepatitis C in diabetic patients. Journal of Clinical Endocrinology & Metabolism. 2011;**96**(8):2601-2608

[63] Lee MS, Hsu CC, Wahlqvist ML, Tsai HN, Chang YH, Huang YC. Type 2 diabetes increases and metformin reduces total, colorectal, liver and pancreatic cancer incidences in Taiwanese: A representative population prospective cohort study of 800,000 individuals. BMC Cancer. 2011;**11**:20

[64] Chen TM, Lin CC, Huang PT, Wen CF. Metformin associated with lower mortality in diabetic patients with early stage hepatocellular carcinoma after radiofrequency ablation. Journal of Gastroenterology and Hepatology. 2011;**26**(5):858-865

[65] Donadon V, Balbi M, Valent F, Avogaro A. Glycated hemoglobin and antidiabetic strategies as risk factors for hepatocellular carcinoma. World Journal of Gastroenterology. 2010;**16**(24):3025-3032

[66] Zhang X, Harmsen WS, Mettler TA, Kim WR, Roberts RO, Therneau TM, et al. Continuation of metformin use after a diagnosis of cirrhosis significantly improves survival of patients with diabetes. Hepatology. 2014;**60**(6):2008-2016

[67] Chojkier M, Elkhayat H, Sabry D, Donohue M, Buck M. Pioglitazone decreases hepatitis C viral load in overweight, treatment naïve, genotype 4 infected-patients: A pilot study. PLoS One. 2012;**7**(3):e31516

[68] Khattab M, Emad M, Abdelaleem A, Eslam M, Atef R, Shaker Y, Hamdy L. Pioglitazone improves virological response to peginterferon alpha-2b/ribavirin combination therapy in hepatitis C genotype 4 patients with insulin resistance. Liver International. 2010 March;**30**(3):447-454

[69] Harrison SA, Hamzeh FM, Han J, Pandya PK, Sheikh MY, Vierling JM. Chronic hepatitis C genotype 1 patients with insulin resistance treated with pioglitazone and peginterferon alpha-2a plus ribavirin. Hepatology. 2012;**56**(2):464-473

[70] Marks KM, Kitch D, Chung RT, Hadigan C, Andersen J, Tien P, et al. Pilot study of pioglitazone before HCV retreatment in HIV/HCV genotype 1-infected subjects with insulin resistance and previous nonresponse to peginterferon and ribavirin therapy: A5239. Journal of Acquired Immune Deficiency Syndromes. 2014;**65**(3):345-349

[71] Sumie S, Kawaguchi T, Kawaguchi A, Kuromatsu R, Nakano M, Satani M, et al. Effect of pioglitazone on outcome following curative treatment for hepatocellular carcinoma in patients with hepatitis C virus infection: A prospective study. Molecular and Clinical Oncology. 2015;**3**(1):115-120

[72] Bonkovsky HL, Azar R, Bird S, Szabo G, Banner B. Severe cholestatic hepatitis caused by thiazolidinediones: Risks associated with substituting rosiglitazone for troglitazone. Digestive Diseases and Sciences. 2002;**47**(7):1632-1637

[73] Valverde I, Villanueva-Peñacarrillo ML, Malaisse WJ. Pancreatic and extrapancreatic effects of GLP-1. Diabetes & Metabolism. 2002;**28**(6 Pt 2):3S85-3S89 discussion 3S108-12

[74] Drucker DJ, Sherman SI, Gorelick FS, Bergenstal RM, Sherwin RS, Buse JB. Incretin-based therapies for the treatment of type 2 diabetes: Evaluation of the risks and benefits. Diabetes Care. 2010;**33**(2):428-433

[75] Itou M, Kawaguchi T, Taniguchi E, Sumie S, Oriishi T, Mitsuyama K, et al. Altered expression of glucagon-like peptide-1 and dipeptidyl peptidase IV in patients with HCV-related glucose intolerance. Journal of Gastroenterology and Hepatology. 2008;**23**(2):244-251

[76] Liu J, Wang G, Jia Y, Xu Y. GLP-1 receptor agonists: Effects on the progression of non-alcoholic fatty liver disease. Diabetes/Metabolism Research and Reviews. 2015;**31**(4):329-335

[77] Arase Y, Kawamura Y, Seko Y, Kobayashi M, Suzuki F, Suzuki Y, et al. Efficacy and safety in sitagliptin therapy for diabetes complicated by non-alcoholic fatty liver disease. Hepatology Research. 2013;**43**(11):1163-1168

[78] Kawaguchi T, Taniguchi E, Morita Y, Shirachi M, Tateishi I, Nagata E, et al. Association of exogenous insulin or sulphonylurea treatment with an increased incidence of hepatoma in patients with hepatitis C virus infection. Liver International. 2010;**30**(3):479-486

[79] Donadon V, Balbi M, Mas MD, Casarin P, Zanette G. Metformin and reduced risk of hepatocellular carcinoma in diabetic patients with chronic liver disease. Liver International. 2010;**30**(5):750-758

[80] Singh S, Singh PP, Singh AG, Murad MH, Sanchez W. Anti-diabetic medications and the risk of hepatocellular cancer: A systematic review and meta-analysis. American Journal of Gastroenterology. 2013;**108**(6):881-891 quiz 92

Chapter 11

Neuropathological and Neuropsychiatric Determinants in HCV-Infected Patients

Vanja Vojnović

Additional information is available at the end of the chapter

http://dx.doi.org/10.5772/intechopen.70670

Abstract

Chronic hepatitis C virus (HCV) infection is a growing global health problem. HCV is a leading cause of chronic hepatitis, cirrhosis, and hepatocellular carcinoma (HCC) and is associated with more than 30 extrahepatic manifestations (EHMs). Although cryoglobulinemia is the main pathological cause of neurologic EHMs, HCV viral replication in the brain itself must also be taken into consideration. The most significant neurological manifestations of HCV chronic infection are stroke, leukoencephalopathy, encephalomyelitis/myelitis, and peripheral neuropathy. The most significant neuropsychological manifestations of HCV infection are fatigue, depression, anxiety, and cognitive dysfunction. Antiviral HCV treatment should be the first-line treatment for managing mild-to-moderate vascular and neurologic symptoms; most of EHMs improve or even resolve if antiviral treatment starts on time.

Keywords: hepatitis C virus, extrahepatic manifestations, cryoglobulinemia, neurological manifestations, neuropsychological manifestations, antiviral treatment

1. Introduction

Chronic hepatitis C virus (HCV) infection is a growing global health problem affecting an estimated 185 million people (a prevalence rate of 2.8%) [1]. HCV is a leading cause of chronic hepatitis, cirrhosis, and hepatocellular carcinoma (HCC) and is associated with more than 30 extrahepatic manifestations (EHMs) [2].

EHMs are immunologic and rheumatologic in their pathophysiology: they are caused by B-cell proliferation, which produce monoclonal and polyclonal autoantibodies and then activate rheumatoid factor or have cryoglobulin properties.

Cryoglobulinemia is the most frequent and best-studied EHM of HCV infection. It is detected in up to 50% of HCV-infected patients. Cryoglobulins (CGs) are cold-precipitable immunoglobulins, which make vascular deposits and then cause inflammation and occlusion of small- and medium-size blood vessels. Typical clinical manifestations of cryoglobulinemia are cutaneous purpura, arthralgias, and membranous proliferative glomerulonephritis. Also, up to 17–60% of patients with cryoglobulinemia develop peripheral neuropathy. Central nervous system (CNS) involvement occurs in approximately 6% of cases. CGs are also a risk factor for carotid plaque formation, hepatic fibrosis, and liver steatosis [3].

Although cryoglobulinemia is the main pathological cause of neurologic EHMs, special consideration must be given to HCV viral replication in brain itself. It is believed that there are specific brain HCV variants that cause neurotoxicity (induce apoptosis). So far, it has been hypothesized that microglial cells (CNS macrophages) are the main targets for HCV entry into the CNS. Detection of replicative intermediate forms of HCV RNA and viral proteins within the CNS has led to this conclusion. Furthermore, sequence analysis of HCV residing in liver and brain has suggested an evolutionary path of a virus to infect the CNS [4].

2. Neurological manifestations

HCV-related CNS complications encompass a wide spectrum of disorders ranging from cerebrovascular events to autoimmune syndromes.

1. Acute cerebrovascular events can sometimes be the initial manifestation of HCV infection.
2. Acute or subacute encephalopathic syndromes have been associated with diffuse involvement of the white matter in HCV chronically infected patients with CG and/or circulating anticardiolipin antibodies.
3. The occurrence of an immune-mediated process induced by HCV causes inflammatory disorders such as acute encephalitis, encephalomyelitis, and meningoradiculitis/polyradiculitis; there are reports of patients with rapidly evolving acute leukoencephalitis or fatal progressive acute encephalomyelitic syndromes [3].
4. HCV has been connected with the metabolic syndrome so HCV infection represents an independent risk factor for increased carotid wall thickness and plaque formation, thus contributing to significant cerebrovascular mortality [3].

Neurological manifestations are most often caused by occlusive vasculopathy (due to mixed cryoglobulinemia), ANCA-associated CNS vasculitis or anti-phospholipid associated syndrome. In addition, HCV infection may increase the risk of atherosclerosis and earlier stroke through predisposition to metabolic diseases such as type 2 diabetes [5].

3. Neuropsychological manifestations

Fatigue, cognitive dysfunction, and mood alterations display a profound effect on social and physical function of HCV-infected subjects, thus impacting health-related quality of life (HRQL).

http://dx.doi.org/10.5772/intechopen.70670

Chronic fatigue (often called "brain fog") is perceived as a sensation of physical and mental exhaustion, and when severe, it is accompanied by deficits of attention tasks, anomia, and word-finding difficulties, in the absence of verbal memory or cognitive ability impairments [6].

It has been found that 28% of chronically HCV-infected subjects have depression [7]. The occurrence of depression has been attributed to psychological factors, or to specific determinants, including immune mechanisms, derangement of the blood–brain-barrier integrity, viral replication within the CNS, iatrogenic factors, or altered dopaminergic and serotoninergic transmission [7]. It is very important to diagnose such manifestations because in moderate-to-severe depression it is mandatory to reduce or discontinue interferon treatment.

Investigation of a large population of patients with chronic HCV infection has disclosed the occurrence of subclinical cognitive dysfunction (alterations in verbal and learning skills, concentration, attention, working memory) in 18% of subjects [8].

4. Peripheral neuropathies

In patients with HCV, the involvement of the peripheral nervous system (PNS) ranges from 26 to 86% in accordance with the disease stage [9]. Peripheral neuropathies occur mostly in the presence of circulating CG which causes ischemic nerve changes, as a consequence of small vessel vasculitis, or, less frequently, necrotizing arteritis of medium-sized vessels [9].

In patients without CG, immune complexes or HCV-induced autoimmune mechanisms may play a pathogenetic role in inducing vascular and perivascular inflammation, which may be driven by an intrinsic nerve population of immunocompetent and potentially phagocytic cells [10].

Many patients develop a symmetrical sensory or sensorimotor axonal-type polyneuropathy, with sensory loss and weakness in distal regions of limbs [11]. Others present with mononeuropathies and mononeuropathy multiplex or the asymmetrical sensory variants such as large-fiber sensory neuropathy (LFSN) and small-fiber sensory polyneuropathy (SFSN) [12]. Cranial nerves are usually spared.

One must also take into consideration that HCV-infected patients can have multiple neurological/neuropsychological manifestations.

5. Impact of HCV treatment on neurological/neuropsychiatric disorders

Antiviral HCV treatment is the first-line treatment for managing mild-to-moderate neurologic/neuropsychologic symptoms. However, patients on interferon (IFN) therapy should be monitored as IFN therapy may aggravate the symptoms of peripheral neuropathies (IFN can create the pathogenic inflammatory environment for neuropathy) [4].

Tricyclic antidepressants, local anesthetics, and opioids may be required to the standard antiviral therapy for treatment of acute pain attacks [4].

Rituximab is also useful in treating neuropathic pain, as it acts by inhibiting cryoglobulin production and its pathogenic cascade [4].

If EHMs do not improve after antiviral treatment, the use of immunosuppressants is also a treatment possibility, but only as a last resort in patients not responding to antiviral treatment or with refractory disease (because of possible worsening of viral infection) [4].

Also, when discussing neuropathological and neuropsychiatric manifestations in HCV-infected patients, it is very important to distinguish between neuropsychiatric diseases caused by the virus itself and those caused by the treatment.

There are many neurological side effects of HCV treatment: up to 70% of HCV patients treated with IFN may develop depression [13]. Neurovegetative symptoms like loss of appetite, fatigue, sexual impairment, and psychosomatic symptoms start to occur within 4 weeks of IFN treatment [13]. The confusional state induced by IFN is associated with psychomotor retardation, disorientation, Parkinsonism, psychosis, and manic disorder [14]. As mentioned above, IFN therapy can also aggravate the symptoms of peripheral neuropathies.

6. Conclusions

Sometimes EHMs can be the first clinical manifestation of HCV infection. This is why in the diagnostic work-up of a patient with the above reported neurological/psychiatric disorders without more obvious causes, clinicians should always consider screening for HCV infection.

Antiviral HCV treatment should be the first-line treatment for managing mild-to-moderate vascular and neurologic symptoms. Persistence or relapse of neurologic symptoms despite viral clearance suggest the presence of other diseases, so further diagnostic work-up should be undertaken.

Author details

Vanja Vojnović[1,2]*

*Address all correspondence to: vanja_vojnovic@yahoo.com

1 Faculty of Medicine, Josip Juraj Strossmayer University, Osijek, Croatia

2 Department of Neurology, University Hospital Dubrava, Zagreb, Croatia

References

[1] Mohd Hanafiah K, Groeger J, Flaxman AD, Wiersma ST. Global epidemiology of hepatitis C virus infection: New estimates of age-specific antibody to HCV seroprevalence. Hepatology. 2013;**57**:1333-1342. DOI: 10.1002/hep.26141 23172780

[2] Jacobson IM, Cacoub P, Dal Maso L, Harrison SA, Younossi ZM. Manifestations of chronic hepatitis C virus infection beyond the liver. Clinical Gastroenterology and Hepatology. 2010;**8**(12):1017-1029

[3] Monaco S, Ferrari (S), Gajofatto A, Zanusso G, Mariotto S. HCV-Related Nervous System Disorders. Clinical and Developmental Immunology, vol. 2012, Article ID 236148, 9 pages, 2012. doi:10.1155/2012/236148

[4] Mathew S, Faheem M, Ibrahim SM, Iqbal W, Rauff B, Fatima K, Qadri I. Hepatitis C virus and neurological damage. World Journal of Hepatology. 2016;**8**(12):545-556. DOI: 10.4254/wjh.v8.i12.545

[5] Adinolfi LE, Nevola R, Lus G, Restivo L, Guerrera B, Romano C, Zampino R, Rinaldi L, Sellitto A, Giordano M, Marrone A. Chronic hepatitis C virus infection and neurological and psychiatric disorders: An overview. World Journal of Gastroenterology. 2015;**21**(8):2269-2280. DOI: 10.3748/wjg.v21.i8.2269

[6] Goh J, Coughlan B, Quinn J, O'Keane JC, Crowe J. Fatigue does not correlate with the degree of hepatitis or the presence of autoimmune disorders in chronic hepatitis C infection. European Journal of Gastroenterology and Hepatology. 1999;**11**(8):833-838

[7] Carta MG, Angst J, Moro MF, et al. Association of chronic hepatitis C with recurrent brief depression. Journal of Affective Disorders. 2012;**141**:361-366

[8] Kramer L, Bauer E, Funk G, et al. Subclinical impairment of brain function in chronic hepatitis C infection. Journal of Hepatology. 2002;**37**(3):349-354

[9] Vital C, Vital A, Canron MH, et al. Combined nerve and muscle biopsy in the diagnosis of vasculitic neuropathy. A 16-year retrospective study of 202 cases. Journal of the Peripheral Nervous System. 2006;**11**(1):20-29

[10] Bonetti B, Monaco S, Giannini C, Ferrari S, Zanusso GL, Rizzuto N. Human peripheral nerve macrophages in normal and pathological conditions. Journal of the Neurological Sciences. 1993;**118**(2):158-168

[11] Authier FJ, Bassez G, Payan C, et al. Detection of genomic viral RNA in nerve and muscle of patients with HCV neuropathy. Neurology. 2003;**60**(5):808-812

[12] Bant A, Hurowitz B, Hassan N, Van Thiel DU, Nadir A. Complex regional pain syndrome (Reflex sympathetic dystrophy) in a patient with essential mixed cryoglobulinemia and chronic hepatitis C. Journal of the Pakistan Medical Association. 2007;**57**(2):96-98

[13] Mariotto S, Ferrari S, Monaco S. HCV-related central and peripheral nervous system demyelinating disorders. Inflammation & Allergy: Drug Targets. 2014;**13**:299-304 [PMID: 25198705. DOI: 10.2174/1871528113666140908113841]

[14] Rifai MA, Gleason OC, Sabouni D. Psychiatric Care of the Patient With Hepatitis C: A Review of the Literature. Primary Care Companion to The Journal of Clinical Psychiatry. 2010;**12**(6):PCC.09r00877. doi:10.4088/PCC.09r00877whi

Chapter 12

HCV and Work Ability Assessment

Milan Milošević, Jelena Jakab, Lucija Kuna and Martina Smolić

Additional information is available at the end of the chapter

http://dx.doi.org/10.5772/intechopen.70774

Abstract

Modifications to work and work ability assessment are required to prevent occupational transmission of hepatitis C virus (HCV). This is usually required in the health care setting, where exposure-prone procedures (EPPs) should not be carried out by infectious carriers of HCV. The risk of an individual surgeon acquiring HCV has been estimated at 0.001–0.032% per annum. Even in an area with a high prevalence of HCV among its population, the risk of acquiring HCV through occupational exposure is low. Rates of viral clearance with treatment of acute HCV infection are considerably higher than treatment of chronic HCV infection. Consequently, it is imperative that health care workers follow universal precautions and promptly report all exposures to blood or body fluid exposures according to their local policy. Health care workers who embark on, or transfer to, a career that requires EPP (exposure-prone procedures and dialysis work) should be assessed to ensure that they are free from infection with HCV. If the HCV antibodies are positive, the health care worker should be tested for HCV RNA PCR. If the HCV RNA PCR is negative on two separate occasions, the health care worker may be permitted to perform EPPs. If the HCV RNA PCR is positive, the health care worker should not be allowed to perform EPPs. Health care workers who already perform EPPs and who believe they may have been exposed to HCV infection should be advised to seek advice from their occupational health department for confidential advice on whether they should be tested.

Keywords: HCV, work ability assessment, fitness for work

1. Introduction

Work ability assessment or fitness to work refers to the process of ensuring that an employee can complete a task safely without presenting a risk to themselves, their colleagues, the company, or a third party. This term also refers to the impact of sickness and absence of employees in order to assess the possibility of having an employee return to work quickly and safely.

Work ability assessments are most often performed to determine medical fitness after an illness or injury, sometimes at the request of an employer after an offer of employment or as a condition of a job transfer.

Fitness to work assesses the capacity of an individual to perform physical and psychological work tasks according to the demands of the job. This demand may be directly associated with a task (e.g., carrying loads) or may be associated with a location that will impact the individual's health. Therefore, fitness to work addresses both the task and the location of the work to be done.

Reduced work productivity (WP) is a measure of the impact of illness and treatment burden in patients diagnosed with chronic diseases [1]. Patient's WP in the setting of a chronic condition presents a complex phenomenon that cannot be understood only by obtaining patient's clinical information. It is also important to collect patient-reported outcomes, especially ones that capture patients' energy and physical components. Hepatitis C (HCV) infection has a considerable negative impact on patient-reported outcomes (PRO) and patients' WP [2]. Numerous manifestations of HCV lead to an economic burden related to the complications and extrahepatic manifestation, thus decreasing WP [3]. For that reason, it is important to collect information that can help caregivers to develop a plan for maintaining patients' employment. Targeting important aspects of PROs has a substantial positive impact on patients' well-being as well as their WP, which results in notable economic benefits for the whole society [4].

2. Impact of HCV infection on work ability and productivity

Chronic HCV is a global health problem affecting 130–170 million people worldwide (80% of patients with acute HCV infections will develop chronic HCV). Every year, 3–4 million people are infected, and approximately 9 million patients have HCV infection in Europe, with greater prevalence in the southern and eastern European regions [5]. Around 2.7–4.1 million people have chronic HCV (HCV) in the United States. While frequently believed of as an asymptomatic disease, numerous studies have shown that those with chronic HCV experience increased work impairment revealed as decreased WP and increased absenteeism and presenteeism (attending work while being impaired) [6]. Risk factors identified included blood transfusion, injection drug use, employment in patient care or clinical laboratory work, exposure to a sex partner or household member who has had a history of hepatitis, exposure to multiple sex partners, and low socioeconomic level. These studies reported no association with military service or exposures resulting from medical, surgical, or dental procedures, tattooing, acupuncture, ear piercing, or foreign travel. If transmission from such exposures does occur, the frequency might be too low to detect [7].

Working in the health care, emergency medical (e.g., emergency medical technicians and paramedics), and public safety sectors (e.g., fire-service, law-enforcement, and correctional facility personnel) who have exposure to blood in the workplace are at high risk for being infected with bloodborne pathogens. Nevertheless, occurrence of HCV infection among health-care workers, including surgeons, is no greater than the general population, averaging 1–2%, and is 10 times lower than that for HBV infection [8]. In a single study that evaluated risk factors for infection, a history of unintentional needle-stick injury was the only occupational risk factor independently associated with HCV infection [9].

Among health care workers, the prevalence of HCV infection is about the same as that of the general population: 1.5%. Following percutaneous exposure of health care workers to infected blood, the risk of HCV seroconversion ranges from 0 to 10%, with an average of 1.8% [7].

HCV infection is a major cause of fatigue, muscle and joint pain, depression, and other psychological disorders, which decrease patient health-related quality of life (HRQL) and health utility [10]. Patients with chronic HCV infection demonstrated lower HRQL compared with the general population. Recently, investigators have turned their interest to the impact of HCV infection on absenteeism, work force participation, and overall work impairment.

Even if patients are employed, the complete participation productivity may be limited. Worker productivity is measured through two key concepts: presenteeism and absenteeism. Absenteeism is related to the percentage of work time missed, while presenteeism is related to the percentage of impairment experienced at work time missed because of one's health [6].

To date, numerous studies have demonstrated the impact of HCV on health care costs. Previous studies have evaluated health care costs associated with HCV to be $2470 per patient during the period from 1997 to 1999 [11, 12]. However, direct medical costs present only part of the societal burden of HCV infection. On the other hand, indirect costs related to work impairment have been ignored in the HCV literature for a long time. Previous models have omitted work impairment completely [13] or have evaluated productivity losses only in the premature mortality and disability as a consequence of projected late stage liver disease. Direct costs associated with HCV are fundamental. Also, indirect economic and humanistic costs are major and arise from the reduction of HRQL owing to both the disease and HCV treatments; this is related on the patient work, daily activities, and lifestyle [14].

Recent investigation has recognized a significant burden of HCV infection on work productivity, with infected patients missing 9% of working hours in the working week and reporting an average of 27% impairment while at work. Also, database study reported that HCV patients were 7.5% less productive based on work units per hour [15].

For better understanding of the societal impact of HCV, the association between the virus and work force participation and WP loss must be observed. It is also essential to investigate potential confusing variables that may contribute to a relationship between HCV and workplace activity. Nowadays, different studies have reviewed the impact comorbidities, and health behaviors may have on health outcomes among HCV patients, including psychiatric illness, fibrosis, fatigue, and depressive symptoms [16].

It would be educative and significant for some employers with a short-term focus to utilize a time series approach to document WP changes pre and post-HCV diagnosis. Although using a regression approach and a propensity scoring approach ensured a numerous series of results, other methodologies may be significant, especially when evaluating economic costs associated with HCV [16].

Patients with HCV infection have reduced WP, in terms of both presenteeism (impairment in WP while working) and absenteeism (productivity loss due to absence from work). The most important drivers of WP in HCV are impairment of physical aspects of PROs and clinical history of depression, anxiety, fatigue, and cirrhosis [4]. Some authors emphasize the impact of eradicating HCV virus on the WP of chronic HCV (CH-C) patients. Sensitivity analyses assessed the possibility that CH-C patients' labor costs were lower than the general populations and presented results by fibrosis stage. Before initiation of treatment, EU patients with CH-C genotype 1 (GT1) exhibited absenteeism and presenteeism impairments of 3.54 and 9.12%, respectively [17]. About 91.8% of EU patients in the ION trials achieved SVR and improved absenteeism and presenteeism impairments by 16.3 and 19.5%, respectively. Weighted average per-employed patient gains from treatment are projected to be higher in cirrhotic than in noncirrhotic patients. CH-C results in a significant economic burden to European society. Due to improvements in WP, sustained virologic response with treatment could provide substantial economic gains, partly offsetting the direct costs related to its widespread use [17].

HCV infection is generally considered an asymptomatic disease. However, studies have shown that HCV has a substantial negative impact on patients' quality of life and functioning. Su et al. [15] evaluated a total number of near 340,000 subjects. Workers with HCV had significantly more lost workdays per worker compared to the control cohort, including sick leave, short-term disability, and long-term disability. HCV-infected workers had 4.15 more days of absence per worker compared to the control cohort. Efficiency was measured by units of work processed per hour and workers with HCV processed 7.5% fewer units per hour than employees without HCV. All health care costs among HCV workers were significantly higher compared to the same costs among workers without HCV. This study provides evidence that there is a considerable secondary burden of disease and labels an association between HCV infection, efficiency, increased absenteeism, and higher health care benefit costs [15].

Gifford et al. [18] showed that at least 50% of the men had symptoms of HCV infection. Tiredness was the most common symptom, followed by nausea and pain in the liver. Men ignored symptoms of disease in higher percentage compared women. Thirty-five percent of men rated their health as 'fair' or 'poor' compared to 18% of men in the general population. Many were concerned about their ability to work and financial income, and more than half were worried about being unable to have a drink with their friends. Coughlan et al. presented a Dublin study documenting psychological well-being, mental health, and quality of life in 93 women diagnosed with medically acquired HCV infection. Overall, the women had significantly lower quality of life than the healthy female population. No significant difference was found between women who had a past or current HCV virus infection; they reported having low energy, poor health, and problems with work and other daily activities. Reduced quality of life can be related to the diagnostic process rather than HCV infection as such. While HCV have a significant physiological effect on the quality of life, it is imperative not to undervalue the social and psychological costs of being identified with a stigmatized chronic disease that has an unknown progression and outcome [19]. Gill et al. found that HCV compared to divorce, loss of source of income, or a move to another city diagnosis is a way more stressful. The authors suggested that pre-and post-test counseling and psychosocial support could help to decrease the stress related with HCV diagnosis [20]. HCV infection has a significant influence on the quality of life. Not only do symptoms such as fatigue lessen effective functioning but also living with a chronic stigmatized disease with an indeterminate future creates problems around expose, retrieving care, and satisfying confidence, employment, and relations.

3. The impact of the HCV antiviral therapy on work ability

A patient's ability to tolerate and adhere to HCV treatment has an impact to WP during the course of HCV treatment. This is important concern for patients considering treatment initiation because they will have to deal with the possibility of temporary reduced work participation during treatment [17].

Eradication of HCV may improve many different components of PRO, including HRQL and WP [21]. It is important that evaluation of new regimens for treatment of chronic hepatitis C (CHC) includes not only efficacy and safety reports but also data related to important PROs such as fatigue, HRQL, and WP [14]. The dual function of PRO is to represent patient experience with treatment and assess the indirect cost of treatment related to lower WP [22].

Treatment of HCV infection with the combination of peginterferon plus ribavirin (pegIFN/RBV) is a process with significant and sometimes dose-limiting adverse events. Those adverse effects further exacerbate the patient's already compromised productivity and consequently increase economic burden [17]. Brook et al. found that patients who received pegIFN/RBV took more sick leave, more long-term disability, and more workers' compensation than those without HCV treatment [3]. Perillo et al. designed a randomized control study and found that during treatment with peginterferon-alpha 2a, patients showed less impairment across all measures of work functioning and productivity when compared to patients who were treated with combination of interferon-alpha 2b plus ribavirin [23]. In a study conducted by McHutchison et al., randomly assigned patients who responded to therapy of IFN/RBV showed improvements across all measures of work functioning and productivity, in contrast with patients who received placebo. In addition, sustained responders work functioning and productivity decreased temporarily in approximately 46% of patients [14]. Patients who do not achieve an SVR are more likely to miss work or other commitments due to HCV infection or its treatment than those who achieve SVR. Aggrawal et al. confirmed that employed patients with genotype 1 chronic HCV infection receiving treatment have reduced work hours and reduced WP levels due to hepatitis or its treatment. This decline was observed early during the course of treatment, with return to baseline levels by week 72 post-treatment initiation, suggesting that WP losses can be considered a short-term outcome of HCV treatment [1].

To improve the tolerability and efficacy profile of anti-HCV treatment, a number of interferon-free regimens, such as sofosbuvir, have been developed. In a study by Younossi et al., subjects treated with the interferon-free regimen completely recovered by the end of 12 weeks of follow-up, their PRO scores returned to baseline values and showed further improvement. The impact on WP, especially presenteeism, was significantly more profound with the interferon-containing regimen than with the interferon-free regimen. Also, subjects who received the interferon-free regimen experienced substantially less fatigue compared with the subjects receiving interferon-containing regimens [22]. Another study by Younossi et al. showed that interferon and ribavirin-free regimen are associated with significant gains in most aspects of HRQL during treatment regardless of the stage of liver disease [24]. Expanding the access to a highly effective cure for all HCV-infected patients will improve the clinical outcomes but also patient-reported outcomes such as HRQL and work productivity, resulting in a superb comprehensive benefit to patients and society.

In conclusion, successful treatment and achieving SVR regardless of therapy have been associated with better economic outcomes [25]. For that reason, there is a strong evidence that this improvement can positively impact the indirect economic burden of HCV by improving WP.

4. Conclusions

In general, work-related activities should not pose a risk to patient with chronic liver disease [26]. The exception would be:

1. Patients with hepatic encephalopathy for whom certain task such as driving and operating heavy machinery may be risky due to impaired judgment and cognitive defects.
2. Working with hepatotoxic chemical such as carbon tetrachloride, vinyl chloride, and polychlorinated biphenyls (PCBs).

Patients with advanced liver disease have decreased exercise capacity from anemia, ascites, renal failure, or hepato-pulmonary syndrome, and work limitations are advised [26].

Modifications to work and work ability assessment are required to prevent occupational transmission of HCV. This is usually only required in the health care setting, where infectious carriers of HCV should not carry out exposure-prone procedures (EPP). Even in an area with a high prevalence of HCV among its population, the risk of acquiring HCV through occupational exposure is low—the risk of an individual surgeon acquiring the HCV has been estimated at 0.001–0.032% per annum [26, 27]. Rates of viral clearance with treatment of acute HCV infection are considerably higher than treatment of chronic HCV infection. Consequently, it is imperative that health care workers follow universal precaution and promptly report all exposures to blood or body fluid exposures according to their local policy.

Health care workers who embark on, or transfer to, a career that requires EPP (exposure-prone procedures and dialysis work) should be assessed to ensure that they are free from infection with HCV. Members of staff known to have been exposed to the blood of a HCV-positive patient through sharps injury should continue to work normally, but it is necessary to do the following procedure [26] that is also shown at **Figure 1**:

1. HCV RNA polymerase chain reaction test 6 weeks after exposure.
2. Twelve weeks after exposure, HCV RNA polymerase chain reaction test should be taken again, together with HCV antibody testing.

http://dx.doi.org/10.5772/intechopen.70774

3. Six months after exposure, additional HCV antibody testing should be commenced (repeated negative testing designates infection absence).

Those who have positive test results should stop undertaking EPPs instantly and should be taken as soon as possible for specialist assessment by a gastroenterologist and/or infectologist. Health care workers who already perform EPPs and who believe they may have been exposed to HCV infection should be advised to seek advice from their occupational health department for confidential advice on whether they should be tested.

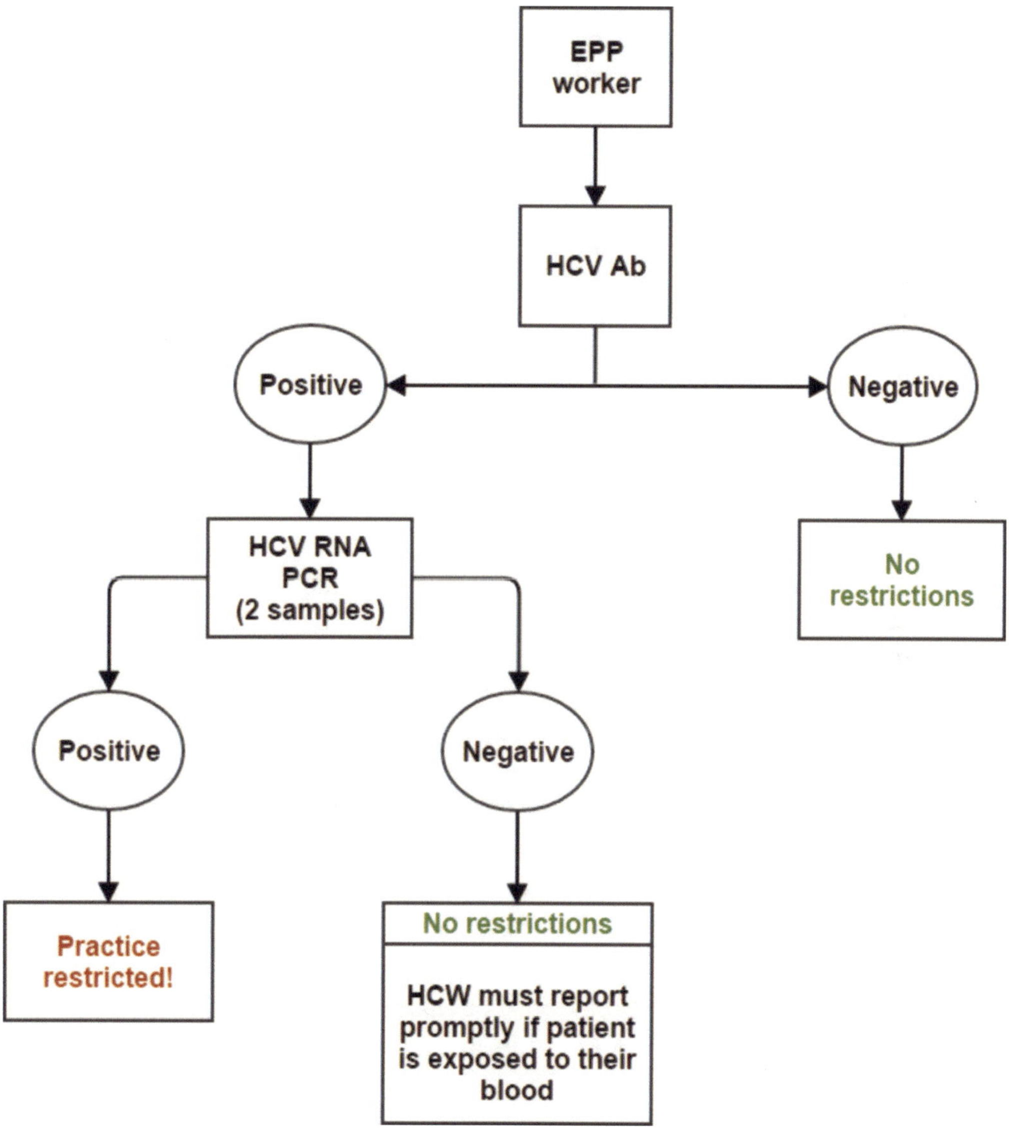

Figure 1. Investigation of HCV status in a worker performing exposure-prone procedures (Modified after Palmer et al. [26]).

Those health care workers who had HCV infection and have been treated with antiviral treatment may return to EPPs if they have tested negative to HCV RNA for at least 6 months after cessation of treatment. They should have one additional check for HCV RNA 6 months later. Present standard laboratory tests cannot demonstrate complete clearance of virus but can state that the virus is undetectable. In these situations, infectivity is likely to be so low that it is safe to return to EPPs and reactivation of infection is unlikely so no further testing is required. There is indication that infection remains within hepatocytes and can be reactivated following treatment with monoclonal antibodies (such as Rituximab) and other immunosuppressants (such as TNF-α inhibitors) including cancer chemotherapy. Recent data suggest that rituximab-based chemotherapy increases HCV expression in hepatic cells, can become a mark for a cell-mediated immune response after the treatment removal and the renewal of the immune control. Some studies have examined the incidence of HCV reactivation and related hepatic flare in patients with oncohematological diseases receiving R-CHOP (rituximab, cyclophosphamide, doxorubicin, vincristine, and prednisone). These studies suggest that the hepatic flares are often asymptomatic, but life-threatening liver failure occurs in closely 10% of cases [28].

Author details

Milan Milošević[1]*, Jelena Jakab[2], Lucija Kuna[2] and Martina Smolić[2]

*Address all correspondence to: milan.milosevic@snz.hr

1 University of Zagreb, School of Medicine, Andrija Stampar School of Public Health, WHO Collaborative Centre for Occupational Health, Zagreb, Croatia

2 Josip Juraj Strossmayer University of Osijek, Faculty of Medicine, Osijek, Croatia

References

[1] Aggarwal J, Vera-Llonch M, Donepudi M, Suthoff E, Younossi Z, Goss TF. Work productivity among treatment-naive patients with genotype 1 chronic hepatitis C infection receiving telaprevir combination treatment. Journal of Viral Hepatitis. 2015;**22**(1):8-17. DOI: 10.1111/jvh.12227

[2] Younossi Z, Henry L. Systematic review: Patient-reported outcomes in chronic hepatitis C – the impact of liver disease and new treatment regimens. Alimentary Pharmacology & Therapeutics. 2015;**41**(6):497-520. DOI: 10.1111/apt.13090

[3] Brook RA, Kleinman NL, Su J, Corey-Lisle PK, Iloeje UH. Absenteeism and productivity among employees being treated for hepatitis C. The American Journal of Managed Care. 2011;**17**(10):657-664

[4] Younossi ZM, Stepanova M, Henry L, Younossi I, Weinstein A, Nader F, Hunt S. Association of work productivity with clinical and patient-reported factors in patients

infected with hepatitis C virus. Journal of Viral Hepatitis. 2016;**23**(8):623-630. DOI: 10.1111/jvh.12528

[5] Vietri J, Prajapati G, El Khoury AC. The burden of hepatitis C in Europe from the patients' perspective: A survey in 5 countries. BMC Gastroenterology. 2013;**13**:16. DOI: 10.1186/1471-230X-13-16

[6] Manne V, Sassi K, Allen R, Saab S. Hepatitis C and work impairment: A review of current literature. Journal of Clinical Gastroenterology. 2014;**48**(7):595-599. DOI: 10.1097/MCG.0000000000000080

[7] Centers for Disease Control and Prevention. Recommendations for prevention and control of hepatitis C virus (HCV) infection and HCV-related chronic disease. MMWR – Recommendations and Reports. 1998;**47**(RR-19):1-39

[8] Cooper BW, Krusell A, Tilton RC, Goodwin R, Levitz RE. Seroprevalence of antibodies to hepatitis C virus in high-risk hospital personnel. Infection Control and Hospital Epidemiology. 1992;**13**(2):82-85

[9] Polish LB, Tong MJ, Co RL, Coleman PJ, Alter MJ. Risk factors for hepatitis C virus infection among health care personnel in a community hospital. American Journal of Infection Control. 1993;**21**(4):196-200

[10] Chong CA, Gulamhussein A, Heathcote EJ, Lilly L, Sherman M, Naglie G, Krahn M. Health-state utilities and quality of life in hepatitis C patients. The American Journal of Gastroenterology. 2003;**98**(3):630-638

[11] Leigh JP, Bowlus CL, Leistikow BN, Schenker M. Costs of hepatitis C. Archives of Internal Medicine. 2001;**161**(18):2231-2237

[12] Armstrong EP, Charland SL. Burden of illness of hepatitis C from a managed care organization perspective. Current Medical Research and Opinion. 2004;**20**(5):671-679. DOI: 10.1185/030079904125003485

[13] Touzet S, Kraemer L, Colin C, Pradat P, Lanoir D, Bailly F, Coppola RC, Sauleda S, Thursz MR, Tillmann H, Alberti A, Braconier JH, Esteban JI, Hadziyannis SJ, Manns MP, Saracco G, Thomas HC, Trépo C. Epidemiology of hepatitis C virus infection in seven European Union countries: A critical analysis of the literature. HENCORE group (Hepatitis C European Network for Co-operative Research). European Journal of Gastroenterology & Hepatology. 2000;**12**(6):667-678

[14] McHutchison JG, Ware JE, Bayliss MS, Pianko S, Albrecht JK, Cort S, Yang I, Neary MP, H I T Group. The effects of interferon alpha-2b in combination with ribavirin on health related quality of life and work productivity. Journal of Hepatology. 2001;**34**(1): 140-147

[15] Su J, Brook RA, Kleinman NL, Corey-Lisle P. The impact of hepatitis C virus infection on work absence, productivity, and healthcare benefit costs. Hepatology. 2010;**52**(2):436-442. DOI: 10.1002/hep.23726

[16] DiBonaventura M, Wagner JS, Yuan Y, L'Italien G, Langley P, Ray Kim W. The impact of hepatitis C on labor force participation, absenteeism, presenteeism and non-work activities. Journal of Medical Economics. 2011;**14**(2):253-261. DOI: 10.3111/13696998.2011.566294

[17] Younossi Z, Brown A, Buti M, Fagiuoli S, Mauss S, Rosenberg W, Serfaty L, Srivastava A, Smith N, Stepanova M, Beckerman R. Impact of eradicating hepatitis C virus on the work productivity of chronic hepatitis C (CH-C) patients: An economic model from five European countries. Journal of Viral Hepatitis. 2016;**23**(3):217-226. DOI: 10.1111/jvh.12483

[18] Gifford SM, O'Brien ML, Smith A, Temple-Smith M, Stoove M, Mitchell D, Jolley D. Australian men's experiences of living with hepatitis C virus: Results from a cross-sectional survey. Journal of Gastroenterology and Hepatology. 2005;**20**(1):79-86. DOI: 10.1111/j.1440-1746.2004.03514.x

[19] Coughlan B, Sheehan J, Hickey A, Crowe J. Psychological well-being and quality of life in women with an iatrogenic hepatitis C virus infection. British Journal of Health Psychology. 2002;**7**(Pt 1):105-116. DOI: 10.1348/135910702169394

[20] Gill ML, Atiq M, Sattar S, Khokhar N. Psychological implications of hepatitis C virus diagnosis. Journal of Gastroenterology and Hepatology. 2005;**20**(11):1741-1744. DOI: 10.1111/j.1440-1746.2005.04061.x

[21] Kamal SM, Ahmed A, Mahmoud S, Nabegh L, El Gohary I, Obadan I, Hafez T, Ghoraba D, Aziz AA, Metaoei M. Enhanced efficacy of pegylated interferon alpha-2a over pegylated interferon and ribavirin in chronic hepatitis C genotype 4A randomized trial and quality of life analysis. Liver International. 2011;**31**(3):401-411. DOI: 10.1111/j.1478-3231.2010.02435.x

[22] Younossi ZM, Stepanova M, Henry L, Gane E, Jacobson IM, Lawitz E, Nelson D, Gerber L, Nader F, Hunt S. Effects of sofosbuvir-based treatment, with and without interferon, on outcome and productivity of patients with chronic hepatitis C. Clin Gastroenterol Hepatol. 2014;**12**(8):1349-1359.e13. DOI: 10.1016/j.cgh.2013.11.032

[23] Perrillo R, Rothstein KD, Rubin R, Alam I, Imperial J, Harb G, Hu S, Klaskala W. Comparison of quality of life, work productivity and medical resource utilization of peginterferon alpha 2a vs the combination of interferon alpha 2b plus ribavirin as initial treatment in patients with chronic hepatitis C. Journal of Viral Hepatitis. 2004;**11**(2):157-165

[24] Younossi ZM, Stepanova M, Afdhal N, Kowdley KV, Zeuzem S, Henry L, Hunt SL, Marcellin P. Improvement of health-related quality of life and work productivity in chronic hepatitis C patients with early and advanced fibrosis treated with ledipasvir and sofosbuvir. Journal of Hepatology. 2015;**63**(2):337-345. DOI: 10.1016/j.jhep.2015.03.014

[25] John-Baptiste AA, Tomlinson G, Hsu PC, Krajden M, Heathcote EJ, Laporte A, Yoshida EM, Anderson FH, Krahn MD. Sustained responders have better quality of life and productivity compared with treatment failures long after antiviral therapy for hepatitis C. The American Journal of Gastroenterology. 2009;**104**(10):2439-2448. DOI: 10.1038/ajg.2009.346

[26] Palmer KT, Brown I, Hobson J. Fitness for Work: The Medical Aspects. 5th ed. Oxford: Oxford University Press; 2013

[27] Yazdanpanah Y, De Carli G, Migueres B, Lot F, Campins M, Colombo C, Thomas T, Deuffic-Burban S, Prevot MH, Domart M, Tarantola A, Abiteboul D, Deny P, Pol S, Desenclos JC, Puro V, Bouvet E. Risk factors for hepatitis C virus transmission to health care workers after occupational exposure: A European case-control study. Clinical Infectious Diseases. 2005;**41**(10):1423-1430. DOI: 10.1086/497131

[28] Sagnelli E, Pisaturo M, Sagnelli C, Coppola N. Rituximab-based treatment, HCV replication, and hepatic flares. Clinical & Developmental Immunology. 2012;**2012**:945950. DOI: 10.1155/2012/945950

Chapter 13

Health-Related Quality of Life in Antiviral-Treated Chronic Hepatitis C Patients

Aleksandar Včev, Jelena Jakab, Lucija Kuna and Martina Smolić

Additional information is available at the end of the chapter

http://dx.doi.org/10.5772/intechopen.70766

Abstract

Chronic hepatitis C has a profound negative impact on both physical and mental well-being, thus decreasing health-related quality of life (HRQL). The most common complaints include symptoms such as fatigue, depression, and neurocognitive deficits. The burden of chronic HCV infections is multiplied by emotional and psychological issues that affect patients' functional health and work ability. Treatment of chronic HCV infection may at the beginning cause worse HRQL rates, as a result of common adverse effects like fatigue, muscle aches, and depression. However, the relationship between sustained virologic response (SVR) and improvement in HRQL is well known. Treatment-related adverse effects may discourage patients from starting therapy and reduce their adherence to treatment. Novel agents, with improved adverse effect profiles and SVR rates, allow more patients the opportunity to achieve improvements in HRQL during and after treatment.

Keywords: chronic hepatitis C, HCV treatment, adverse effects, health-related quality of life

1. Introduction

Life expectancy and causes of death have been used as key indicators of population health. Although these indicators provide information about the health status of populations, they do not offer any evidence about the quality of the physical, mental, or social functioning. To date, health is systematically included as a significant aspect of quality of life. Health-related quality of life (HRQL) measures have been developed to evaluate numerous aspects of an individual's subjective experience that cover health, disease, and different disabilities [1]. Despite the huge interest in quality of life, agreement is lacking on the definition and measurement of quality of life. Therefore, quality of life is used as a generic designation to describe a range of different physical and psychosocial variables [2].

2. Health-related quality of life (HRQL)

At the beginning of the 1990s, the World Health Organization (WHO) accepted the importance of evaluating and improving people's quality of life and developed a project in order to create a cross-cultural instrument of quality of life assessment: the World Health Organization Quality of Life (WHOQOL) [3]. WHO started its own project for several reasons. One of the reasons was to develop an international quality of life evaluation. Also, it was important to include a consideration of patients' quality of life in treatment decisions, approval of new pharmaceuticals, and policy research. Hence, having an international quality of life assessment as WHOQOL makes it possible to follow up quality of life research in different cultural settings and to directly compare results obtained in these different placements [4].

Likewise, clinicians and public health professionals have used health-related quality of life (HRQL) to evaluate the effects of the chronic diseases, treatments, and different disabilities. Institutes at the National Institutes of Health (NIH): for instance, the National Cancer Institute (NCI) and centers within the Centers for Disease Control and Prevention (CDC) have involved the evaluation and improvement of HRQL as a public health preference [5].

There are two potential explanations for the increasing interest in the assessment of quality of life in health care. The first explanation is an increased life expectancy as a result of improved medical care. Diagnostic and therapeutic treatments have increasingly advanced prognoses and management of many diseases, also increasing the life expectancy of individuals affected by these diseases. Consequently, many more patients are diagnosed with chronic, clinically manageable diseases than terminal diseases [2]. This evolution has led to the conclusion that health care interventions can no longer be evaluated solely on the basis of mortality or morbidity. Indeed, the impact of a disorder on a patient's life must also be observed [6]. The second explanation is referred to as the proliferation of improved medical and surgical technologies. Quality of life is included in the evaluation of the benefits of different treatment options.

HRQL aims at measuring disabilities related to specific diseases and also on effectiveness of treatment. Studies on HRQL focus on quality of life components that can be impacted by specific diseases. For example, measures of well-being typically evaluate the positive aspects of a person's life such as positive emotions. Therefore, numerous studies evaluate the quality and outcome of provided health care [2, 5].

It is important to emphasize that in HRQL, the experience of patients is most important. However, not only patient's estimation of their level of functioning is significant, for instance, cognitive process, but also the level of satisfaction in the different scopes, for instance, emotional process [7]. Investigators focused on HRQL may overestimate the impact of health-related factors. In addition, they could seriously underestimate the importance of nonmedical phenomena [8]. Some analyses of quality of life that have been undertaken have recognized this idea. Therefore, the majority of analyses have demonstrated that quality of life is most properly defined in patient satisfaction [9]. Finally, health should be observed as significant indicator as well as an important contributor to better quality of life.

3. HRQL measurements

Assessment of HRQL is related to functioning and well being in physical, mental, and social parts of life. Moreover, it shows importance in screening for disability and in improving communication between patients and clinicians [10, 11].

Common HRQL profile measures use multiple points to evaluate each of multiple parts of health and to decrease response burden. For that purpose, short-form HRQL measures, such as short-form 36 (SF-36), are widely used. Their briefness makes short-form measures practical for use as only 7 to 10 minutes are required to complete the form [12]. To provide the briefest possible measure of HRQL, the Dartmouth Cooperative Functional Assessment Charts (COOP) were designed. They consist of global items representing every single domain of health. These items are managed using five response choices: *Excellent, Very good, Good, Fair, Poor,* and COOP charts are original examples of global health items to evaluate multiple HRQL domains [13]. The NIH Patient-Reported Outcomes Measurement Information System (PROMIS) assesses global physical, mental, and social HRQL. It also designs, develops, validates, and standardizes item banks to measure patient-reported outcomes (PROs) relevant across common medical conditions. PRO is a 10-question measure which was developed through PROMIS, a NIH Roadmap electronic system designed to collect self-reported HRQL data from different populations with different types of chronic diseases [14]. The PROMIS global measure includes questions that evaluate self-rated health, physical HRQL, mental HRQL and evaluate for fatigue, pain, emotional distress, and their effects on different types of social activities. Recent investigations showed that psychometric evaluation of the PROMIS global health questions identified global physical and mental health summary scales but also separate scoring for global health, social activities, and numerous roles. Since it has been demonstrated, individual questions can be used to assess physical and mental HRQL, and social questions are included to assess social HRQL [14]. The PROMIS global health measure is scheduled to be managed on the National Health Interview Survey (NHIS) every 5 years. Analysis of summary scores and individual questions are expected to provide useful results and information. Their results are also expected to be reported every 5 years.

Well-being measures evaluate the positive aspects of people's lives. These measures have an association with their health and satisfaction, the quality of their relationships, positive emotions, their resiliency, and also with the realization of their potential. Well-being indicators measure when people feel very healthy and satisfied with life. Therefore, these characteristics representing well-being are associated with different benefits related to health, work, family, and economics. For instance, positive emotions are associated with decreased risk of disease and injury, as well as better immune functioning, which includes faster recovery time and increased longevity [15]. Measures of well-being can helpful for the public because they track results, such as meaningful work, relationships, satisfaction, and happiness. These outcomes are personally significant, easily understood, and can motivate change or modification [15, 16].

Participation measures reflect individual's assessments of the impact of their health on their social involvement within their environment. Participation includes education, employment, civic, social, and leisure activities. The principle behind participation measures is that an individual with a functional limitation can live a long and productive life and enjoy a good quality of life [17]. Hence, this approach of the measurement of participation is a significant supplement to the evaluation of quality of life. Participation is measured in the context of a person's health state and within his current social and physical ambiences [18].

Three scales are often used to measure HRQL among patients living with HCV: the SF-36 questionnaire, a generic instrument used to assess HRQL, Functional Assessment of Chronic Illness Therapy-Fatigue (FACIT-F) questionnaire, and Chronic Liver Disease Questionnaire–Hepatitis C Virus (CLDQ-HCV) instrument [19].

FACIT-F is a generic core questionnaire which involves 27 items that are divided into four parts: functional well-being, physical, social, or family and emotional [20]. The above items, as well as a fatigue subscale, range from 0 (worst) to 160 (best) [21]. No information regarding the validity of FACIT-F or its minimal clinically important difference (MCID) in hepatitis C patients were found.

SF-36 is a generic health instrument that has been used for assessment of HRQL and also in clinical trials to study the impact of chronic disease on HRQL. SF-36 uses eight scales: physical functioning, pain, vitality, social functioning, role emotional, role physical, general health perceptions (GH), and mental health. SF-36 also predicts two constituent summaries: the first one is physical component summary (SF-36 PCS), and the second is mental component summary (SF-36 MCS) [20]. The SF-36 PCS, SF-36 MCS, and other eight scales are measured on a scale of 0 to 100 [21].

The CLDQ is a HRQL assessment for patients with chronic liver disease and involves 29 items divided into six different parts: abdominal symptoms, fatigue, systemic symptoms, activity, emotional function, and worry. For each item, the patient allocates a score of 1 (all the time) to 7 (none of the time). Finally, the domain score is divided by the number of items in the domain; therefore, scores are represented on a 1 to 7 scale. Consequently, it is important to emphasize that higher numbers indicate the best potential function [22].

4. Socioeconomic burden of HCV infection and HRQL

Chronic liver disease is a major medical and public health problem worldwide. Reports from the European Center for Disease Prevention and Control indicate that the prevalence of chronic hepatitis B virus (HBV) infection in the general population ranges from 0.2% to over 7% in the different European countries, while the prevalence of hepatitis C virus (HCV) varies from 0.4% to over 3% in Mediterranean countries [23].

Hepatitis C virus is a blood-borne disease that infects approximately 160 million people worldwide [24]. The infection has been transmitted through blood transfusions, contaminated injections during medical treatments, and through needle-sharing by injection drug users [25]. Combined efforts to educate the injection drug use population and anticipate different methods by which they can acquire sterile needles are indispensable and relatively economical, especially in countries where prevention and support programs for substance abusers are developed [26, 27]. Testing populations at high risk for HCV infection reduce economic burden by identifying patients with HCV infection and anticipating early therapy, hence potentially preventing progression to more serious and costly complications.

Nevertheless, HCV is asymptomatic, and nowadays, most new cases go undiscovered and approximately 75% become chronic conditions [23] which increases risk for cirrhosis, liver failure, and hepatocellular carcinoma (HCC) [28]. Economic burden is multiplied by the impact of HCV on HRQL resulting from complications of some liver diseases such as encephalopathy, variceal hemorrhage, ascites, and need for liver transplantation [29].

The recognition that the burden of HCV expands beyond its economic impact corresponds with recommendations by the NIH to conduct studies that measure not only traditional biological results in HCV, such as HCV RNA, liver enzyme levels, liver histology, but also patient-oriented results [30]. However, clinicians often do not use HRQL in HCV, and patient-oriented results may fail to resonate with clinicians in the same way as long-established practice. In light of the disconnect between the growing significance of measuring HRQL in the HCV population and the incompetence of clinicians to interpret HRQL differences, it is crucial to establish the clinical importance of HRQL score differences by anchoring them to changes in clinically familiar results [31]. In conclusion, public health officials, physicians, and patients should also discuss the impact of HCV infection on HRQL when considering treatment strategies [32].

5. HCV infection impact on HRQL

Patients with chronic hepatitis C have a decreased HRQL compared to the general population. The impact of HCV infection on physical well-being is comparable to other chronic diseases or some stressful life events [33]. Many symptoms of chronic HCV infection negatively affect patients' functional health, psychological well-being, and self-perceived health (**Figure 1**). HCV patients commonly experience physical and psychiatric symptoms as a direct consequence of chronic infection and its sequelae.

HCV causes both hepatic and extrahepatic manifestations. The clinical outcomes of the hepatic manifestations include hepatocellular carcinoma and cirrhosis, which are the primary indications for liver transplantation. HCV infection is also associated with a range of extrahepatic manifestations including mixed cryoglobulinemia, vasculitis, arthritis, thyroid disease, and type 2 diabetes [34]. Somatic symptoms of chronic HCV infection include fatigue, nausea, anorexia, headache, irritability, abdominal discomfort, and muscle aches [35, 38]. Fatigue is among the most frequent and disabling complaints of chronic

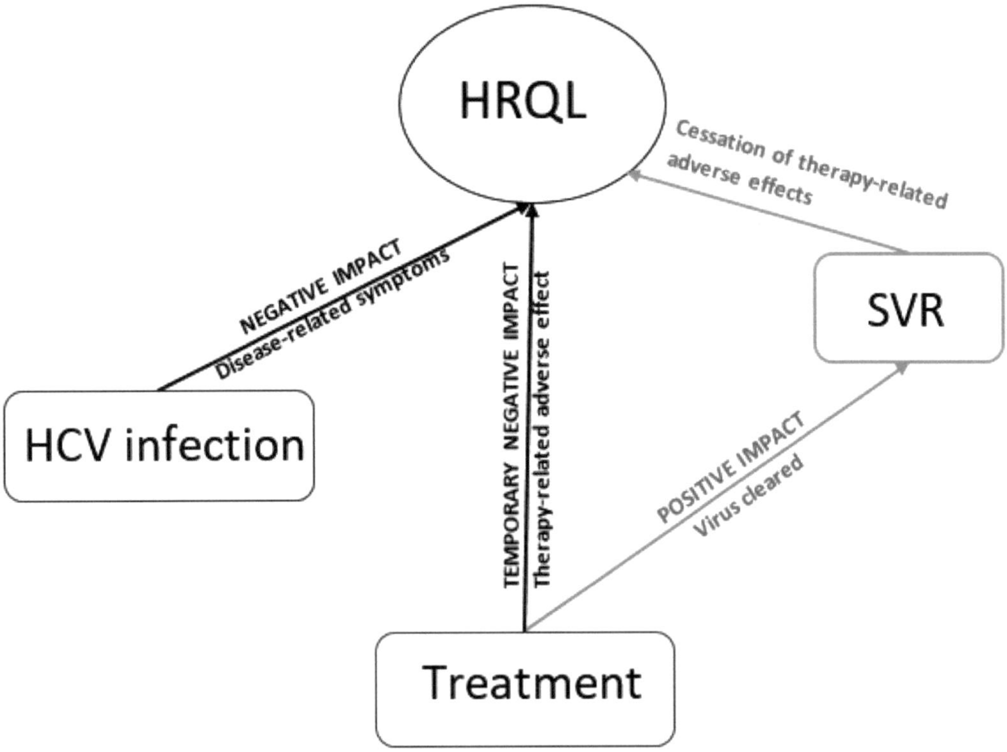

Figure 1. Chronic infection with hepatitis C compromises HRQL due to disease-related symptoms. Antiviral therapy affects HRQL negatively through side effects, but successful treatment of CHC improves HRQL because of cessation of treatment-related adverse effects and also due to disease eradication and virus clearance.

hepatitis C, and it serves as an independent predictor of low HRQL. Neuropsychological symptoms and hepatic encephalopathy can be found among patients with chronic hepatitis C, as well as mild cognitive deficits. Those symptoms may be the result of released inflammatory cytokines and altered neurotransmission [35]. Depression is another common feature of chronic hepatitis C which has been shown to be associated with lower work and social adjustment, lower acceptance of illness, and higher rates of subjective physical symptoms [36]. It is possible that mood-related aspects of HRQL are mediated by HCV colonization of brain microglia.

Poor baseline HRQL is partly psychosocial in origin, relating to the psychiatric comorbidity associated with acquisition of HCV, stigma of illness, and history of illicit drug use [37]. Patients with HCV infection are stigmatized in society which affects their HRQL but may also be a barrier to treatment, resulting in decreased social support [36]. Chronic hepatitis C as a disease with uncertain outcome raises serious concerns about future health status and presents significant emotional and psychological burden. Patients with chronic HCV infection aware of their diagnosis had worse HRQL scores as compared with unaware seropositive patients, suggesting the psychological impact of diagnosis awareness.

HCV patients who experience greater physical and psychiatric symptoms and have poorer HRQL are more likely to discontinue treatment prematurely. These issues highlight the importance of investigating the physical and psychosocial experiences and HRQL of patients chronically infected with HCV [38].

6. HCV treatment impact on HRQL

Patient-reported outcome (PRO) measures are important to evaluate the impact of chronic infection, willingness for treatment and assessment of HRQL during and post treatment. These measures ensure that patient preferences are taken into consideration when deciding between treatment options. While antiviral treatment can eradicate the virus and prevent liver-related death, associated toxicity can have effect on HRQL by decreasing physical, social, and emotional functioning [39].

In recent years, treatment options for HCV infection have moved from the use of interferon with low efficacy and significant toxicity to first-generation direct antiviral agents (DAAs) which were more efficient but still toxic to interferon-free regimens with high efficacy and minimal toxicity [40].

Besides HRQL burden of HCV infection, the previous anti-HCV treatment with interferon and ribavirin had further negative impact on patients' HRQL due to substantial side effects. Well documented side effects of interferon include fever, myalgias, and headache, often described as influenza-like illness. IFN-mediated myelosuppression may lead to decreases in erythrocyte, leukocyte, and platelet counts. Neuropsychiatric side effects include irritability, depression, anxiety, and fatigue. Fatigue is the most commonly reported adverse effect which occurs as a part of neurovegetative symptoms during the first 3 months of treatment [41]. Anorexia, nausea, vomiting, and diarrhea are gastrointestinal adverse effect [36]. Adding RBV to interferon improves SVR, but it substantially impairs physical functioning, which may be the result of hemolytic anemia, occasional rash, and additional fatigue [42]. The use of peg-IFN and RBV is associated with less fatigue and bodily pain than standard IFN and RBV, but it is also characterized by considerable toxicity, neuropsychiatric side-effects, lethargy, and influenza-like symptoms [43]. The side effects of HCV therapy increase the likelihood that patients will discontinue treatment, and because of that, adjunctive therapy must be considered to treat those side effects. Fatigue, depression, and anemia are more difficult to control so addressing those symptoms is of major importance for patients' adherence to therapy [36].

However, successful clearance of the virus after treatment results in certain HRQL improvement in patients who respond well to therapy. Patient-reported outcomes, including HRQL, fatigue, and work productivity improved in patients after achieving sustained virologic response (SVR) with interferon and ribavirin-containing regimens [44]. Therefore, reaching SVR is crucial in achieving long-term HRQL in patients with chronic HCV infection.

The first-generation direct antiviral agents (DAA) shifted the treatment focus to protease inhibitors (PI). A triple combination therapy (PEG-IFN + ribavirin + a protease inhibitor) increased SVR rates but decreased HRQL. Along with the pegylated interferon and RBV side effects, PIs carried plenty of additional side effects. Telaprevir treatment causes nausea, rectal burning, diarrhea, and recently, it has been connected to decrease renal function. Lower glomerular filtration rate led to decreased renal elimination of RBV. Boceprevir has been associated with nausea, headache, and anemia. Furthermore, these regimens had significant drug–drug interactions (DDIs) [41]. However, symptom alleviation after successful treatment can improve HRQL, having economic and social benefits and resulting in removal of social stigma [39].

The next generation of DAAs focused on different targets: HCV viral replication in the cytoplasm. These new drugs, given without concomitant interferon, can result in SVR in over 90% of cases. Additionally, toxicity is reduced in comparison with second generation triple combinations, although response is influenced by genotype, stage of hepatic fibrosis, and drug-resistant mutations [39]. Shortly after initiation of treatment, there is an improvement in PRO scores which correlates with viral suppression. Furthermore, therapy with the new generation of DAAs maximizes PRO rates during treatment as well as after achieving SVR [40]. Most of the data about HRQL come from sofosbuvir (SOF)-based treatment options. Analysis showed that the PRO profile of interferon-free regimens (SOF/RBV) was significantly better compared to peg-IFN/RBV regimens. However, RBV-containing regimens still carry important HRQL impairment, possibly due to hemolytic anemia and mental health side effects of RBV. When both RBV and interferon are removed from the regimen, improvements in HRQL, work productivity, and other PROs were noted 2 weeks after starting treatment (**Figure 1**) [41].

7. The road to success: future directions to improve HCV HRQL

Regardless of the regimen, there are significant improvements in PRO scores after achieving SVR. Still, these improvements are more noticeable in patients who achieve SVR with DAAs. It is shown in multivariate analysis that receiving a regimen that contained IFN and RBV was the strongest negative predictor of HRQL during treatment [45]. On the other hand, IFN- and RBV-free was the only regimen independently associated with improved HRQL during treatment. Moreover, DAAs remained the only independent predictor of HRQL improvement after achieving SVR [46]. However, there are still unanswered questions in terms of DAA safety, and we require data from real-world settings. For example, postauthorization studies would be useful to identify and characterize safety profiles of the new DAAs [47].

8. Conclusions

Chronic HCV infection causes a decline in HRQL measures through a broad spectrum of clinical complaints. The impact on HRQL affects physical, social, and mental health domains. SVR is associated with improvement in HRQL, thereby indicating that treatment of HCV may

http://dx.doi.org/10.5772/intechopen.70766

improve PRO rates in patients who respond well to therapy. Considering low efficacy and significant toxicity of IFN/RBV regimens, treatment options are shifting to the new DAAs which offer improved SVR rates with less toxicity, leading to improvements in HRQL in patients with chronic hepatitis C.

Author details

Aleksandar Včev[1,2]*, Jelena Jakab[2], Lucija Kuna[2] and Martina Smolić[2,3]

*Address all correspondence to: aleksandar.vcev@mefos.hr

1 Department of Medicine, Faculty of Medicine Osijek, University of Osijek, Osijek, Croatia

2 Department of Integrative Medicine, Faculty of Medicine Osijek, University of Osijek, Osijek, Croatia

3 Department of Pharmacology, Faculty of Medicine Osijek, University of Osijek, Osijek, Croatia

References

[1] Coletta SL. Adults with congenital heart disease: Utilizing quality of life and Husted's nursing theory as a conceptual framework. Critical Care Nursering Quarterly. 1999;**22**(3): 1-11

[2] Moons P. Why call it health-related quality of life when you mean perceived health status? European Journal of Cardiovascular Nursing. 2004;**3**(4):275-277

[3] Canavarro MC, Serra AV, Simões MR, Rijo D, Pereira M, Gameiro S, et al. Development and psychometric properties of the World Health Organization quality of life assessment instrument (WHOQOL-100) in Portugal. International Journal of Behavioral Medicine. 2009;**16**(2):116-124

[4] Diener Ed, Seligman M.E.P. Beyond money: toward an economy of well-being. Psychological Science in the Public Interest. 2004;**5**(1):1-31

[5] The WHOQOL Group. The World Health Organization Quality of Life assessment (WHOQOL): position paper from the World Health Organization. Soc Sci Med. 1995; **41**(10):1403-9

[6] Colin M. Respondent-generated quality of life measures: Useful tools for nursing or more fool's gold? Journal of Advanced Nursing. 2000;**32**(2):375-382

[7] Kamphuis M, Zwinderman KH, Vogels T, Vliegen HW, Kamphuis RP, Ottenkamp J, et al. A cardiac-specific health-related quality of life module for young adults with congenital heart disease: Development and validation. Quality of Life Research. 2004;**13**(4):735-745

[8] Gill TM, Feinstein AR. A critical appraisal of the quality of quality-of-life measurements. Journal of the American Medical Association. 1994;**272**(8):619-626

[9] Ferrans CE. Development of a conceptual model of quality of life. Scholarly Inquiry for Nursing Practice. 1996;**10**(3):293-304

[10] McHorney CA. Health status assessment methods for adults: Past accomplishments and future challenges. Annual Review of Public Health. 1999;**20**:309-335

[11] Velikova G, Booth L, Smith AB, Brown PM, Lynch P, Brown JM, et al. Measuring quality of life in routine oncology practice improves communication and patient well-being: A randomized controlled trial. Journal of Clinical Oncology. 2004;**22**(4):714-724

[12] Coons SJ, Rao S, Keininger DL, Hays RD. A comparative review of generic quality-of-life instruments. PharmacoEconomics. 2000;**17**(1):13-35

[13] Nelson EC, Wasson JH, Johnson DJ, Hays RD. Dartmouth COOP Functional Health Assessment Charts: Brief measures for clinical practice. in: B Spilker (Ed.) Quality of Life and Pharmacoeconomics in Clinical Trials. ed 2. Lippincott-Raven, Philadelphia, PA; 1996

[14] Cella D, Yount S, Rothrock N, Gershon R, Cook K, Reeve B, et al. The patient-reported outcomes measurement information system (PROMIS): Progress of an NIH roadmap cooperative group during its first two years. Medical Care. 2007;**45**(5 Suppl 1):S3-S11

[15] Lyubomirsky S, King L, Diener E. The benefits of frequent positive affect: Does happiness lead to success? Psychological Bulletin. 2005;**131**(6):803-855

[16] Ed D. Well-Being for Public Policy. New York: Oxford University Press. Oxford Scholarship Online; 2010

[17] Albrecht GL, Devlieger PJ. The disability paradox: High quality of life against all odds. Social Science & Medicine. 1999;**48**(8):977-988

[18] Ronald DM. Healthy People 2010: national health objectives for United States. BMJ. 1998;**317**(7171):1513-1517

[19] Smith-Palmer J, Cerri K, Valentine W. Achieving sustained virologic response in hepatitis C: A systematic review of the clinical, economic and quality of life benefits. BMC Infectious Diseases. 2015;**15**:19

[20] Webster K, Cella D, Yost K. The functional assessment of chronic illness therapy (FACIT) measurement system: Properties, applications, and interpretation. Health and Quality of Life Outcomes. 2003;**1**:79

[21] Younossi ZM, Stepanova M, Henry L, Gane E, Jacobson IM, Lawitz E, et al. Effects of sofosbuvir-based treatment, with and without interferon, on outcome and productivity of patients with chronic hepatitis C. Clinical Gastroenterology and Hepatology. 2014;**12**(8): 1349-1359 e13

[22] Younossi ZM, Guyatt G, Kiwi M, Boparai N, King D. Development of a disease specific questionnaire to measure health related quality of life in patients with chronic liver disease. Gut. 1999;**45**(2):295-300

[23] Luciana S. The societal burden of chronic liver diseases: results from the COME study. BMJ Open Gastroenterol. 2015;**2**(1):e000025. Published online 2015 Mar 30. DOI:10.1136/bmjgast-2014-000025

[24] Lavanchy D. Evolving epidemiology of hepatitis C virus. Clinical Microbiology and Infection. 2011;**17**(2):107-115

[25] Van Herck K, Vorsters A, Van Damme P. Prevention of viral hepatitis (B and C) reassessed. Best Practice & Research. Clinical Gastroenterology. 2008;**22**(6):1009-1029

[26] NIH Consensus Statement on management of hepatitis C: 2002. NIH Consensus and State-of-The-Science Statements. 2002;**19**(3):1-46

[27] Edlin BR, Kresina TF, Raymond DB, Carden MR, Gourevitch MN, Rich JD, et al. Overcoming barriers to prevention, care, and treatment of hepatitis C in illicit drug users. Clinical Infectious Diseases. 2005;**40**(Suppl 5):S276-S285

[28] McHutchison JG, Bacon BR, Owens GS. Making it happen: Managed care considerations in vanquishing hepatitis C. The American Journal of Managed Care. 2007;**13**(Suppl 12): S327-S336 quiz S37-40

[29] Chong CA, Gulamhussein A, Heathcote EJ, Lilly L, Sherman M, Naglie G, et al. Health-state utilities and quality of life in hepatitis C patients. The American Journal of Gastroenterology. 2003;**98**(3):630-638

[30] Seeff LB, Hoofnagle JH. National Institutes of Health consensus development conference: Management of hepatitis C: 2002. Hepatology. 2002;**36**(5 Suppl 1):S1-S2

[31] Spiegel BMR. Impact of hepatitis C on health related quality of Life: A systematic review and quantitative assessment. Hepatology. 2005;**41**:790-800

[32] El Khoury AC, Vietri J, Prajapati G. Health-related quality of life in patients with hepatitis C virus infection in Brazil. Revista Panamericana de Salud Pública. 2014;**35**(3):200-206

[33] Bezemer G, Van Gool AR, Verheij-Hart E, Hansen BE, Lurie Y, Esteban JI, et al. Long-term effects of treatment and response in patients with chronic hepatitis C on quality of life. An international, multicenter, randomized, controlled study. BMC Gastroenterology. 2012;**12**:11

[34] Kallman J, O'Neil MM, Larive B, Boparai N, Calabrese L, Younossi ZM. Fatigue and health-related quality of life (HRQL) in chronic hepatitis C virus infection. Digestive Diseases and Sciences. 2007;**52**(10):2531-2539

[35] Vera-Llonch M, Martin M, Aggarwal J, Donepudi M, Bayliss M, Goss T, et al. Health-related quality of life in genotype 1 treatment-naïve chronic hepatitis C patients receiving telaprevir combination treatment in the ADVANCE study. Alimentary Pharmacology & Therapeutics. 2013;**38**(2):124-133

[36] Younossi ZM, Kallman J, Kincaid J. The effects of HCV infection and management on health-related quality of life. Hepatology. 2007;**45**(3):806-816

[37] Isaacs D, Abdelaziz N, Keller M, Tibble J, Haq I. Measuring the response of extrahepatic symptoms and quality of life to antiviral treatment in patients with hepatitis C. Hepatitis Research and Treatment. 2013;**2013**:910519

[38] Dan AA, Martin LM, Crone C, Ong JP, Farmer DW, Wise T, et al. Depression, anemia and health-related quality of life in chronic hepatitis C. Journal of Hepatology. 2006;**44**(3):491-498

[39] Armstrong AR, Herrmann S, Carrieri P, Chassany O, Duracinsky M. The international development of PROQOL-HCV: An instrument to assess the health-related quality of life of persons living with the Hepatitis C virus. BMC Infectious Diseases. 2016;**16**(443):1-11

[40] Younossi ZM, Stepanova M, Feld J, Zeuzem S, Sulkowski M, Foster GR, et al. Sofosbuvir and Velpatasvir Combination Improves Patient-reported Outcomes With HCV Infection, Without or With Compensated or Decompensated Cirrhosis. Clin Gastroenterol Hepatol. 2016;**15**(3):421-430

[41] Raison CL, Demetrashvili M, Capuron L, Miller AH. Neuropsychiatric adverse effects of interferon-α. CNS Drugs. 2005;**19**(2):105-123

[42] Lam BP, Jeffers T, Younoszai Z, Fazel Y, Younossi ZM. The changing landscape of hepatitis C virus therapy: Focus on interferon-free treatment. Therapeutic Advances in Gastroenterology. 2015;**8**(5):298-312

[43] Doyle JS, Grebely J, Spelman T, Alavi M, Matthews GV, Thompson AJ, et al. Quality of Life and Social Functioning during Treatment of Recent Hepatitis C Infection: A Multi-Centre Prospective Cohort. PLoS ONE. 2016;**11**(6):e0150655. https://doi.org/10.1371/journal.pone.0150655

[44] Younossi ZM, Stepanova M, Afdhal N, Kowdley KV, Zeuzem S, Henry L, et al. Improvement of health-related quality of life and work productivity in chronic hepatitis C patients with early and advanced fibrosis treated with ledipasvir and sofosbuvir. Journal of Hepatology. 2015;**63**(2):337-345

[45] Younossi ZM, Stepanova M, Henry L, Nader F, Hunt S. An in-depth analysis of patient-reported outcomes in patients with chronic hepatitis C treated with different anti-viral regimens. The American Journal of Gastroenterology. 2016;**111**:808-816

[46] Younossi ZM, Stepanova M, Nader F, Lam B, Hunt S. The patient's journey with chronic hepatitis C from interferon plus ribavirin to interferon- and ribavirin-free regimens: A study of health-related quality of life. Alimentary Pharmacology & Therapeutics. 2015;**42**(3):286-295

[47] Scavone C, Sportiello L, Rafaniello C, Mascolo A, Sessa M, Rossi F, et al. New era in treatment options of chronic hepatitis C: Focus on safety of new direct-acting antivirals (DAAs). Expert Opinion on Drug Safety. 2016;**15**(Suppl 2):85-100

Section 4

From Scientific Concepts to the Cure

Chapter 14

Pharmacogenomic Testing in the Era of Patient-Tailored HCV Treatment

Martina Smolić, Tea Omanović, Ivana Božić,
Ines Bilić-Ćurčić, Robert Smolić and Aleksandar Včev

Additional information is available at the end of the chapter

http://dx.doi.org/10.5772/intechopen.70794

Abstract

Hepatitis C affects approximately 180 million people worldwide, with 3–4 million newly infected each year. Hepatitis C virus (HCV) has been classified into seven different genotype categories, wherein HCV genotype 1 (HCV-1) is the most prevalent. To date, there is still no vaccine available against HCV infection. Until recently, combination therapy of pegylated interferon-a (PegIFN) and ribavirin (RBV) has been the standard of care. Nevertheless, for many patients, particularly those infected with HCV genotype 1 (HCV-1), this treatment has resulted with unsatisfactory treatment response rates and high adverse drug reaction (ADR) rates. Many clinical factors, including pharmacogenetics, influence the treatment response rate. This review focuses on the association between pharmacogenetics and HCV antiviral therapy in patients infected with HCV genotype 1 and other genotypes (GT); patients reinfected with HCV after liver transplantation; and patients coinfected with HCV and human immunodeficiency virus. Data considering triple therapy in HCV-infected patients are also reviewed. Additionally, various genetic polymorphisms, with an emphasis to IL-28B, and their association with pharmacogenetic testing in HCV are discussed.

Keywords: hepatitis C virus, pharmacogenetics, pegylated interferon and ribavirin, direct-acting antiviral agents, genetic polymorphisms, IL-28B, ITPA

1. Introduction

1.1. Clinical background of HCV infection

Infection with hepatitis C virus (HCV), an enveloped single-stranded RNA virus of the *Flaviviridae* family, affects over 2% of the worldwide population and it is estimated that the number of people with a chronic HCV infection is over 180 million, representing an important public health issue [1, 2]. Epidemiological studies have shown that 46.2% of all hepatitis C cases are caused by HCV GT1, making GT1 the most prevalent genotype [3]. Even though most of the patients initially do not experience any symptoms, about 75% are not able to spontaneously clear the virus from the organism, and develop a chronic HCV infection [4]. HCV causes progressive liver injury in those patients, which in approximately 16% progress to liver cirrhosis and ultimately in 1–5%, within two decades from acute infection, to hepatocellular carcinoma. Therefore, HCV infection is one of the most common reasons for liver failure and an indication for liver transplantation procedures worldwide [5–7]. HCV has been classified into seven different genotype categories, having nucleotide differences of greater than 30% among genotypes (GT). Due to that fact, the task to produce pan-genotypic drugs has been very demanding [8]. Accordingly, the response of HCV infection to treatment regimens and its duration can vary depending on viral genotype [9].

1.2. Changes in the HCV treatment goals and HCV treatment timeline development

The search for optimal hepatitis C treatment has been ongoing even before the HCV had been cloned in 1989 [10, 11]. The ultimate goal of every standard-of-care treatment from that point in history was the cure of hepatitis C, in particular, the removal of the virus from the organism and prevention of further liver damage due to HCV. A patient is considered to be cured when sustained virological response (SVR) is reached, defined as undetectable HCV RNA viral load 24 or 12 weeks post-therapy [12, 13]. Formerly, SVR had been determined 6 months (24 weeks) after completion of treatment with interferon-cased therapy. However, with direct-acting agents, that are so much more potent, it has been shown that the viral clearance can be assessed 12 weeks after therapy. Thus, SVR12 is the currently advised standard [14, 15]. At the time when interferon (IFN)-α was approved as the first anti-HCV drug in the SVR, it was only achieved in 2–7% of treated patients [16]. The addition of ribavirin (RBV) and the later change of IFN-α to its pegylated form (PegIFN (pegylated interferon-a)) in the therapeutic regimen increased the SVR marginally. Even though the dual therapy containing PegIFN-RBV showed to be a considerably effective treatment for patients who were infected with HCV GT2 or GT3, achieving SVR in up to 80% of the treated patients, the success in curing patients infected with HCV GT1 was still izbaciti R skroz below 50% despite treatment prolongation up to 72 weeks [17, 18]. Also, many treated patients suffered from severe and potentially life threatening adverse drug reactions (ADRs) such as influenza-like syndrome, anemia, leukopenia, thrombocytopenia, depression, concentration issues, gastrointestinal ADRs, etc., which often led to preterm therapy dismissal [19]. Consequently, there was a great need to develop novel targeted drugs, with higher efficacy and fewer ADRs. In order to develop such drugs, scientific progress in the fields of virology, molecular biology, and biochemistry and an understanding of the individual steps in the HCV replication cycle had to be determined. This led to the discovery of contributing viral proteins such as NS3/4A protease, NS5A polymerase, and NS5B replication complex as possible therapeutic targets [20]. The development of ciluprevir (Biln 2061), the first NS3 protease inhibitor (PI), in 2002 was the first attempt to develop direct-acting antivirals (DAA) and influence the HCV replication

http://dx.doi.org/10.5772/intechopen.70794

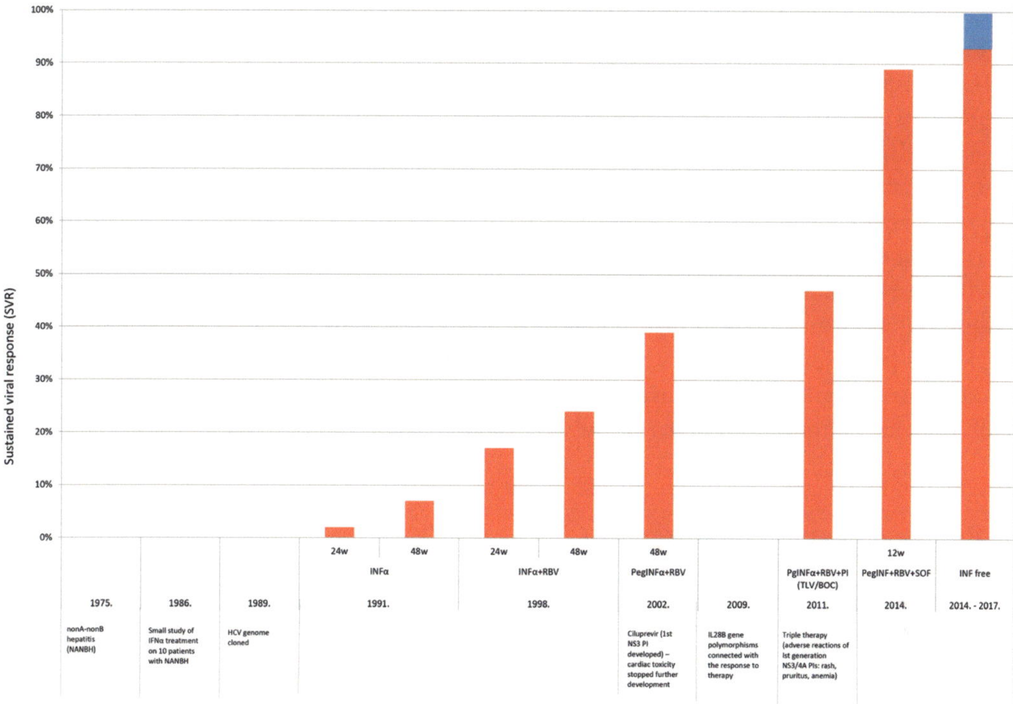

Figure 1. Timeline of discoveries in the history of HCV and the dynamics of SVR through time depending on the standard-of-care treatment. SVR rates did improve greatly since 1991, when IFN-α got approved as the first drug for patients with hepatitis C. Nowadays, the therapy with DAAs made chronic hepatitis C a curable disease with SVR rates over 93%.

cycle (**Figure 1**). Even though ciluprevir was found to perform rapid antiviral activity, the clinical trials had to be discontinued due to cardiac toxicity and this drug was never approved for use [21–23]. Telaprevir (TLV) and boceprevir (BOC) were approved in combination with PegIFN and ribavirin (RBV) for the treatment of HCV GT1 infections by the FDA in May 2011. These were the first DAAs to reach the market [24–26]. Whereas, the so-called triple therapy, containing one of the two NS3/4A inhibitors TLV or BOC with PegIFN and RBV, markedly increased the number of patients with HCV GT1 infections achieving SVR in >70%, severe ADRs often led to discontinuation of therapy [27–29]. Indeed, since the triple therapy also involved PegIFN and RBV, some adverse effects induced by those drugs were persistent compared with the previous treatment regimen. However, the addition of NS3/4A protease inhibitor (PI) not only intensified some of the IFN-induced ADRs such as anemia, but also led to novel side effects like skin rashes, gastrointestinal disorders and dysgeusia [18, 30]. In November 2013, simeprevir (SMV), as a second generation NS3/4A inhibitor was approved by the FDA, which contrary to prior developed drugs in this class, was more convenient regarding dosing and had fewer ADRs [31, 32]. Subsequently, the first HCV NS5B polymerase inhibitor sofosbuvir (SOF) was approved. The combination of SOF with PegIFN and RBV shortened the treatment to 12 weeks and achieved SVR in 90% of the treated patients [33].

Finally, in 2014, a great step forward was made regarding pharmacotherapy of HCV-infected patients by the approval of first all-oral IFN-free regimens. The first IFN-free regimens, 3D-combination dasabuvir (DSV) plus ombitasvir (OBV) plus paritaprevir/ritonavir (PTV/r) +/− RBV (whereby OBV has been the first approved drug in the class of NS5A inhibitors), as well as ledipasvir (LDV) plus sofosbuvir (SOF were marketed in 2014 [34, 35]. Moreover, in July 2015, daclatasvir (DCL) and the fixed combination of OBV plus paritaprevir plus ritonavir became FDA approved, followed by elbasvir plus grazoprevir as well as velpatasvir plus sofosbuvir in 2016 [36–39]. Presently, as a result of IFN-free DAA treatment regimens, 92–100% of treatment naïve patients infected with HCV GT1 achieve SVR [40]. Provided that with IFN-free treatments shortage of therapy duration, improvements in efficacy and fewer ADRs are possible, the prospect of HCV eradication became a real opportunity rather than an unachievable goal [41]. However, the extremely high costs of IFN-free regimens combined with limited healthcare resources hinder accessibility of this valuable therapy worldwide.

2. Pharmacogenetic testing

During the past decades, much effort has been applied toward improvement of the safety and efficiency of drugs used for the treatment of many diseases, including hepatitis C. Adverse drug reactions (ADRs) are a significant cause of morbidity and mortality in patients. However, existing evidence considering individualization of pharmacotherapeutic regimens based on the patient genetic information indicate that ADRs could be at least partially overcome by the application of pharmacogenetics and pharmacogenomics. Pharmacogenetics is a scientific field for studying differences in drug response and the occurrence of adverse drug reactions due to the genetic impact of variations in individual genes, whereas pharmacogenomics studies the impact of the whole genome on drug response, nowadays using genome-wide association studies (GWAS) as successful tools [42–44].

Pharmacogenomics is a rapidly emerging and promising scientific field, used to improve drug safety by avoiding specific drugs to susceptible individuals who are likely to develop ADRs [45]. Although there are still challenges remaining, with the improvement of study designs and the establishment of international cooperation pharmacogenomic study results could be validated and pharmacogenetic testing could become a clinical reality [45, 46]. Additional studies with even more participants are likely to yield results in the near future, which could enhance the number of clinical implementations of pharmacogenetic test results and make another step toward personalized medicine [46]. The cost-effectiveness of drugs is likely to improve by the implementation of pharmacogenomic tests, since the drugs should be used only to treat patients expected to experience a satisfactory therapeutic effect, with minimal risk for morbidity and mortality [47–50]. Furthermore, it is of enormous significance to educate clinicians on data interpretation of pharmacogenetic test results, so that they could gain the required knowledge to accurately stratify patients into high risk or low risk groups regarding drug toxicity. Consequently, therapeutic outcome would be improved without putting susceptible patients at risk of predictable life threatening ADRs. Therefore, new user-friendly and up-to-date guidelines should be made for clinicians, which could help the future implementation of pharmacogenomic study results into the clinical daily routine [45, 51–53].

3. HCV pharmacogenetic testing in the IFN era

As previously mentioned, combination of PegIFN and RBV had been the standard-of-care for patients with chronic hepatitis C for more than a decade [9]. Notwithstanding, many patients still did not respond to therapy and could not achieve SVR or developed adverse events [54]. It has been noticed that many clinical factors, including pharmacogenetics, could influence the treatment response rate [9]. Both virological factors (such as HCV genotype, quasispecies diversity, and baseline viremia) and host factors (age, gender, race-ethnicity, fibrosis stage, obesity, hepatic steatosis, low-density lipoprotein cholesterol, insulin resistance, and genetic variances) played an important role in predicting the natural course of hepatitis C and IFN response to therapy [7, 55–57]. Pharmacogenetic testing could play very important role in optimizing HCV therapy by identifying variations in response to treatment, considering ethnic variations in response to therapy, enlightening the molecular mechanism of current and future therapies, and advancement of innovative genetic tools that will enable physicians to individualize drug therapy, adjust dosages, and reduce the possibility of adverse drug reactions and therapeutic costs (**Table 1**) [54, 58]. Over 40 genes have been linked to modulation of anti-HCV therapy affecting either adverse drug events or response to treatment [59, 60].

Genetic polymorphism	Mechanism of action	Favorable genotypes	Use in predicting treatment outcomes	Use in predicting adverse drug events
IL28B rs8099917 IL28B rs12979860	Triggers JAK-STAT pathway and activates ISG	rs8099917 TT rs12979860 CC	HCV 1, HCV 4 infection, liver transplantation, HIV-HCV coinfection	NO
ITPA rs1127354 ITPA rs7270101	Reduced ITPA activity advances the accumulation of ITP in erythrocytes, reduces ATP depletion and protects against hemolytic anemia caused by RBV	rs1127354 AA/AC rs7270101 CC/CA	NO	HCV 1 infection, HIV-HCV coinfection
G protein b3 unit (GNB3) C825T	Transmits signals via the G protein-coupled receptors, consequently advancing immune response	rs5443 TT	HIV-HCV coinfection	NO
LDLR rs14158	Decreases HCV entry into hepatocytes	rs14158 CC rs12979860 CC	HCV-1 infection, HIV-HCV coinfection	NO
CTLA4 A49G	Decreases suppression of T-cell proliferation, adjusts the threshold of T-cell activation	rs231775 GG	HCV-1 infection, HIV-HCV coinfection	NO
IL 6* C174G	Involved in liver regeneration and in protection against hepatic injury	rs1800795 GG	HCV-1 infection, HIV-HCV coinfection	NO

Abbreviations: IL28B, interleukin 28B; ITPA, inosinetriphosphatase; LDLR, low-density lipoprotein receptor; CTLA, cytotoxic lymphocyte antigen 4; IL 6, interleukin 6.

Note: Data for IL28B from Kamal [54], for ITPA, G protein b3 unit, LDLR, CTLA4 and for IL 6 from Kawaguchi-Suzuki and Fyre [9].

Table 1. Most important host genetic polymorphisms associated with HCV pharmacogenetic testing in the IFN era.

3.1. IL 28B polymorphisms in prediction of HCV infection treatment outcome

IL 28B gene belongs to the type III IFN family named IFN-λ located on the human chromosome 19, and corresponds to IFN-$\lambda 3$ [7]. Viral infection induces the corresponding cytokines and their antiviral activity is mediated by triggering JAK–STAT pathway [61–63]. ISGs (interferon stimulated genes), which are known to cause apoptosis, growth inhibition, and inhibition of viral replication, are activated by JAK–STAT pathway [64].

3.1.1. IL 28B polymorphisms and HCV1 infection

Several GWAS have demonstrated the role of SNPs near the interleukin 28B (IL 28B) gene in predicting PegIFN/RBV treatment outcome and spontaneous clearance of HCV infection [7, 55]. Two bi-allelic SNPs were most strongly associated with favorable response in HCV genotype 1 (HCV-1) infected patients: rs8099917 located 8 kb downstream of the IL28B gene (favorable response TT genotype, and unfavorable GT/GG genotypes) and rs12979860 located 3 kb upstream of the IL28B gene (favorable response CC genotype, and unfavorable CT/TT genotypes) [7]. Other SNPs of IL28B (rs8105790, rs11881222, rs28416813, rs4803219, and rs7248668) have been also identified in HCV genotype 1-infected patients, but they have not yet been strongly associated with the treatment outcome [55]. It has been shown that unfavorable IL28B genotypes expressed higher baseline ISGs levels compared with the favorable genotype, which could indicate an exhaustion of innate immunity prior to treatment in patients with unfavorable IL28B genotype [65–67]. In contrast, rs12979860 CC and rs8099917 TT genotypes were associated with low ISG expression at baseline, which led to greater ISG expression upon IFN treatment and better treatment responses [68]. Differences in the SVR rates were large and clinically significant with a ~2-fold increase in SVR (70–80% vs. 40%) observed in patients carrying the favorable IL28B rs12979860 CC genotype [9]. Independent studies confirmed the association of the IL28B genotype with SVR in various populations from Asia, Europe, and Latin America [9]. The IL28B favorable genotype also indicates an increased likelihood of achieving SVR among a pediatric population [69]. These treatment response findings were confirmed in different populations: HCV GT1 patients, HCV GT4 patients, patients with a recent HCV infection, adults and children with a spontaneous HCV clearance, HCV/HIV co-infected patients and patients with a recurrent HCV infection after orthotopic liver transplantation [7].

3.1.2. IL28B polymorphisms and HCV2/3 infection

Studies have shown different results which relate to association of IL28B SNP and HCV 2/3 genotype infection. Mangia et al. showed that IL28B SNP rs12979860 was significantly associated with SVR to PEG-IFN/ribavirin therapy in chronic HCV genotype 2/3 [70]. Other studies demonstrated that the difference in the SVR rates between the IL28B genotypes was generally smaller in HCV-2/3 infections than in genotype 1 infection, which could indicate that IL28B has less value in predicting SVR in genotype 2 and 3 infections [9]. It is also possible that some studies did not achieve statistical significance because the SVR rates were generally high among patients infected with HCV-2/3 [9].

3.1.3. IL28B polymorphisms and liver transplantation

HCV reinfection after liver transplantation can occur in most patients and had represented the primary reason for death and graft loss in the pre-DAA era [71]. The cause of the reinfection of the new liver is residual HCV, and IL28B genotype was shown to be an important predictor of SVR for liver transplant recipients reinfected with HCV [9]. The rs12979860 CC and rs8099917 TT genotypes of the recipient were notably associated with higher SVR rates, and the same trend was detected with the donor genotype [72]. Although, both donor and recipient IL28B genotypes have been associated with treatment response, it has not yet been confirmed which genotype is the better indicator of SVR, but it is clear that having both genotypes would be most informative [9]. Most of the study participants were infected with HCV-1, with scarce evidence for HCV non-genotype 1 infections [9]. Considering that this is a complicated patient population, other clinical factors should not be ignored while therapeutic decisions are made [9].

3.1.4. IL28B polymorphisms and HIV-HCV coinfection

Several studies have confirmed the association between IL28B genotypes and treatment response in HIV/HCV coinfected patients [9]. rs12979860 CC genotype and rs8099917 TT genotype have been demonstrated as strong predictors of SVR in HIV/HCV coinfection [9, 68]. This association was observed in patients infected with genotype 1 and 4, but less obvious in patients with genotype 2 and 3 [9, 54, 68, 73]. SVR rates were generally higher among HCV-2 or 3-infected patients than those with HCV-1 or 4. Therefore, HCV2/3 genotype itself indicated good response to treatment [9]. Favorable rs12979860 CC genotype was associated with a higher SVR rate in a study of patients coinfected with HIV/HCV-1 or 4, even if patients were previous nonresponders to PegIFN/RBV therapy [73]. IL28B genotypes remained a good indicator of SVR, but they were not proven to affect HIV outcomes [73]. Consequently, IL28B genotypes should be interpreted only for the HCV outcomes, focusing on IFN-based treatment of patients coinfected with HIV/HCV-1 or 4.

3.2. ITPA in prediction of adverse drug reactions

Hemolytic anemia is a very common side effect of RBV-based HCV therapy [9, 55]. In clinical trials, 30% of treatment-naïve patients experienced anemia on PegIFN/RBV therapy, and most likely the major cause of anemia is ribavirin-induced hemolysis [68, 74]. Furthermore, in more than 15% of cases it is a cause of RBV dose reduction or premature discontinuation of RBV therapy, which may have had a deleterious impact on SVR [74, 75]. RBV depletes guanosine triphosphate (GTP) and causes a relative deficiency of ATP in human erythrocytes consequently inhibiting the ATP-dependent oxidative metabolism [7]. Depletion of erythrocyte ATP content leads to oxidative damage to the erythrocyte membranes, consequently causing extravascular hemolysis by the reticuloendothelial system [76–78]. ITPA gene encodes inosine-triphosphatase which is a protein that hydrolyses inosine triphosphate (ITP). A reduced ITPA activity advances the accumulation of ITP in erythrocytes allowing substitution of ITP for GTP in ATP biosynthesis which reduces ATP depletion and protects against hemolytic anemia [79–82]. Two functional SNPs (rs1127354 and rs7270101) in the ITPA gene, responsible for ITPA deficiency, were identified in two large GWAS [83, 84]. Consequently, the AA/$AC_{rs1127354}$ (for rs1127354, the wild-type and variant alleles are the C and A alleles) protective genotypes, as well as the $CC/CA_{rs7270101}$ (for rs7270101, the A allele is the wild type, and the C allele is the variant) protective genotypes, led to a decrease in hemolytic side effects from RBV therapy of HCV-1 infection [7]. Additionally, various studies showed an association between SNP ITPA and lower rates of clinically significant hemoglobin reduction among HIV/HCV coinfected patients [85–88]. Nevertheless, SNP ITPA does not predict SVR and was not associated to treatment outcomes [89]. However, considering that anemia is one of the main ADRs leading to premature withdrawal of therapy, any marker able to predict the risk of severe anemia before treatment would be of extreme importance [7]. For this purpose, two studies have designed predictions models incorporating *ITPA* genotype along with creatinine clearance, baseline hemoglobin and quantitative hemoglobin decline at week 2 of treatment [90, 91]. Further validation before entering these algorithms into clinical practice is necessary [7].

4. HCV pharmacogenetic testing in the IFN-free era

Since pharmacogenomics played a very important role in the era of IFN-based therapy, questions arose as to whether pharmacogenomic markers would still have a meaningful place in IFN-free treatment regimens involving DAA +/− ribavirin. Even though some studies suggested that HCV patients with the IL28B TT genotype had reduced therapeutic efficacy of some DAA regimens, IL28B genotyping did lose importance in the IFN-free era [15, 29, 92]. Furthermore, in African-American patients infected with HCV GT1a, ribavirin is recommended to be added to ombitasvir plus paritaprevir/ritonavir or dasabuvir treatment regimens to improve cure rates [93]. Even though IL28B is not as important for IFN-free treatments as it was before, genotyping is still being routinely performed in some countries in order to identify patients likely to be cured with older drugs at significantly lower cost.

While new, effective, and well-tolerated drugs with fewer ADRs and minimal monitoring requirements are on the market, the high treatment price is reducing accessibility, leading to compromises in the price-effectiveness area. The high cost of IFN-free treatment regimens leads to a resource-guided therapy assessment in countries with a lower national affordability for expensive DAAs [94]. The reason for further IL28B genotype determination in the era of available IFN-free treatments lies in the fact that patients with the interferon-favorable CC allele combination achieve SVR in 70–80% when treated with PegIFN plus ribavirin, which makes this treatment regimen only a relatively acceptable alternative for those patients in countries with deficient resources for new and expensive treatments [9, 94]. While in high-income countries like the USA as well as in most Northern and Western European countries, IFN-free treatments became first-line therapy for all patients with chronic HCV infections, in lower- or middle-income countries, which represent around 85% of the HCV related global health burden. This is still inaccessible for socioeconomic reasons [95–97]. In resource-limited countries, treatment naïve patients with IL28B CC allele, a viral load below 400,000–800,000 IU/ml and a low stage liver fibrosis (F1 and F2), are considered as good responders to a 24-week IFN-based therapy with SVR rates up to 80%with PegIFN plus ribavirin treatment [94, 95, 97]. However, even though patients with IL28B non-CC allele or a higher viral load are not considered easy-to-cure, the initial therapy in Croatia is PegIFN plus ribavirin for patients suffering from low stage liver fibrosis (F1 or F2), with a treatment duration of 24–48 weeks if rapid virological response (RVR, defined as not detectable HCV RNA 4 weeks after treatment start) is achieved [98, 99]. In patients where RVR is not achieved, simeprevir or sofosbuvir are added to the treatment [98]. However, priority for obtaining IFN-free treatment for treatment naïve patients is accessed by evaluation of the liver fibrosis stage according to Metavir classification (whereas, F3 and F4 stages as well as decompensated liver cirrhosis, where contraindications for IFN-based regimens exist, are being prioritized for DAA treatments). Also, patients with greater risk for disease progression, with the existence of extrahepatic manifestations of the HCV infection, those who are at higher risk of viral transmission, with a presence of HIV-HCV coinfection or in the case of prior liver transplantation should be receive priority [98, 100]. However, for socioeconomic reasons, patients with liver fibrosis stages F1, F2, or F3 with relapse or only partial response to previous therapy are being treated with PegIFN plus ribavirin plus sofosbuvir/simeprevir in Croatia [98].

5. Conclusion

We have witnessed remarkable improvement in HCV therapy options, resulting from cutting-edge discoveries. Treatment of HCV infection has been challenging since 1989, when HCV was first discovered and published [101]. After approval of interferon in 1992, great progress has been made. Consequently, many drugs have been introduced to clinical practice for HCV therapy [101]. In the late 2000s, another class of drugs, DAAs, was approved for use in combination therapy [101]. DAAs have been shown to be very effective HCV therapy, with high SVR rates and enhanced treatment safety. Nevertheless, barriers still remain in making these therapies accessible worldwide. Drug pricing, screening and disease assessment, and public health prioritization represent the biggest issues associated with DAAs treatment accessibility [102, 103]. Development of pharmacogenetic testing in the IFN-ribavirin era has been remarkable, leading to the discovery of various genetic polymorphisms associated with treatment outcome predictions. Although application of pharmacogenetic testing in IFN-free DAA era has been doubtful, it could play an important role in concept of "resource-guided therapy," where peginterferon/ribavirin might be applied for easy-to-treat interferon-eligible patients in resource-constrained areas [94]. Although treatment efficacy of HCV infection has increased dramatically, the goal of making the therapy available to everyone in need remains a major challenge.

Author details

Martina Smolić[1,2,3]*, Tea Omanović[1], Ivana Božić[1], Ines Bilić-Ćurčić[1,3,4], Robert Smolić[1,4] and Aleksandar Včev[2,3,4]

*Address all correspondence to: martina.smolic@mefos.hr

1 Department of Pharmacology, Faculty of Medicine, Josip Juraj Strossmayer University of Osijek, Osijek, Croatia

2 Department of Integrative Medicine, Faculty of Medicine, Josip Juraj Strossmayer University of Osijek, Osijek, Croatia

3 Department of Mineral Research, Faculty of Medicine, Josip Juraj Strossmayer University of Osijek, Osijek, Croatia

4 Department of Internal Medicine, University Hospital Center Osijek, Osijek, Croatia

References

[1] Baron S, editor. Medical Microbiology. 4th ed. University of Texas Medical Branch at Galveston; 1996

[2] Mohd Hanafiah K, Groeger J, Flaxman AD, Wiersma ST. Global epidemiology of hepatitis C virus infection: New estimates of age-specific antibody to HCV seroprevalence. Hepatology. 2013;**57**(4):1333-1342

[3] Messina JP, Humphreys I, Flaxman A, Brown A, Cooke GS, Pybus OG, et al. Global distribution and prevalence of hepatitis C virus genotypes. Hepatology. 2015;**61**(1):77-87

[4] Wang CC, Krantz E, Klarquist J, Krows M, McBride L, Scott EP, et al. Acute hepatitis c in a contemporary US cohort: Modes of acquisition and factors influencing viral clearance. Journal of Infectious Diseases. 2007;**196**(10):1474-1482

[5] Wise M, Bialek S, Finelli L, Bell BP, Sorvillo F. Changing trends in hepatitis C-related mortality in the United States, 1995-2004. Hepatology. 2008;**47**(4):1128-1135

[6] Thein HH, Yi QL, Dore GJ, Krahn MD. Estimation of stage-specific fibrosis progression rates in chronic hepatitis C virus infection: A meta-analysis and meta-regression. Hepatology. 2008;**48**(2):418-431

[7] Gatselis NK, Zachou K, Saitis A, Samara M, Dalekos GN. Individualization of chronic hepatitis C treatment according to the host characteristics. World Journal of Gastroenterology. 2014;**20**(11):2839-2853

[8] Smith DB, Bukh J, Kuiken C, Muerhoff AS, Rice CM, Stapleton JT, et al. Expanded classification of hepatitis C virus into 7 genotypes and 67 subtypes: Updated criteria and genotype assignment web resource. Hepatology. 2014;**59**(1):318-327

[9] Kawaguchi-Suzuki M, Frye RF. The role of pharmacogenetics in the treatment of chronic hepatitis C infection. Pharmacotherapy. 2014;**34**(2):185-201

[10] Hoofnagle JH, Mullen KD, Jones DB, Rustgi V, Di Bisceglie A, Peters M, et al. Treatment of chronic non-A, non-B hepatitis with recombinant human alpha interferon. A preliminary report. The New England Journal of Medicine. 1986;**315**(25):1575-1578

[11] Choo QL, Kuo G, Weiner AJ, Overby LR, Bradley DW, Houghton M. Isolation of a cDNA clone derived from a blood-borne non-A, non-B viral hepatitis genome. Science. 1989;**244**(4902):359-362

[12] Smith-Palmer J, Cerri K, Valentine W. Achieving sustained virologic response in hepatitis C: A systematic review of the clinical, economic and quality of life benefits. BMC Infectious Diseases. 2015;**15**:19

[13] Pearlman BL, Traub N. Sustained virologic response to antiviral therapy for chronic hepatitis C virus infection: A cure and so much more. Clinical Infectious Diseases. 2011;**52**(7):889-900

[14] Martinot-Peignoux M, Stern C, Maylin S, Ripault MP, Boyer N, Leclere L, et al. Twelve weeks posttreatment follow-up is as relevant as 24 weeks to determine the sustained virologic response in patients with hepatitis C virus receiving pegylated interferon and ribavirin. Hepatology. 2010;**51**(4):1122-1126

[15] Yoshida EM, Sulkowski MS, Gane EJ, Herring RW, Ratziu V, Ding X, et al. Concordance of sustained virological response 4, 12, and 24 weeks post-treatment with sofosbuvir-containing regimens for hepatitis C virus. Hepatology. 2015;**61**(1):41-45

[16] McHutchison JG, Gordon SC, Schiff ER, Shiffman ML, Lee WM, Rustgi VK, et al. Interferon alfa-2b alone or in combination with ribavirin as initial treatment for chronic hepatitis C. Hepatitis Interventional Therapy Group. The New England Journal of Medicine. 1998;**339**(21):1485-1492

[17] Zeuzem S, Berg T, Moeller B, Hinrichsen H, Mauss S, Wedemeyer H, et al. Expert opinion on the treatment of patients with chronic hepatitis C. Journal of Viral Hepatitis. 2009;**16**(2):75-90

[18] Macarthur KL, Smolic R, Smolic MV, Wu CH, Wu GY. Update on the development of anti-viral agents against hepatitis C. Journal of Clinical and Translational Hepatology. 2013;**1**(1):9-21

[19] Bagheri H, Fouladi A, Barange K, Lapeyre-Mestre M, Payen JL, Montastruc JL, et al. Follow-up of adverse drug reactions from peginterferon alfa-2b-ribavirin therapy. Pharmacotherapy. 2004;**24**(11):1546-1553

[20] Adinolfi LE, Guerrera B. All-oral interferon-free treatments: The end of hepatitis C virus story, the dream and the reality. World Journal of Hepatology. 2015;**7**(22):2363-2368

[21] Reiser M, Hinrichsen H, Benhamou Y, Reesink HW, Wedemeyer H, Avendano C, et al. Antiviral efficacy of NS3-serine protease inhibitor BILN-2061 in patients with chronic genotype 2 and 3 hepatitis C. Hepatology. 2005;**41**(4):832-835

[22] Hinrichsen H, Benhamou Y, Wedemeyer H, Reiser M, Sentjens RE, Calleja JL, et al. Short-term antiviral efficacy of BILN 2061, a hepatitis C virus serine protease inhibitor, in hepatitis C genotype 1 patients. Gastroenterology. 2004;**127**(5):1347-1355

[23] Macrocycles in Drug Discovery: The Royal Society of Chemistry; 2015.

[24] Ghany MG, Nelson DR, Strader DB, Thomas DL, Seeff LB. Diseases AAfSoL. An update on treatment of genotype 1 chronic hepatitis C virus infection: 2011 practice guideline by the American Association for the Study of Liver Diseases. Hepatology. 2011;**54**(4):1433-1444

[25] FDA. FDA approved drugs: INCIVEK (TELAPREVIR) 2011. Available from: http://www.accessdata.fda.gov/drugsatfda_docs/label/2011/201917lbl.pdf.

[26] FDA. FDA approved drugs: VICTRELIS (BOCEPREVIR) 2011. Available from: http://www.accessdata.fda.gov/drugsatfda_docs/label/2011/202258lbl.pdf.

[27] Zeuzem S, Andreone P, Pol S, Lawitz E, Diago M, Roberts S, et al. Telaprevir for retreatment of HCV infection. The New England Journal of Medicine. 2011;**364**(25):2417-2428

[28] Poordad F, Bronowicki JP, Gordon SC, Zeuzem S, Jacobson IM, Sulkowski MS, et al. Factors that predict response of patients with hepatitis C virus infection to boceprevir. Gastroenterology. 2012;**143**(3):608.e1-5-618.e1-5

[29] Jacobson IM, McHutchison JG, Dusheiko G, Di Bisceglie AM, Reddy KR, Bzowej NH, et al. Telaprevir for previously untreated chronic hepatitis C virus infection. The New England Journal of Medicine. 2011;**364**(25):2405-2416

[30] Gordon SC, Muir AJ, Lim JK, Pearlman B, Argo CK, Ramani A, et al. Safety profile of boceprevir and telaprevir in chronic hepatitis C: Real world experience from HCV-TARGET. Journal of Hepatology. 2015;**62**(2):286-293

[31] Solbach P, Wedemeyer H. The new era of interferon-free treatment of chronic hepatitis C. Viszeralmedizin. 2015;**31**(4):290-296

[32] FDA. FDA approved drugs: OLYSIO (SIMEPREVIR) 2013. Available from: http://www.accessdata.fda.gov/scripts/cder/daf/index.cfm?event=BasicSearch.process.

[33] FDA. FDA approved drugs: SOFOSBUVIR 2013. Available from: http://www.accessdata.fda.gov/drugsatfda_docs/label/2014/204671s001lbl.pdf.

[34] FDA. FDA approved drugs: VIEKIRA PAK (DASABUVIR SODIUM, OMBITASVIR, PARITAPREVIR, RITONAVIR) 2014. Available from: http://www.accessdata.fda.gov/scripts/cder/daf/index.cfm?event=overview.process&ApplNo=206619.

[35] FDA. FDA approved drugs: HARVONI (LEDIPASVIR + SOFOSBUVIR) 2014. Available from: http://www.accessdata.fda.gov/drugsatfda_docs/label/2014/205834s000lbl.pdf.

[36] FDA. FDA approved drugs: DACLINZA (DACLATASVIR) 2015. Available from: http://www.accessdata.fda.gov/drugsatfda_docs/label/2015/206843Orig1s000lbl.pdf.

[37] FDA. FDA approved drugs: TECHNIVIE (OMBITASVIR, PARITAPREVIR, RITONAVIR) 2015. Available from: https://www.accessdata.fda.gov/drugsatfda_docs/label/2015/207931s001lbl.pdf.

[38] FDA. FDA approved drugs: ZEPATIER (ELBASVIR, GRAZOPREVIR) 2016. Available from: http://www.accessdata.fda.gov/drugsatfda_docs/label/2016/208261Orig1s000lbl.pdf.

[39] FDA. FDA approved drugs: EPCLUSA (SOFOSBUVIR, VELPATASVIR) 2016. Available from: http://www.accessdata.fda.gov/drugsatfda_docs/label/2016/208341s000lbl.pdf.

[40] Mauss S, Berg T, Rockstroh J, Sarrazin C, Wedemeyer H. Hepatology—A Clinical Textbook. 6th ed. 2015. http://www.liver.ca/files/Professional_Education___Partnerships/Information___Resources_for_HCP/Hepatology_2015_-_A_Clinical_Textbook.pdf.

[41] Mishra P, Murray J, Birnkrant D. Direct-acting antiviral drug approvals for treatment of chronic hepatitis C virus infection: Scientific and regulatory approaches to clinical trial designs. Hepatology. 2015;**62**(4):1298-1303

[42] Severino G, Del Zompo M. Adverse drug reactions: Role of pharmacogenomics. Pharmacological Research. 2004;**49**(4):363-373

[43] Ritter JM, Lewis LD, Mant TG, Ferro A. A Textbook for Clinical Pharmacology and Therapeutics. 5th ed. London: Hodder Arnold; 2008

[44] Aneesh TP, Sonal Sekhar M, Jose A, Chandran L, Zachariah SM. Pharmacogenomics: The right drug to the right person. Journal of Clinical Medicine Research. 2009;**1**(4):191-194

[45] Bozic I, Omanovic T, Kuna L, Kizivat T, Smolic R, Vcev A, Smolic M. Pharmacogenomics: Sex differences and application in pediatrics. Southeastern European Medical Journal. 2017;**1**:108-120

[46] Caudle KE, Klein TE, Hoffman JM, Muller DJ, Whirl-Carrillo M, Gong L, et al. Incorporation of pharmacogenomics into routine clinical practice: The Clinical Pharmacogenetics Implementation Consortium (CPIC) guideline development process. Current Drug Metabolism. 2014;**15**(2):209-217

[47] Lazarou J, Pomeranz BH, Corey PN. Incidence of adverse drug reactions in hospitalized patients: A meta-analysis of prospective studies. Journal of the American Medical Association. 1998;**279**(15):1200-1205

[48] Kongkaew C, Noyce PR, Ashcroft DM. Hospital admissions associated with adverse drug reactions: A systematic review of prospective observational studies. The Annals of Pharmacotherapy. 2008;**42**(7):1017-1025

[49] Ernst FR, Grizzle AJ. Drug-related morbidity and mortality: Updating the cost-of-illness model. Journal of the American Pharmaceutical Association (Washington, DC). 2001;**41**(2):192-199

[50] Meisel C, Gerloff T, Kirchheiner J, Mrozikiewicz PM, Niewinski P, Brockmöller J, et al. Implications of pharmacogenetics for individualizing drug treatment and for study design. Journal of Molecular Medicine (Berlin). 2003;**81**(3):154-167

[51] Abaji R, Krajinovic M. Current perspective on pediatric pharmacogenomics. Expert Opinion on Drug Metabolism & Toxicology. 2016;**12**(4):363-365

[52] Moran C, Thornburg CD, Barfield RC. Ethical considerations for pharmacogenomic testing in pediatric clinical care and research. Pharmacogenomics. 2011;**12**(6):889-895

[53] Siest G, Marteau JB, Visvikis-Siest S. Personalized therapy and pharmacogenomics: Future perspective. Pharmacogenomics. 2009;**10**(6):927-930

[54] Kamal SM. Pharmacogenetics of hepatitis C: Transition from interferon-based therapies to direct-acting antiviral agents. Hepatic Medicine. 2014;**6**:61-77

[55] Ansaldi F, Orsi A, Sticchi L, Bruzzone B, Icardi G. Hepatitis C virus in the new era: Perspectives in epidemiology, prevention, diagnostics and predictors of response to therapy. World Journal of Gastroenterology. 2014;**20**(29):9633-9652

[56] Chuang WL, Yu ML. Host factors determining the efficacy of hepatitis C treatment. Journal of Gastroenterology. 2013;**48**(1):22-30

[57] Asselah T, Estrabaud E, Bieche I, Lapalus M, De Muynck S, Vidaud M, et al. Hepatitis C: Viral and host factors associated with non-response to pegylated interferon plus ribavirin. Liver International. 2010;**30**(9):1259-1269

[58] Afdhal NH, McHutchison JG, Zeuzem S, Mangia A, Pawlotsky JM, Murray JS, et al. Hepatitis C pharmacogenetics: State of the art in 2010. Hepatology. 2011;**53**(1):336-345

[59] Schlecker C, Ultsch A, Geisslinger G, Lötsch J. The pharmacogenetic background of hepatitis C treatment. Mutation Research. 2012;

[60] Estrabaud E, Vidaud M, Marcellin P, Asselah T. Genomics and HCV infection: Progression of fibrosis and treatment response. Journal of Hepatology. 2012;**57**(5):1110-1125

[61] Kotenko SV, Gallagher G, Baurin VV, Lewis-Antes A, Shen M, Shah NK, et al. IFN-lambdas mediate antiviral protection through a distinct class II cytokine receptor complex. Nature Immunology. 2003;**4**(1):69-77

[62] Sheppard P, Kindsvogel W, Xu W, Henderson K, Schlutsmeyer S, Whitmore TE, et al. IL-28, IL-29 and their class II cytokine receptor IL-28R. Nature Immunology. 2003; **4**(1):63-68

[63] Zhang L, Jilg N, Shao RX, Lin W, Fusco DN, Zhao H, et al. IL28B inhibits hepatitis C virus replication through the JAK-STAT pathway. Journal of Hepatology. 2011;**55**(2):289-298

[64] Maher SG, Sheikh F, Scarzello AJ, Romero-Weaver AL, Baker DP, Donnelly RP, et al. IFNalpha and IFNlambda differ in their antiproliferative effects and duration of JAK/STAT signaling activity. Cancer Biology & Therapy. 2008;**7**(7):1109-1115

[65] Urban TJ, Thompson AJ, Bradrick SS, Fellay J, Schuppan D, Cronin KD, et al. IL28B genotype is associated with differential expression of intrahepatic interferon-stimulated genes in patients with chronic hepatitis C. Hepatology. 2010;**52**(6):1888-1896

[66] Dill MT, Duong FH, Vogt JE, Bibert S, Bochud PY, Terracciano L, et al. Interferon-induced gene expression is a stronger predictor of treatment response than IL28B genotype in patients with hepatitis C. Gastroenterology. 2011;**140**(3):1021-1031

[67] Raglow Z, Thoma-Perry C, Gilroy R, Wan YJ. IL28B genotype and the expression of ISGs in normal liver. Liver International. 2013;**33**(7):991-998

[68] Cariani E, Villa E, Rota C, Critelli R, Trenti T. Translating pharmacogenetics into clinical practice: Interleukin (IL)28B and inosine triphosphatase (ITPA) polymophisms in hepatitis C virus (HCV) infection. Clinical Chemistry and Laboratory Medicine. 2011; **49**(8):1247-1256

[69] Domagalski K, Pawłowska M, Tretyn A, Halota W, Pilarczyk M, Smukalska E, et al. Impact of IL-28B polymorphisms on pegylated interferon plus ribavirin treatment response in children and adolescents infected with HCV genotypes 1 and 4. European Journal of Clinical Microbiology & Infectious Diseases. 2013;**32**(6):745-754

[70] Mangia A, Thompson AJ, Santoro R, Piazzolla V, Tillmann HL, Patel K, et al. An IL28B polymorphism determines treatment response of hepatitis C virus genotype 2 or 3 patients who do not achieve a rapid virologic response. Gastroenterology. 2010;**139**(3): 821-827

[71] Rosen HR. Clinical practice. Chronic hepatitis C infection. The New England Journal of Medicine. 2011;**364**(25):2429-2438

[72] Coto-Llerena M, Pérez-Del-Pulgar S, Crespo G, Carrión JA, Martínez SM, Sánchez-Tapias JM, et al. Donor and recipient IL28B polymorphisms in HCV-infected patients undergoing antiviral therapy before and after liver transplantation. American Journal of Transplantation. 2011;**11**(5):1051-1057

[73] Clark PJ, Thompson AJ. Host genomics and HCV treatment response. Journal of Gastroenterology and Hepatology. 2012;**27**(2):212-222

[74] Jacobson IM, Kowdley KV, Kwo PY. Anemia management in the era of triple combination therapy for chronic HCV. Gastroenterology & Hepatology (New York). 2012;**8**(9 Suppl 6):1-16

[75] Soriano V, Poveda E, Vispo E, Labarga P, Rallón N, Barreiro P. Pharmacogenetics of hepatitis C. The Journal of Antimicrobial Chemotherapy. 2012;**67**(3):523-529

[76] De Franceschi L, Fattovich G, Turrini F, Ayi K, Brugnara C, Manzato F, et al. Hemolytic anemia induced by ribavirin therapy in patients with chronic hepatitis C virus infection: Role of membrane oxidative damage. Hepatology. 2000;**31**(4):997-1004

[77] Russmann S, Grattagliano I, Portincasa P, Palmieri VO, Palasciano G. Ribavirin-induced anemia: Mechanisms, risk factors and related targets for future research. Current Medicinal Chemistry. 2006;**13**(27):3351-3357

[78] Homma M, Hosono H, Hasegawa Y, Kohda Y. Morphological transformation and phosphatidylserine exposure in erythrocytes treated with ribavirin. Biological & Pharmaceutical Bulletin. 2009;**32**(11):1940-1942

[79] Sumi S, Marinaki AM, Arenas M, Fairbanks L, Shobowale-Bakre M, Rees DC, et al. Genetic basis of inosine triphosphate pyrophosphohydrolase deficiency. Human Genetics. 2002;**111**(4-5):360-367

[80] Cao H, Hegele RA. DNA polymorphisms in ITPA including basis of inosine triphosphatase deficiency. Journal of Human Genetics. 2002;**47**(11):620-622

[81] Stepchenkova EI, Tarakhovskaya ER, Spitler K, Frahm C, Menezes MR, Simone PD, et al. Functional study of the P32T ITPA variant associated with drug sensitivity in humans. Journal of Molecular Biology. 2009;**392**(3):602-613

[82] Hitomi Y, Cirulli ET, Fellay J, McHutchison JG, Thompson AJ, Gumbs CE, et al. Inosine triphosphate protects against ribavirin-induced adenosine triphosphate loss by adenylosuccinate synthase function. Gastroenterology. 2011;**140**(4):1314-1321

[83] Fellay J, Thompson AJ, Ge D, Gumbs CE, Urban TJ, Shianna KV, et al. ITPA gene variants protect against anaemia in patients treated for chronic hepatitis C. Nature. 2010;**464**(7287):405-408

[84] Ochi H, Maekawa T, Abe H, Hayashida Y, Nakano R, Kubo M, et al. ITPA polymorphism affects ribavirin-induced anemia and outcomes of therapy—A genome-wide study of Japanese HCV virus patients. Gastroenterology. 2010;**139**(4):1190-1197

[85] Naggie S, Rallon NI, Benito JM, Morello J, Rodriguez-Novoa S, Clark PJ, et al. Variants in the ITPA gene protect against ribavirin-induced hemolytic anemia in HIV/HCV-coinfected patients with all HCV genotypes. The Journal of Infectious Diseases. 2012;**205**(3):376-383

[86] Rallón NI, Morello J, Labarga P, Benito JM, Rodríguez-Nóvoa S, Vispo E, et al. Impact of inosine triphosphatase gene variants on the risk of anemia in HIV/hepatitis C virus-coinfected patients treated for chronic hepatitis C. Clinical Infectious Diseases. 2011;**53**(12):1291-1295

[87] Domingo P, Guardiola JM, Salazar J, Torres F, Mateo MG, Pacho C, et al. Association of ITPA gene polymorphisms and the risk of ribavirin-induced anemia in HIV/hepatitis C virus (HCV)-coinfected patients receiving HCV combination therapy. Antimicrobial Agents and Chemotherapy. 2012;**56**(6):2987-2993

[88] Osinusi A, Naggie S, Poonia S, Trippler M, Hu Z, Funk E, et al. ITPA gene polymorphisms significantly affect hemoglobin decline and treatment outcomes in patients coinfected with HIV and HCV. Journal of Medical Virology. 2012;**84**(7):1106-1114

[89] Macías J, Vispo E, Pineda JA, Soriano V. Host genetics. Current Opinion in HIV and AIDS. 2011;**6**(6):491-500

[90] Tsubota A, Shimada N, Abe H, Yoshizawa K, Agata R, Yumoto Y, et al. Several factors including ITPA polymorphism influence ribavirin-induced anemia in chronic hepatitis C. World Journal of Gastroenterology. 2012;**18**(41):5879-5888

[91] Kurosaki M, Tanaka Y, Nishida N, Sakamoto N, Enomoto N, Matsuura K, et al. Model incorporating the ITPA genotype identifies patients at high risk of anemia and treatment failure with pegylated-interferon plus ribavirin therapy for chronic hepatitis C. Journal of Medical Virology. 2013;**85**(3):449-458

[92] Kanda T, Nakamoto S, Yokosuka O. Is the use of IL28B genotype justified in the era of interferon-free treatments for hepatitis C? World Journal of Virology. 2015;**4**(3):178-184

[93] Vierling J, Puoti M, Bernstein D. Efficacy by race or geographic region in HCV genotype 1- infected patients treated with ABT-450/ritonavir/ombitasvir and dasabuvir, with or without ribavirin (Abstract 1968). 65th Annual Meeting of the American Association for the Study of Liver Diseases (AASLD). November 7-11, 2014. Boston, MA. 2014

[94] Hepatitis YML, Treatment C. From "Response-guided" to "Resource-guided" therapy in the transition era from IFN-containing to IFN-free regimens. Journal of Gastroenterology and Hepatology. 2017;

[95] AASLD. Recommendations for Testing, Managing, and Treating Hepatitis C. 2016. http://www.hcvguidelines.org/

[96] AFEF AFEF. Guidelines: Management of hepatitis C. Virus. 2015. http://www.afef.asso.fr/ckfinder/userfiles/files/actualites/veille/French-HCV-guidelines-June-2015.pdf

[97] Sarrazin C, Berg T, Buggisch P, Dollinger MM, Hinrichsen H, Hofer H, et al. Aktuelle Empfehlung zur Therapie der chronischen Hepatitis C. Zeitschrift für Gastroenterologie. 2015;**53**(4):1-44

[98] CfIDD*FM*. Preporuke za liječenje hepatitisa C 2016. Available from: http://www.bfm.hr/page/hepatitis-c.

[99] Poordad F, Reddy KR, Martin P. Rapid virologic response: A new milestone in the management of chronic hepatitis C. Clinical Infectious Diseases. 2008;**46**(1):78-84

[100] Pawlotsky J. EASL Recommendations on Treatment of Hepatitis C 2015. Journal of Hepatology. 2014;**61**:373-395

[101] PP Inc. A Proposal for Managing the Harvoni Wave. 2015. http://www.personalizedprescribing.com/wp-content/uploads/2015/06/hepatitis-c-%E2%80%93-white-paper-2015.pdf

[102] Lynch SM, Hepatitis WGY, Virus C. A review of treatment guidelines, cost-effectiveness, and access to therapy. Journal of Clinical and Translational Hepatology. 2016;**4**(4):310-319

[103] Dore GJ, Feld JJ. Hepatitis C virus therapeutic development: In pursuit of "perfectovir". Clinical Infectious Diseases. 2015;**60**(12):1829-1836

Chapter 15

Progress in Vaccine Development for HCV Infection

Ashraf Tabll, Reem El-Shenawy and Yasmine El Abd

Additional information is available at the end of the chapter

http://dx.doi.org/10.5772/intechopen.70649

Abstract

Hepatitis C virus (HCV) is a blood-transmitted disease that spreads among 3% of the world's population causing seriously increasing mortality rates. The HCV prevalence in Egypt in October 2008 was 14.7% and declined to 6.3% in the survey carried out in October 2015. Nowadays, the new direct-acting antivirals (DAAs) show amazing results especially with regard to HCV genotype 1, but there is still a great necessity to produce a vaccine to avoid this viral infection. Additionally, neutralizing anti-HCV antibodies could be utilized in combination with DAAs empowering their effect. A powerful candidate HCV vaccine should create comprehensively cross-receptive T cells CD4 and CD8 and effectively neutralizing antibodies to successfully clear the virus. The current clinical trials for HCV vaccines comprise synthetic peptides, DNA-based vaccines, or recombinant protein vaccines. Several preclinical vaccine studies are under research including cell culture-derived HCV (HCVcc), HCV-like particles, and recombinant adenoviral vaccines. This mini-review will discuss the prevalence of HCV worldwide and in Egypt. We will present the recent progress in basic research and preclinical and clinical studies for HCV vaccine. Finally, it will present the phenomena of spontaneous clearance of HCV without treatment as a model for study of HCV vaccine development.

Keywords: HCV vaccine, cell culture-derived HCV, HCV-like particles, spontaneous clearance, neutralizing antibodies

1. Introduction

Hepatitis C virus (HCV) infection is the main health problem worldwide and in Egypt. Until now there is no prophylactic or therapeutic vaccine for HCV. The development of a protective vaccine is essential in combating the global HCV epidemic. Understanding the immune response in those who spontaneously resolve HCV infections versus those who develop chronic infection is the key to the development of prophylactic or therapeutic vaccine. In this mini review, we will discuss the recent and more promising progress in the HCV vaccine development.

2. Prevalence of HCV in the world

HCV is a worldwide predominant pathogen with very high mortality rates [1]. Sub-Saharan Africa accounts for almost one-fifth of worldwide infections; in Southeast Asia, approximately 32.2 million people have chronic HCV infection, and over 6 million infected people are in Latin America [2]. In [3], it is reported that 2.8% people equating more than 185 million are infected by HCV worldwide. Egypt was from the countries with the high prevalence rates (14.7%), followed by Pakistan (4.8%) and China (3.2%). Constant HCV disease is connected with the advancement of liver fibrosis, liver cirrhosis, hepatocellular malignancy, and death [3]. Although the HCV occurrence rate is clearly diminishing in the developing countries, Razavi et al. [4] reported that over the next 20 years the mortality from liver diseases secondary to HCV will keep on rising.

3. Prevalence of HCV in Egypt

The 2015 Egypt Health Issues Survey conducted on behalf of the Ministry of Health and Population by El-Zanaty and Associates (http://www.dhsprogram.com) showed that the prevalence of HCV antibodies was 6.3% of the tested individuals (n = 26,027) in cases with ages 1–59 years, while prevalence of HCV RNA was 4.4%. In 2008, according to the health survey carried out, the prevalence of HCV antibodies was 14.7% (number of examined individuals was 11,126) and that of HCV RNA was 9.8% (as shown in **Figure 1**). Interestingly, a

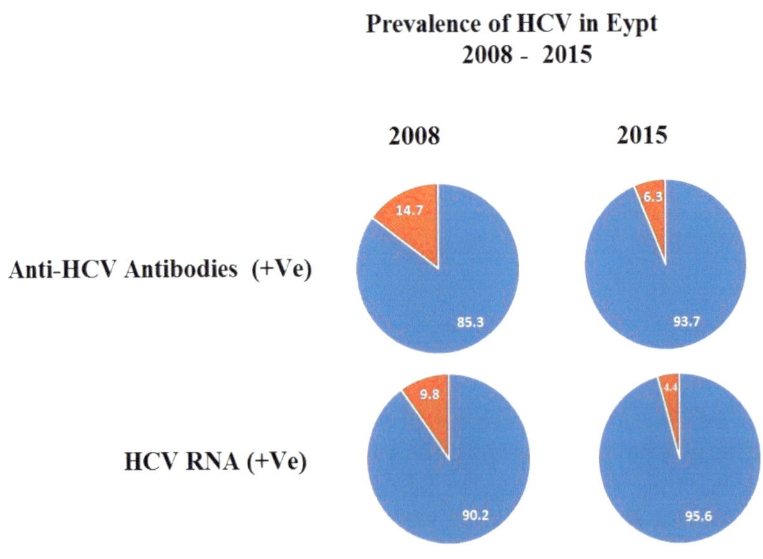

Figure 1. Prevalence of HCV in Egypt according to health survey carried out at 2008 and 2015 in cases aged from 1 to 59 years (male and females).

promising finding of the 2015 survey is that the prevalence of HCV antibodies was 0.7 and HCV RNA was 0.3 among cases with age 10–14, while the percentage of HCV antibodies in cases with ages 50–59 years ($n = 627$) was 30.5–41.9%, and that of HCV RNA was 23.7–27.8%. This means that low prevalence of HCV infection is expected among the future generation. The decline of prevalence of HCV antibodies and HCV RNA is due to single usage of syringes and needles, sterilization of medical, dental and dialysis instruments, regular check-up, testing of blood donors, and also activity of Egyptian National Control Strategy for viral hepatitis.

4. Barriers that limit HCV vaccine development

HCV is the world's most common blood-borne viral infection for which there is no vaccine [5, 6]. Most acute HCV infections are asymptomatic, and viral persistence is established in the majority of infected subjects. Vaccine development is fundamental to globally eliminate HCV infection through prevention, representing a public health priority. Generally, a good vaccine must induce cellular and humoral immunity, during early phase of viral infection, before the virus gets the opportunity to trigger its numerous immune escape mechanisms [7]. Also a new vaccine should be affordable, safe, not inducing autoimmunity or hypersensitivity, and finally providing long-lasting immunity. Progress in HCV vaccine development is hampered due to the high level of genetic diversity among different HCV strains resulting from the absence of proofreading activity for the NS5B RNA-dependent polymerase [8], which led to the production of genetically distinct but closely related variants within the same genotype designated quasi species [9]. Also, the high viral mutation rate enabled the viral persistence by evading the cellular and humoral immune control [10], either by binding low-density lipoproteins or infecting surrounding cells through cell-to-cell contact mediated by CD81 and Claudin-1 and inducing interfering antibodies by continuous mutation [11]. Also the barriers that challenges vaccine research against HCV is the lack of small and suitable animal models for studying HCV pathogenesis and protective specific immunity. Nowadays, the chimpanzee is the only suitable infectious animal model with lots of ethical and financial obstacles to acquire [12]. Progression to chronic liver disease results from the ineffective weak immune response against the virus. In summary, many barriers occur for HCV vaccine development such as the presence of several HCV genotypes, restricted accessibility of animal models, and the complicated nature of the immunological response to HCV. Neutralizing antibody (Nab) and cellular immune responses to $CD4^+$ and $CD8^+$ T cells are essential for HCV clearance [13]. Some reports suggest that the highly changeable, quasi-species' nature of HCV and the continuous emergence of resistant strains are reasons for the HCV resistance attitude. However, the HCV resistance in the presence of circulating antibodies cannot be completely explained by the continuous and rapid acquired viral genetic variability alone.

5. HCV vaccine strategies

The target of all strategies is to activate a long-lasting T-cell response involving both helper $CD4^+$ and $CD8^+$ rather than only adaptive immune response. HCV is vastly mutable, thus developing an effective vaccine is very challenging. In 2013 [14], scientists from Scripps Research Institute reported that the virus uses HCV E2 envelope glycoprotein as the key protein to invade liver cells. Discovering that E2 binds to the CD81 receptor on the liver cells through a relatively conserved binding region will empower designing of a vaccine which triggers effective antibody responses to various HCV genotypes. Previous studies focused on certain peptide sequences from envelope regions 1 and 2 of HCV as a candidate vaccine. They found that peptide region E1 (aa 315–323) and peptide regions from HCV E2 (aa 412–219) and HCV E2 (aa 517–531) had capability to introduce neutralizing antibodies in mice, rabbits, and goats, while peptide sequence from HCV E2 (aa 430–447) produced nonneutralizing antibodies, which are known interference antibodies [15–22]. Another strategy is to use viral vectors inducing T-cell responses against HCV-infected cells, e.g., adenoviral vectors that have big areas of the HCV genome itself. Early vaccines targeted only genotypes 1a and 1b, accounting for more than 60% of chronic HCV infections worldwide, while subsequent vaccines might target other genotypes by prevalence [23].

Various HCV candidate vaccines were described, comprising synthetic peptides [24], recombinant E1 and E2 proteins [25, 26], recombinant adenoviral and prime-boost strategies with modified vaccinia Ankara (MVA) vaccines or recombinant E1 and E2 glycoproteins [27–30]. However, only few proceeded to phases I and II using recombinant poxvirus [31], DNA vaccines [29, 32], synthetic peptide-based vaccines [33], and MVA vaccines and adenoviral [34, 35]. Recently, Teimourpour et al. [36] successfully cloned structural viral genes in pCDNA3.1 (+) vector and expressed them in eukaryotic expression system facilitating the development of new DNA vaccines against HCV. These candidate vaccines produced robust cross-reactive HCV-specific cellular responses, and HCV viral load was reduced.

On the other hand, plant-based vaccine is a new approach for making an inexpensive and easily producible HCV vaccine. Infecting plants with a genetically engineered tobacco mosaic virus (TMV) produced the hyper variable region 1 (HVR1) peptide fused to the B subunit of cholera toxin CTB. The plant-derived HVR1/CTB reacted with specific antibodies acquired from HCV-infected individuals [37].

6. HCV-like particles and cell culture-derived HCV (HCVcc)

Special focus will be drawn on candidate vaccine HCV-like particles and HCVcc, which is expected to boom in the next years. Virus-like particle consists of some of the structural viral proteins. These proteins self-assemble into particles which resemble the virus but lack viral nucleic acid; thus, they are not infectious. Viral-like particles (VLP) are typically more immunogenic because of their highly repetitive and multivalent structure.

6.1. HCV-viral like particles (VLP)

HCV VLP vaccine is very promising for the development of a prophylactic vaccine. VLP are vectors for gene delivery that closely resemble the mature HCV. Hence, using a single VLP-based vaccine, neutralizing antibodies and T-cell responses against many epitopes can be induced. Hepatitis B virus (HBV) and human papillomavirus (HPV) have licensed VLP vaccines [38]. Baumert et al. [39] generated HCV-LPs using a recombinant baculovirus containing the complementary DNA for HCV structural proteins in insect cells.

Recently, results of Kumar et al. [40] suggested that the combined regimen of HCV viral-like particles followed by recombinant adenovirus could more effectively inhibit HCV infection, endorsing the novel vaccine strategy.

HCV-LPs were used to immunize four chimpanzees, and all developed HCV-specific T-cell and proliferative lymphocyte responses against core, E1, and E2 proteins. Challenging with infectious HCV, one chimpanzee developed transitory viremia, and the other three displayed higher levels of viremia, but after 10 weeks, their viral levels became immeasurable as reported by Elmowalid et al. [41]. Technique for high-capacity purification of HCV VLPs was defined by Earnest-Silveira et al. [42]. The structural HCV protein coding sequences of genotypes 1a, 1b, 2a, or 3a were coexpressed using a recombinant adenoviral expression system in Huh7 cell line. Using iodixanol ultracentrifugation and Stirred cell ultrafiltration, the structural proteins self-assembled into VLPs which were purified from Huh7 cell lysates. VLPs of the different genotypes are morphologically similar as revealed by electron microscopy. Results showed that it is feasible to produce big quantities of individual HCV genotype VLPs, making this approach an alternative for the manufacture of a quadrivalent mammalian cell-derived HCV VLP vaccine. HCV-specific neutralizing antibodies (Nabs) recognize quaternary structures [43, 44]. The particulate structure of HCV VLPs makes them an attractive vaccine candidate [45–47].

6.2. Cell culture-derived HCV (HCVcc)

Kato and Wakita [48] introduced the HCV infection system in cell culture using clone JFH-1, taken from a fulminant HCV-infected Japanese patient. JFH-1 replicates well in hepatic cancer cells and releases infectious virion in the cells' media. Understanding how hosts react to HCV infection and how the viruses escape from host immune reactions was studied using HCVcc systems. Although it is difficult to understand the mechanisms underlying the HCV infection outcomes, innate immune responses seem to have a crucial effect on HCV infection outcomes. Later, robust production of HCVcc particles was obtained by introducing a few specific mutations in JFH-1 structural proteins [49].

Also, Akazawa et al. [50] showed that a protective vaccine can be developed from inactivated HCV particles derived from cultured cells that protected chimeric liver uPA(+/+)-SCID mice against HCV infection. Also, Gottwein and Bukh [51] cultured virus particles constituting the antigen in most antiviral vaccines.

Recently, Yokokawa evaluated neutralizing antibody induction and cellular immune responses following the immunization of a nonhuman primate model with (HCVcc) in [52]. This preclinical study demonstrated that the vaccine included both HCVcc and K3-SPG-induced humoral and cellular immunity in marmosets. Vaccination with this combination resulted in the production of antibodies exhibiting cross-neutralizing activity against multiple HCV genotypes. Based on these findings, the vaccine created in this study represents a promising, potent, and safe prophylactic option against HCV.

Generally, we can conclude the comparison between the two strategies of candidate vaccines of HCVcc and HCV VLP in **Table 1**.

Subject	HCV VLP	HCVcc
Component	Structural core + E1 + E2	Structural and nonstructural
Induction	Induced humoral and cellular immunity	Induced humoral and cellular immunity
Large production	Large production	Not yet
RNA	Lack RNA (noninfectious)	With RNA (infectious particles)
Clinical trail	Not yet	Not yet

Table 1. Comparison between candidate vaccines derived from cell culture-derived HCV (HCVcc) and HCV viral-like particles (VLP).

7. Clinical trails

Fifty-five studies were conducted on HCV vaccine and were registered for the clinical trial webs, most of them in United States and in Europe (https://clinicaltrials.gov). Yet, one study only (ClinicalTrials.gov NCT01436357) revealed encouraging results for population at risk. The study used a replicative defective simian adenoviral vector (ChAd3) and a modified vaccinia Ankara (MVA) vector that encodes HCV genotype 1b proteins, the NS3, NS4, NS5A, and NS5B. It was a placebo-controlled double-blind study with HCV-uninfected male and females aged 18–45 years. In phase I, 68 subjects were enrolled and then an interim analysis of safety data was carried out. Additional 382 volunteers were enrolled in phase II. Very high levels of HCV-specific T cells targeting various HCV antigens were produced giving a persistent memory and effector T cell. Kelly et al. [53] studied the specific HCV immune responses and T-cell cross-reactivity to endogenous virus in chronically HCV-infected genotype 1 patients who were vaccinated using heterologous adenoviral vectors (ChAd3-NSmut and Ad6-NSmut) encoding nonstructural HCV proteins in escalating dose,

ClinicalTrials.gov Identifier	NCT00500747	NCT01436357
Antigen	Envelop (E1 and E2)	Nonstructure (NS3-NS4a-NS4b-NS5a-NS5b)
Composition	Subunit glycoproteins (oil:water adjuvant)	Recombinant virus vectors (Ad and MVA)
Immunity	Neutralizing antibodies and $CD4^+$ T cells	$CD4^+$ and CD8 T cells
Objective	Neutralize infectivity and prevent persistence	Prevent persistence
Name of company	Chiron (Novartis)	Okairos (GlaxoSmithKline)

Table 2. Comparing two candidate HCV vaccines in clinical trial stages.

prime-boost regimen, with and without concomitant pegylated interferon-a/ribavirin therapy. This study concluded that there is a major challenge of overcoming T-cell exhaustion in the context of persistent antigen exposure as the vaccination with potent adenoviral HCV-vectored vaccine was only effective when there is genetic mismatch between immunogen vaccine and endogenous virus.

All trials in **Table 2** are obtained from www.clinicaltrials.gov and Ogholikhan and Schwarz [54].

8. Studying spontaneous clearance of HCV as a model for developing HCV vaccine

Studying the immune response in subjects who spontaneously resolve HCV infections is the key to the development of a prophylactic vaccine. Recently, we studied the role of circulating neutralizing antibodies in the spontaneous clearance of HCV in infected blood donors and answered the question of why some anti-HCV-positive donors clear viremia while others do not [19]. Human plasma immunoglobulins targeting HCV E1 region (aa 315–323) and HCV E2 (aa 412–419) and HCV E2, (aa 517–531) in blood donors positive for HCV antibodies were studied. Antibodies targeting HCV E1 region (aa 315—323) and HCV E2 (aa 412–419) and HCV E2 (aa 517–531) possessed cross-neutralizing activity [16, 19].

Spontaneous clearance of HCV is only achieved with early and effective T-cell responses that are entirely efficient with respect to cytolytic capacity, reflected by granzyme and cytokine production [55]. To elaborate the role of cell-mediated immune response in achieving spontaneous clearance, it was documented that patients with hypogammaglobulinemia had the ability to spontaneously clear HCV infection; thus, T-cell responses might be responsible for the protection against HCV [56].

9. General conclusion

HCV is still health problem worldwide and in Egypt, although the prevalence started to decline. HCV vaccine development is urgent as prophylactic and therapeutic agents against new HCV infection. HCV-like particles and cell culture-derived HCV (HCVcc) are the promising candidates for HCV vaccine development. Finally, studying spontaneous clearance of HCV without treatment can be used as a model for HCV vaccine development.

Acknowledgements

This work was partially funded by the project STDF 5041 to Dr. Ashraf Tabll.

Author details

Ashraf Tabll*, Reem El-Shenawy and Yasmine El Abd

*Address all correspondence to: Ashraftabll@yahoo.com

Microbial Biotechnology Department, Genetic Engineering and Biotechnology Research Division, National Research Center, Dokki, Giza, Egypt

References

[1] Cooke GS, Lemoine M, Thursz M, Gore C, Swan T, Kamarulzaman A, et al. Viral hepatitis and the Global Burden of Disease: A need to regroup. Journal of Viral Hepatitis. 2013;**20**:600-601. DOI: 10.1111/jvh.12123

[2] Daw MA, Dau AA. Hepatitis C virus in Arab world: A state of concern. The Scientific World Journal. 2012;719494. DOI: 10.1100/2012/534173

[3] Mohd Hanafiah K, Groeger J, Flaxman AD, Wiersma ST. Global epidemiology of hepatitis C virus infection: New estimates of age-specific antibody to HCV seroprevalence. Hepatology. April 2013;**57**(4):1333-1342. DOI: 10.1002/hep.26141

[4] Razavi H, ElKhoury AC, Elbasha E, Estes C, Pasini K, Poynard T, et al. Chronic hepatitis C virus (HCV) disease burden and cost in the United States. Hepatology. 2013;**57**:2164-2170. DOI: 10.1002/hep.26218

[5] Rosen HR. Emerging concepts in immunity to hepatitis C virus infection. Journal of Clinical Investigation. 2013;**123**:4121-4130. DOI: 10.1172/JCI67714

[6] Barnes D, Kunitomi M, Vignuzzi M, Saksela K, Andino R. Harnessing endogenous miRNAs to control virus tissue tropism as a strategy for developing attenuated virus vaccines. Cell Host & Microbe. 2008;**4**:239-248. DOI: 10.1016/j.chom.2008.08.003

[7] Ghasemi F, Rostami S, Meshkat Z. Progress in the development of vaccines for hepatitis C virus infection. World Journal of Gastroenterology. 2015;**21**:11984-12002. DOI: 10.3748/wjg.v21.i42.11984

[8] Duffy S, Shackelton LA, Holmes EC. Rates of evolutionary change in viruses: Patterns and determinants. Nature Reviews Genetics. 2008;**9**:267-276. DOI: 10.1038/nrg2323

[9] Bukh J, Miller RH, Purcell RH. Genetic heterogeneity of hepatitis C virus: Quasispecies and genotypes. Seminars in Liver Diseases. 1995;**15**:41-63. DOI: 10.1055/s-2007-1007262

[10] Bowen DG, Walker CM. Mutational escape fromCD8+ T cell immunity: HCV evolution, from chimpanzees to man. Journal of Experimental Medicine. 2005;**201**:1709-1714. DOI: 10.1084/jem.20050808

[11] Timpe JM, Stamataki Z, Jennings A, Hu K, Farquhar MJ, Harris HJ, Schwarz A, Desombere I, Roels GL, Balfe P, McKeating JA, Hepatitis C. Virus cell-cell transmission in hepatoma cells in the presence of neutralizing antibodies. Hepatology. 2008;**47**:17-24. DOI: 10.1002/hep.21959

[12] Mailly L, Robinet E, Meuleman P, Baumert TF, Zeisel MB. Hepatitis C virus infection and related liver disease: The quest for the best animal model. Frontiers in Microbiology. 2013;**4**:213. DOI: 10.3389/fmicb.2013.00212

[13] Torresi J, Johnson D, Wedemeyer H. Progress in the development of preventive and therapeutic vaccines for hepatitis C virus. Journal of Hepatology. 2011;**54**:1273-1285. DOI: 10.1016/j.jhep.2010.09.040

[14] Kong L, Giang E, Nieusma T, Kadam RU, Cogburn KE, Hua Y, Dai X, Stanfield RL, Burton DR, Ward AB, Wilson IA, Law M. Hepatitis C virus E2 envelope glycoprotein core structure. Science. 2013;**342**(6162):1090-1094. DOI: 10.1126/science.1243876 PMID: 24288331

[15] Tabll A, Khalil S, El-Shenawy R, Esmat G, Helmy A, Attallah A, El-Awady M. Establishment of hybrid cell lines producing monoclonal antibodies to a synthetic peptide from E1 region of the hepatitis C virus. Journal of Immunoassay and Immunochemistry. 2008;**29**:91-104. DOI: 10.1080/15321810701735161

[16] Tabll A, El Abd Y, Bader El Din N, El Shenawy R, Abdelhafez T, El Awady M, El-Mohamady H, Viazov S. Establishment of human clones producing neutralizing human monoclonal antibodies to the envelope E1/E2 protein of hepatitis C virus by EBV immortalization of immune CD22+ B cells. Human Antibodies. 2013;**22**:55-65. DOI: 10.3233/HAB-140271

[17] Tabll A, Moustafa R, El Abd Y, Bader El Din N, El-Shenawy R, Yousef H, Hussein M, Dawood R, Omran M, El-Awady M. Mouse monoclonal antibody towards E1 specific epitope blocks viral entry and intracellular viral replication in vitro. Journal of Immunoassay and Immunochemistry. 2014;**35**:60-73. DOI: 10.1080/15321819.2013.792831

[18] Tabll A, Abbas A, El-Kafrawy S, Wahid A. Monoclonal antibodies: Principles and applications of immmunodiagnosis and immunotherapy for hepatitis C virus. World Journal of Hepatology. 2015;**7**:2369-2383. DOI: 10.4254/wjh.v7.i22.2369

[19] Tabll A, Salem E, El-Abd Y, El-Shenawy R, Saad A, Abdallah O, Dawood R, El-Awady M. Level of human antibodies targeting HCV E1/E2 peptides and spontaneous clearance of HCV in blood donors. Clinical Laboratory. 2016;**62**:1879-1885. DOI: 10.7754/Clin.Lab.2016.160108

[20] El Abd YS, Tabll AA, Bader El Din NG, Hosny AE, Moustafa RI, El-Shenawy R, Atef K, El-Awady MK. Neutralizing activities of caprine antibodies towards conserved regions of the HCV envelope glycoprotein E2. Virology Journal. 2011;**8**:391. DOI: 10.1186/1743-422X-8-391

[21] El-Awady MK, Tabll A, El-Abd Y, Yousif H, Hegab M, Reda M, El-Shenawy R, Moustafa R, Degheidy N, Bader El Din N. Conserved peptides within the E2 region of hepatitis

C virus induce humoral and cellular responses in goats. Virology Journal. 2009;**6**(1):66. DOI: 10.1186/1743-422X-6-66

[22] El-Shenawy R, Tabll A, Bader El Din NG, El Abd Y, Mashaly M, Abdel Malak CA, Dawood R, El-Awady M. Antiviral activity of virocidal peptide derived from NS5A against two different HCV genotypes: An in vitro study. Journal of Immunoassay and Immunochemistry. 2015;**36**:63-79. DOI: 10.1080/15321819.2014.896264

[23] Kong L, Giang E, Nieusma T, Kadam RU, Cogburn KE, Hua Y, Dai X, Stanfield RL, Burton DR, Ward AB, Wilson IA, Law M. Hepatitis C virus E2 envelope glycoprotein core structure. Science. 2013;**342**:1090-1094. DOI: 10.1126/science.1243876

[24] Kong L, Lee DE, Kadam RU, Liu T, Giang E, Nieusma T, Garces F, Tzarum N, Woods Jr. VL, Ward AB, Li S, Wilson IA, Law M. Structural flexibility at a major conserved antibody target on hepatitis C virus E2 antigen. Proceedings of the National Academy of Sciences of the United States of America. October 2016. pii: 201609780. PMID: 27791120

[25] Colombatto P, Brunetto MR, Maina AM, Romagnoli V, Almasio P, Rumi MG, Ascione A, Pinzello G, Mondelli M, Muratori L, Rappuoli R, Rosa D, Houghton M, Abrignani S, Bonino F. *HCV E1E2-MF59* vaccine in chronic hepatitis C patients treated with PEG-IFNα2a and Ribavirin: A randomized controlled trial. Journal of Viral Hepatitis. 2014;21:458-465. DOI: 10.1111/jvh.12163

[26] Houghton M. Prospects for prophylactic and therapeutic vaccines against the hepatitis C viruses. Immunological Reviews. 2011;**239**:99-108. DOI: 10.1111/j.1600-065X.2010.00977

[27] Grubor-Bauk B, Yu W, Wijesundara D, Gummow J, Garrod T, Brennan AJ, Voskoboinik I, Gowans EJ. Intradermal delivery of DNA encoding HCV NS3 and perforin elicits robust cell-mediated immunity in mice and pigs. Gene Therapy. 2016;**23**:26-37. DOI: 10.1038/gt.2015.86

[28] Gummow J, Li Y, Yu W, Garrod T, Wijesundara D, Brennan AJ, Mullick R, Voskoboinik I, Grubor-Bauk B, Gowans EJ. A multiantigenic DNA vaccine that induces broad hepatitis C virus-specific T-cell responses in mice. Journal of Virology. 2015;**89**:7991-8002. DOI: 10.1128/JVI.00803-15

[29] Sällberg M, Frelin L, Weiland O. DNA vaccine therapy for chronic hepatitis C virus (HCV) infection: Immune control of a moving target. Expert Opinion on Biological Therapy. 2009;**9**:805-815. DOI: 10.1517/14712590902988444

[30] Chmielewska AM, Naddeo M, Capone S, Ammendola V, Hu K, Meredith L, Verhoye L, Rychlowska M, Rappuoli R, Ulmer JB, Colloca S, Nicosia A, Cortese R, Leroux-Roels G, Balfe P, Bienkowska-Szewczyk K, Meuleman P, McKeating JA, Folgori A. Combined adenovirus vector and hepatitis C virus envelope protein prime-boost regimen elicits T cell and neutralizing antibody immune responses. Journal of Virology. 2014;**88**:5502-5510. DOI: 10.1128/JVI.03574-13

[31] Habersetzer F, Honnet G, Bain C, Maynard-Muet M, Leroy V, Zarski JP, Feray C, Baumert TF, Bronowicki JP, Doffoël M, Trépo C, Agathon D, Toh ML, Baudin M, Bonnefoy JY,

Limacher JM, Inchauspé G. A poxvirus vaccine is safe, induces T-cell responses, and decreases viral load in patients with chronic hepatitis C. Gastroenterology. 2011;**141**(3):890-899.e1-4. DOI: 10.1053/j.gastro.2011.06.009 PMID: 21699798

[32] Levander S, Sällberg M, Ahlén G, Frelin L. A non-human hepadnaviral adjuvant for hepatitis C virus-based genetic vaccines. Vaccine. 2016;**34**(25):2821-2833. DOI: 10.1016/j.vaccine.2016.04.030

[33] Klade CS, Schuller E, Boehm T, von Gabain A, Manns MP. Sustained viral load reduction in treatment-naive HCV genotype 1 infected patients after therapeutic peptide vaccination. Vaccine 2012;30:2943-2950. DOI: 10.1016/j.vaccine.2012.02.070

[34] Swadling L, Halliday J, Kelly C, Brown A, Capone S, Ansari MA, Bonsall D, Richardson R, Hartnell F, Collier J, Ammendola V, Del Sorbo M, Von Delft A, Traboni C, Hill AV, Colloca S, Nicosia A, Cortese R, Klenerman P, Folgori A, Barnes E. Highly-immunogenic virally-vectored T-cell vaccines cannot overcome subversion of the T-cell response by HCV during chronic infection. Vaccines (Basel). 2016;**4**(3). pii: E27). DOI: 10.3390/vaccines4030027 PMID: 27490575

[35] Swadling L, Capone S, Antrobus RD, Brown A, Richardson R, Newell EW, Halliday J, Kelly C, Bowen D, Fergusson J, Kurioka A, Ammendola V, Del Sorbo M, Grazioli F, Esposito ML, Siani L, Traboni C, Hill A, Colloca S, Davis M, Nicosia A, Cortese R, Folgori A, Klenerman P, Barnes E. A human vaccine strategy based on chimpanzee adenoviral and MVA vectors that primes, boosts, and sustains functional HCV-specific T cell memory. Science Translational Medicine. 2014;**5**(6):261ra153. DOI: 10.1126/scitranslmed.3009185

[36] Teimourpour R, Tajani AS, Askari VR, Rostami S, Meshkat Z. Designing and development of a DNA vaccine based on structural proteins of hepatitis C virus. Iranian Journal of Pathology. 2016;**11**:222-230 PMC5079455

[37] Nemchinov LG, Liang TJ, Rifaat MM, Mazyad HM, Hadidi A, Keith JM. Development of a plant-derived subunit vaccine candidate against hepatitis C virus. Archives of Virology. 2000;**145**:2557-2573 11205105

[38] Roldão A, Mellado MC, Castilho LR, Carrondo MJ, Alves PM. Virus-like particles in vaccine development. Expert Review of Vaccines. 2010;**9**:1149-1176. DOI: 10.1586/erv.10.115

[39] Baumert TF, Vergalla J, Satoi J, Thomson M, Lechmann M, Herion D, Greenberg HB, Ito S, Liang TJ. Hepatitis C virus-like particles synthesized in insect cells as a potential vaccine candidate. Gastroenterology. 1999;**117**:1397-1407 10579981

[40] Kumar A, Das S, Mullick R, Lahiri P, Tatineni R, Goswami D, Bhat P, Torresi J, Gowans EJ, Karande AA, Das S. Immune responses against hepatitis C virus genotype 3a virus-like particles in mice: A novel VLP prime-adenovirus boost strategy. Vaccine. 2016;**34**:1115-1125. DOI: 10.1016/j.vaccine.2015.11.061

[41] Elmowalid GA, Qiao M, Jeong SH, Borg BB, Baumert TF, Sapp RK, Hu Z, Murthy K, Liang TJ. Immunization with hepatitis C virus-like particles results in control of hepatitis

C virus infection in chimpanzees. Proceedings of the National Academy of Sciences of the United States of America. 2007;**104**:8427-8432. DOI: 10.1073/pnas.0702162104

[42] Earnest-Silveira L, Chua B, Chin R, Christiansen D, Johnson D, Herrmann S, Ralph SA, Vercauteren K, Mesalam A, Meuleman P, Das S, Boo I, Drummer H, Bock CT, Gowans EJ, Jackson DC, Torresi J. Characterization of a hepatitis C virus-like particle vaccine produced in a human hepatocyte-derived cell line. Journal of General Virology. 2016;**97**:1865-1876. DOI: 10.1099/jgv.0.000493

[43] Keck ZY, Saha A, Xia J, Wang Y, Lau P, Krey T, Rey FA, Foung SK. Mapping a region of hepatitis C virus E2 that is responsible for escape from neutralizing antibodies and a core CD81-binding region that does not tolerate neutralization escape mutations. Journal of Virology. 2011;**85**:10451-10463. DOI: 10.1128/JVI.05259-11

[44] Giang E, Dorner M, Prentoe JC, Dreux M, Evans MJ, Bukh J, Rice CM, Ploss A, Burton DR, Law M.Human broadly neutralizing antibodies to the envelope glycoprotein complex of hepatitis C virus. Proceedings of the National Academy of Sciences of the United States of America. 2012;109:6205-6210. DOI:10.1073/pnas.1114927109

[45] Elmowalid GA, Qiao M, Jeong SH, Borg BB, Baumert TF, Sapp RK, Hu Z, Murthy K, Liang TJ. Immunization with hepatitis C virus-like particles results in control of hepatitis C virus infection in chimpanzees. Proceedings of the National Academy of Sciences of the United States of America. 2007;104:8427-8432. DOI: 10.1073/pnas.0702162104

[46] Chua BY, Johnson D, Tan A, Earnest-Silveira L, Sekiya T, Chin R, Torresi J, Jackson DC. Hepatitis C VLPs delivered to dendritic cells by a TLR2 targeting lipopeptide results in enhanced antibody and cell-mediated responses. PloS One. 2012;**7**(10):e47492. DOI: 10.1371/journal.pone.0047492

[47] Kumar A, Gupta V, Sharma P, Bansal N, Singla V, Arora A. Association of overt diabetes mellitus with the Non-CC but not the CC genotype of Interleukin-28B in hepatitis C virus infected patients. Journal of Clinical and Translational Hepatology 2016;4:26-31. DOI: 10.14218/JCTH.00040

[48] Kato T, Wakita T. Production of infectious hepatitis C virus in cell culture. Uirusu. 2005;**55**:287-295 16557015

[49] Delgrange D, Pillez A, Castelain S, Cocquerel L, Rouillé Y, Dubuisson J, Wakita T, Duverlie G, Wychowski C. Robust production of infectious viral particles in Huh-7 cells by introducing mutations in hepatitis C virus structural proteins. Journal of General Virology 2007;88:2495-2503. DOI: 10.1099/vir.0.82872-0 DOI:10.1099/vir.0.82872-0

[50] Akazawa D, Moriyama M, Yokokawa H, Omi N, Watanabe N, Date T, Morikawa K, Aizaki H, Ishii K, Kato T, Mochizuki H, Nakamura N, Wakita T. Neutralizing antibodies induced by cell culture-derived hepatitis C virus protect against infection in mice. Gastroenterology. 2013;**145**:447-455. DOI: 10.1053/j.gastro.2013.05.007

[51] Gottwein JM, Bukh J. Viral hepatitis: Cell-culture-derived HCV--a promising vaccine antigen. Nature Reviews Gastroenterology & Hepatology. 2013;10(9):508-509. DOI: 10.1038/nrgastro.2013.136. PMID: 23897287

[52] Yokokawa H, Higashino A, Suzuki S, Moriyama M, Nakamura N, Suzuki T, Suzuki R, Ishii K, Kobiyama K, Ishii KJ, Wakita T, Akari H, Kato T. Induction of humoural and cellular immunity by immunisation with HCV particle vaccine in a non-human primate model. Gut. 2016;26. pii: gutjnl-2016-312208. DOI: 10.1136/gutjnl-2016-312208

[53] Kelly C, Swadling L, Capone S, Brown A, Richardson R, Halliday J, von Delft A, Oo Y, Mutimer D, Kurioka A, Hartnell F, Collier J, Ammendola V, Del Sorbo M, Grazioli F, Esposito ML, Di Marco S, Siani L, Traboni C, Hill AV, Colloca S, Nicosia A, Cortese R, Folgori A, Klenerman P, Barnes E. Chronic hepatitis C viral infection subverts vaccine-induced T-cell immunity in humans. Hepatology 2016;63:1455-1470. DOI: 10.1002/hep.28294

[54] Ogholikhan S, Schwarz KB. Hepatitis vaccines. Vaccines (Basel). 2016;**4**(1). DOI: 10.3390/vaccines4010006

[55] Schulze ZJ, Ciuffreda D, Lewis-Ximenez L, Kasprowicz V, Nolan BE, Streeck H, Aneja J, Reyor LL, Allen TM, Lohse AW, McGovern B, Chung RT, Kwok WW, Kim AY, Lauer GM. Broadly directed virus-specific CD4+ T cell responses are primed during acute hepatitis C infection, but rapidly disappear from human blood with viral persistence. Journal of Experimental Medicine. 2012;**209**:61-75. DOI: 10.1084/jem.201003

[56] Razvi S, Schneider L, Jonas MM, Cunningham-Rundles C. Outcome of intravenous immunoglobulin-transmitted hepatitis C virus infection in primary immunodeficiency. Journal of Clinical Immunology. 2001;**101**:284-288. DOI: 10.1006/clim.2001.5132

Chapter 16

Approaches and Considerations for the Successful Treatment of HCV Infection

Robert Smolić, Jelena Jakab, Lucija Kuna,
Martina Smolić, Martina Kajić, Marinko Žulj and
Aleksandar Včev

Additional information is available at the end of the chapter

http://dx.doi.org/10.5772/intechopen.70780

Abstract

The complexity of the hepatitis C virus (HCV) infection is reflected in its therapy, and great efforts are needed from the patient and the physician to be successful in eliminating the infection. How HCV will progress depends a lot on patient characteristics and social factors, in addition to the timing of initiation, duration, and final results of the therapy. The first treatment approved for patients with chronic hepatitis C was interferon (IFN) which had a sustained viral response (SVR) rate in 20%. Due to side effects, the adherence to this treatment was limited and required a patient-tailored approach with various medical disciplines working together and intervening at the right time to minimize potential obstacles. The introduction of direct-acting antivirals (DAAs) has contributed to the advancement of HCV treatment. However, a major obstacle to wide use of DAAs is their high price which has largely limited access to treatment. Guidelines and recommendations on treatment of hepatitis C have been developed to assist physicians and other health care providers to determine priority. Despite that, the arrival of new oral therapies has been met with enthusiasm as shorter, simpler, safer treatment allows for the possibility of delivering antiviral therapy on a large scale.

Keywords: HCV treatment, patient-tailored approach, treatment development, treatment goals, treatment priority

1. Introduction

Nowadays, the complexity of HCV infection is reflected in its therapy, and great efforts are needed from the patient and the treating physician. As a chronic disease with potential progression to fibrosis and HCV-associated cirrhosis, therapy of HCV in patients with liver disease and post-liver transplant patients represents a challenge for physicians. Initiation, duration, and final results of the therapy depend on various factors such as viral factors, patient characteristics, and numerous social factors. The patient-tailored approach and close patient-physician cooperation as well as the role of various medical disciplines working together and intervening at the right time is important to decrease the potential barrier in the achieving an SVR.

2. HCV infection: complexity of infection

HCV is a single-stranded positive-sense RNA virus which belongs to the genus *Hepacivirus* of the Flaviviridae family. The most significant nonstructural (NS) proteins involved in virus replication include the NS3 helicase, NS3-NS4A serine protease, and the NS5B RNA-dependent RNA polymerase [1]. There are six known genotypes and a single known case of genotype 7 and more than 50 subtypes. Because the highest prevalence of genotype 1 is found in the most of middle-income countries, many DAAs have been primarily developed for use in those countries. Some DAAs are effective against multiple HCV genotypes. They are less effective for genotype 3 and cirrhosis [2].

The most significant clinical problems of chronic hepatitis C (CHC) involve the development of liver cirrhosis, hepatocellular carcinoma (HCC), or the need for liver transplantation [3, 4]. Progression of liver disease is more likely in patients with older age, male sex, longer duration of infection, advanced histologic stage and grade, genotype 1, increased hepatic iron, concomitant liver disorders, HIV infection, and obesity [5]. As many as 74% of people suffer from extrahepatic manifestations, and fatigue is the most common symptom. There are immune complex–mediated extrahepatic complications, glomerulonephritis, lymphoproliferative disorders such as B-cell lymphoma and extrahepatic complications unrelated to immune-complex injury (Sjögren's syndrome, lichen planus, porphyria cutanea tarda, type-II diabetes mellitus, and the metabolic syndrome) [2].

Recurrence of HCV following liver transplant occurs in more than 95% of patients and reinfection occurs within 72 h [2]. Not all patients can receive therapy instantly on the approval of new agents, so priority should be given to those patients with the most urgent necessity [6]. About 80% of patients treated with interferon-based treatment experience adverse effects. Hence, the close monitoring, timely preventive, therapeutic measures, and patient motivation are needed. Furthermore, adverse effects vary between drugs and range from poor general well-being to specific conditions affecting hematopoiesis, skin, behavior, thyroid, eyes, or lungs, and therefore, a multidisciplinary approach is necessary [7].

3. HCV treatment options goals and timeline development

CHC caused by infection with HCV is one of the major causes of liver disease. The goal of hepatitis C treatment is to achieve SVR defined as no detectable HCV in blood at least 12 weeks after finishing treatment. If a durable SVR can be achieved, the risks for liver-related morbidity and mortality are decreased [2].

In infected patients, IFN-mediated immune response is associated with the induction of IFN-stimulated genes (ISGs) in the liver [9] during the first 4–10 weeks of infection. This is followed by an HCV-specific T cell response [8]. However, the virus persists in 80% of infected patients. To boost the immune response, in 1989, interferon-alfa (IFN-α) was first developed, and in the decades that followed IFN-α, monotherapy was the standard therapy for hepatitis C. While developing the best regimen, various doses and durations of treatment were tested, but SVR rates remained modest (15–20%) [8].

The natural history of the HCV does not differ significantly among genotypes. However, HCV genotype 3 induces liver steatosis more often than the other genotypes. Patients with different genotypes can differ in their response to treatment with recombinant IFN-α and DAAs. Treatment efficacy has shown progressive improvement following the pegylation of IFN-α and its effect in combination with other antiviral drugs. However, viral escape mechanisms, IFN-α signaling in the liver, and substantial drug toxicity still restricted the efficacy of this treatment [9]. The restricted efficacy of IFN-α treatments stimulated considerable research efforts of academia and industry with the aim of understanding the mechanisms of nonresponse to IFN-α [10]. Recently, numerous studies showed association between genetic variants near the IFNL3 known as IL28B gene and the response to IFN-α treatments [11]. The molecular mechanisms that link genetic variation in the IFNL3 gene locus to the response to IFN-α remains to be investigated [12].

Combining IFN-α with ribavirin (RBV) became the new standard therapy in 1998. RBV had been used as a monotherapy for CHC in the 1990s, and it was discovered to transiently decrease serum alanine aminotransferase (ALT) levels during therapy [13, 14]. Subcutaneously injected interferon-α2b (INF-α2b) with daily oral RBV achieved an SVR in 38%. SVR was 54–56% after pegylated INF α (PEG-INF) was introduced. Until 2011, when the interferon-free era began, hepatitis C was treated with 6–12 months of weekly PEG-INF injections and twice-daily RBV tablets [2, 8]. Oral DAAs have simplified treatment procurement and delivery and improved HCV treatment outcomes. Numerous trials of interferon-free, oral DAA regimens have reported cure rate of more than 85% regardless of HCV genotype, many in only 12 weeks [5]. To date, it is assumed that high serum concentrations of IFN-α which are obtained after therapy with PEG-INF ensure a crucial advantage compared with nonpegylated forms of recombinant IFN-α [9].

In 2014, four classes of DAAs were described: NS3/4A protease inhibitors, non-nucleoside polymerase inhibitors, nucleoside/tide polymerase inhibitors, and NS5A inhibitors [5]. In general, DAA regimens are better tolerated and more effective than PEG-IFN and RBV. Boceprevir and telaprevir—two HCV protease inhibitors—were developed to be given in combination with RBV and PEG-IFN. This combination prevented emergence of HCV mutants with genetic resistance to the protease inhibitors. For the first time, an SVR could be achieved in more than 75% of individuals that were infected with the HCV genotype 1 [15, 16]. HCV non-nucleoside polymerase inhibitors (dasabuvir) are twice-daily drugs developed primarily for genotype1 [17, 18]. HCV nucleoside/tide polymerase inhibitors, such as sofosbuvir, are taken once daily and generally have a pangenotypic activity, potency, high resistance barrier, and low propensity for drug-drug interactions. HCV NS5A inhibitors

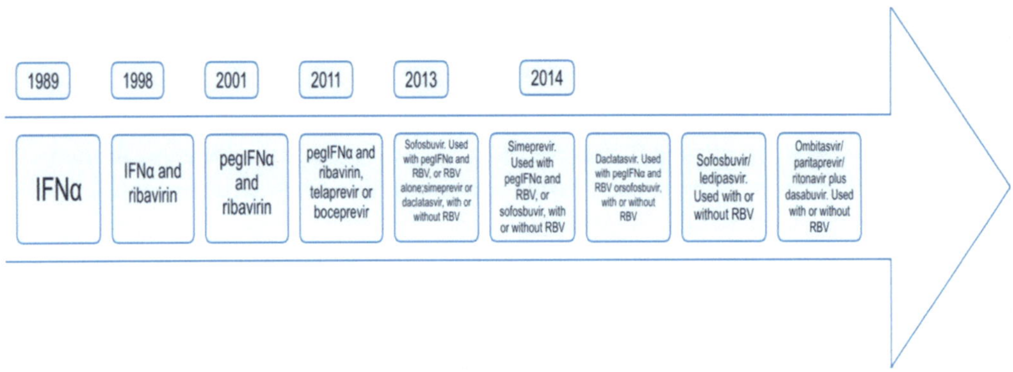

Figure 1. HCV Therapeutic Timeline.

(daclatasvir, ledipasvir, and ombitasvir) are novel drug class that are potent and have low barrier to resistance (**Figure 1**). So further research is needed to prevent or overcome drug resistance. On the other hand, daclatasvir and ledipasvir are pangenotypic and are well suited for combination with other DAAs [16].

4. Approach considerations in the IFN treatment era

Adherence to therapy is one of the most important factors for successful therapy [19]. It is important to reduce side effects and motivate patients to adhere to treatment in favor of optimizing treatment responses [20]. Due in part to the side effects, the adherence to interferon-based HCV treatment was limited, resulting in dosage reduction and sometimes discontinuation of therapy, which led to the frequent virus breakthrough [21]. Historically, the most predominant side effects have consisted of "flu"-like symptoms: fatigue, myalgia, fever, insomnia, and weakness [22]. Although up to two-thirds of patients complained of fatigue, it is important that the clinician distinguishes it from severe anemia, depression, or other metabolic disorders [23]. The "flu"-like symptoms were usually easily managed and did not lead to treatment discontinuation. On the other hand, cytopenias, particularly anemia, were the most troublesome side-effect, causing drug-dose reduction and early treatment discontinuation [24]. In addition, patients with HCV had other conditions that required treatment with medications that could cause hematologic toxicities. For that reason, a multifaceted approach was required, such as pretreatment screening, cardiac, and hematologic consultations when necessary, frequent laboratory monitoring, and dose reductions [25]. Erythropoietin and blood transfusions, as well as aggressive RBV dosage reductions, are effective for managing anemia [26].

Various types of dermatologic manifestations, such as dry skin and pruritus, have been reported during anti-HCV therapy. Dermatologic side effects seriously affect the skin barrier, quality of life, and sleep. A break in the skin can be the point of entry for a bacterial infection. Injection site reactions from interferon-based therapies may occur typically characterized by local tenderness, erythema, and itching [27]. It is wise to eliminate any unnecessary medications before HCV therapy and to recommend good skin hygiene. For patients who develop drug-related rash, use of topical antipruritics or systemic antihistamines can be helpful, but sometimes dermatology consultation is required for further management [28].

Some of the most frequently reported gastrointestinal symptoms include nausea and dysgeusia. Patients may minimize nausea by taking RBV with food; however, antiemetics may be needed [25]. Dysgeusia is treated by sipping water frequently. To maintain salivary flow and oral hygiene, oral ointments and mouth washes are used [29]. Anal discomfort, with or without diarrhea, may respond to barrier creams and hemorrhoidal ointments. Patients presenting with a rectal bleed and abdominal pain should be worked-up for ischemic colitis, which can be diagnosed by CT scan with contrast or colonoscopy [30].

Psychiatric effects of HCV therapy are relatively preventable through symptom monitoring, frequent visits to assess clinical improvement, the use of selective serotonin reuptake inhibitors, and IFN dose reduction when needed. Patients who develop severe depression should be taken off HCV therapy because suicide has been reported on combination therapy [31]. The health care provider should observe symptoms that could be related to depression, such as sleep disturbance, irritability, and decreased memory. Early consultation with a psychiatrist is of great importance for defining a psychiatric diagnosis, selecting a treatment, and educating the patient about treatment expectations [32].

There are many ways a health care provider can help the patient manage side effects of the treatment. A gentle modification of behavior or routine medical therapy is often the first step, followed by dose reduction or adding additional medications. Patients are advised to rest when required and to maintain a regular daily schedule. Also, encouraging physical activity may help maintain emotional balance and promote energy levels [33]. Maintaining hydration is important in boosting a sense of well being. Providing a support network, such as availability of nurses and an after-hours telephone health link, improves adherence to treatment and patient satisfaction. Additionally, the right timing and the adequate injection of the PEG-INF injection can be helpful [29].

Patient quality of life (QOL) during HCV treatment affects medication adherence [34], which is why it is necessary to think broadly about treatment management. In a study conducted by Manos et al., serious financial consequences of the HCV treatment (job loss, decreased work hours, difficulty paying for medications) were reported by 34.8% patients [35]. Over half of the patients reported difficulty attending social functions. When asked to rank how helpful different types of support might be for future patients undergoing treatment, the most highly ranked options were more frequent provider contact by telephone and peer support availability. Overall, patients were more satisfied with a care provided by a nurse or clinical pharmacist rather than by physicians. Others have reported frustration with communication among physicians and communication between the patient and the physician [36]. Furthermore, a common desire among patients was access to multidisciplinary services [35]. Communication quality is impacted by the time limitation of providers. To address such limitations, some healthcare systems rely on nurse practitioners and physician assistants to care for patients with hepatitis C [37]. The importance of nurses in patient QOL during HCV treatment and their support has been rated highly [38]. Mental health providers are also helpful to maintain HCV treatment adherence, and a pilot study suggests effectiveness of the weekly telephone meetings with a mental health professional [39]. Other studies and guidelines suggest that interdisciplinary, integrated care models can help optimizing HCV treatment [40, 41].

In conclusion, the treatment of HCV should be undertaken by physicians with a broad clinical knowledge. Close clinical follow-up of patients is needed for early recognition and appropriate management of most of the side effects. Prescreening patients for potential clinical problems is crucial part of side effects anticipation which leads to involving specialists in a timely manner. The HCV provider is able to address side effects and monitor the efficacy of the regimen when patient visits twice monthly, at least in the beginning of therapy. Moreover, successful adherence to treatment can be enhanced by a strong support network, which includes specially trained hepatitis nurses and a multidisciplinary team consisting of pharmacists, counselors, and social workers.

5. Approach considerations in the IFN-free treatment era

The protease inhibitor boceprevir was approved in 2011, followed by the approval of telaprevir [42]. A third protease inhibitor, simeprevir, was approved in 2013 and is recommended as a part of combination therapy for chronic HCV infection. More recently, NS5B polymerase inhibitor sofosbuvir has emerged as an important component of currently recommended regimens [43]. In 2014, the FDA approved an all-oral regimen of simeprevir plus sofosbuvir for treatment-naïve or treatment-experienced patients [44]. DAAs are effective regardless of race, gender, or HIV status [45, 46]. They have few side effects, short durations of treatment, and high SVRs. Therefore, DAAs have the potential to lower mortality, improve QOL, and reduce long-term costs of complications in HCV infected individuals [47]. This is why every patient with chronic HCV infection should be considered for antiviral treatment with DAA agents, even if previous interferon-based therapy has failed [48].

There are certain settings where limited access to medications forces health practitioner to decide which patient should be treated first. In circumstances like this, practitioners rely on evidence-based medicine and guidelines. Treatment for CHC is based on guidelines from the Infectious Diseases Society of America (IDSA) and the American Associations for the Study of Liver Diseases (AASLD) [49]. Recommendations are evidence based and are constantly updated as new data from peer-reviewed evidence become available. The guidelines propose that treatment priority should be given to those with the most urgent need. The recommendations include the following:

1. The highest priority for treatment should be given to the patients with advanced fibrosis, compensated cirrhosis, and severe extrahepatic hepatitis, as well as liver transplant recipients.

2. Patients with high priority for treatment are the ones at high risk for liver-related complications and severe extrahepatic hepatitis C complications.

3. Certain subgroups of HCV patients, such as men who have high-risk sex with men, active injection drug users, incarcerated persons, and those on hemodialysis are patients whose risk of HCV transmission is high, and in whom, HCV treatment may result in a reduction in

http://dx.doi.org/10.5772/intechopen.70780

transmission. In those patients, treatment decisions should balance the anticipated reduction in transmission versus the likelihood of reinfection.

Although antiviral therapy for CHC should be determined on a case-by-case basis, treatment is widely recommended for patients with elevated ALT levels who meet the following criteria [50]: older than 18 years, positive HCV antibody and serum HCV RNA, compensated liver disease, adequate hematologic and biochemical indices, willingness, and adherence to treatment, without contraindications.

In Europe, EASL Recommendations on Treatment of Hepatitis C assist physicians and other healthcare providers in the clinical decision-making process by providing information about the current optimal management of patients with acute and chronic HCV infections [51]. The recommendations have been based on evidence from existing publications and presentations at international meetings and the expert personal experiences. According to EASL, all treatment-naïve and treatment-experienced patients with compensated or decompensated chronic liver disease related to HCV, who have no contraindications to treatment, must be considered for therapy. The treatment must be available without delay in patients with significant fibrosis or cirrhosis, including decompensated cirrhosis; patients with clinically significant extrahepatic manifestations (e.g., symptomatic vasculitis, mixed cryoglobulinemia, nephropathy, and non-Hodgkin B-cell lymphoma); patients with HCV recurrence after liver transplantation; patients with concurrent comorbidities who are at risk of a rapid evolution of liver disease (non-liver solid organ or stem cell transplant recipients, diabetes); and individuals at risk of transmitting HCV (active injection drug users, men who have sex with men with high-risk sexual practices, women of childbearing age who wish to get pregnant, hemodialysis patients, incarcerated individuals) [51].

Prior to initiating DAA therapy, patients should undergo a thorough pre-treatment evaluation, which includes identifying the genotype of hepatitis C, evidence of cirrhosis, and previous treatment. Comorbid physical or psychological conditions should be optimized before commencing therapy because it will improve compliance. Evaluation for advanced fibrosis is recommended for all persons with HCV infection [49]. Another important consideration before starting therapy is the possibility of drug-drug interactions, as well as severe renal impairment [48].

Treatment of chronic HCV infection has two goals: to achieve SVR and to prevent progression of cirrhosis, hepatocellular carcinoma, and decompensated liver disease which can lead to the liver transplantation [49]. Patients who achieve an SVR experience numerous health benefits, including a decrease in liver inflammation levels, a reduction in the rate of progression of liver fibrosis [52], and reduced symptoms and mortality from severe extrahepatic manifestations [53]. Patients with normal liver function tests after SVR can be managed as if they had never been infected with HCV. Individuals who have failed to achieve SVR must be given an opportunity to pursue further therapeutic options [48].

6. Approach considerations in the near future

Currently, access to treatment for HCV is limited, with only a minority diagnosed patients, and even fewer assessed are initiated on treatment [54]. HCV therapy has the potential to ensure individual and health benefits, but high prices have stopped access to HCV therapy, even in high income countries and to people with advanced liver disease. If DAAs are to stop HCV-related mortality and decrease the global burden of HCV infection in the coming years, current HCV treatment rates of 1% to <5% must be increased [55]. Treating patients with fibrosis will decrease morbidity and mortality of HCV, but unless patients without advanced liver disease are treated too, the epidemic of HCV will continue [56].

7. Conclusion

Key desirable characteristics of the HCV therapy include high efficacy, tolerability, pan-genotypic activity, short duration, oral administration, affordability, and fixed-dose combination. The major reasons for limited treatment access are the cost, complexity, and limited effectiveness of treatment, as well as lack of access to reliable and affordable diagnostics. The improved safety profile and improved efficacy across genotypes of the new DAAs make the pre-treatment screening simple. In the future, HCV treatment could be initiated immediately after confirmation of infection and the presence of viremia, with only an initial assessment of the stage of liver disease. Future development of pan-genotypic regimens with minimal side effects that will be available at an affordable price holds the greatest potential for expanding access to treatment to all HCV patients.

Author details

Robert Smolić[1,2]*, Jelena Jakab[2], Lucija Kuna[2], Martina Smolić[2], Martina Kajić[3], Marinko Žulj[2] and Aleksandar Včev[1,2]

*Address all correspondence to: robert.smolic@mefos.hr

1 University Hospital Center Osijek, Osijek, Croatia

2 Faculty of Medicine, Josip Juraj Strossmayer University of Osijek, Osijek, Croatia

3 Pharmaceutical Company Pliva, Zagreb, Croatia

References

[1] Poustchi H, Esmaili S, Mohamadkhani A, Nikmahzar A, Pourshams A, Sepanlou SG, et al. The impact of illicit drug use on spontaneous hepatitis C clearance: Experience from a large cohort population study. PloS One. 2011;**6**(8):

[2] Longo DL, Kasper DL, Jameson JL, Fauci AS, Hauser SL, Loscalzo J. Harrison's Principles of Internal Medicine. USA: McGraw Hill Medical; 2012.

[3] Lee MH, Yang HI, SN L, Jen CL, You SL, Wang LY, et al. Chronic hepatitis C virus infection increases mortality from hepatic and extrahepatic diseases: A community-based long-term prospective study. The Journal of Infectious Diseases. 2012;**206**(4):469-477

[4] Maasoumy B, Wedemeyer H. Natural history of acute and chronic hepatitis C. Best Practice & Research. Clinical Gastroenterology. 2012;**26**(4):401-412

[5] Swan T. Overview of New Treatments for Hepatitis C Virus: Moving Towards a Public Health Agenda. Geneva: World Health Organization; 2017. Available from: http://www.who.int/selection_medicines/committees/expert/20/reviews/overview-new-treatments-HEP-C

[6] Garcia-Retortillo M, Forns X, Feliu A, Moitinho E, Costa J, Navasa M, et al. Hepatitis C virus kinetics during and immediately after liver transplantation. Hepatology. 2002;**35**(3):680-687

[7] Strazzula L, Pratt DS, Zardas J, Chung RT, Thiim M, Kroshinsky D. Widespread morbilliform eruption associated with telaprevir: Use of dermatologic consultation to increase tolerability. JAMA Dermatology. 2014;**150**(7):756-759

[8] Bigger CB, Brasky KM, Lanford RE. DNA microarray analysis of chimpanzee liver during acute resolving hepatitis C virus infection. Journal of Virology. 2001;**75**(15):7059-7066

[9] Heim MH. 25 years of interferon-based treatment of chronic hepatitis C: An epoch coming to an end. Nature Reviews Immunology. 2013;535-542

[10] Heim MH. Innate immunity and HCV. Journal of Hepatology. 2013;**58**(3):564-574

[11] Rauch A. Genetic variation in IL28B is associated with chronic hepatitis C and treatment failure: A genome-wide association study. Gastroenterology. 2010;1338-1345

[12] Prokunina-Olsson L. A variant upstream of IFNL3 (IL28B) creating a new interferon gene IFNL4 is associated with impaired clearance of hepatitis C virus. Nature Genetics. 2013;**45**(2):164-171

[13] Reichard O, Andersson J, Schvarcz R, Weiland O. Ribavirin treatment for chronic hepatitis C. Lancet. 1991;**337**(8749):1058-1061

[14] Di Bisceglie AM, Shindo M, Fong TL, Fried MW, Swain MG, Bergasa NV, et al. A pilot study of ribavirin therapy for chronic hepatitis C. Hepatology. 1992;**16**(3):649-654

[15] Poordad F, McCone J, Bacon BR, Bruno S, Manns MP, Sulkowski MS, et al. Boceprevir for untreated chronic HCV genotype 1 infection. The New England Journal of Medicine. 2011;**364**(13):1195-1206

[16] Jacobson IM, McHutchison JG, Dusheiko G, Di Bisceglie AM, Reddy KR, Bzowej NH, et al. Telaprevir for previously untreated chronic hepatitis C virus infection. The New England Journal of Medicine. 2011;**364**(25):2405-2416

[17] Everson GTSK, Rodriguez-Torres M. Efficacy of an interferon- and ribavirin-free regimen of daclatasvir, asunaprevir, and BMS-791325 in treatment-naive patients with HCV genotype 1 infection. Gastroenterology. 2014;**146**(2):420-429

[18] Kowdley KVLE, Poordad F, et al. Phase 2b trial of interferon-free therapy for hepatitis C virus genotype 1. The New England Journal of Medicine. 2014;**370**(3):222-232

[19] McHutchison JG, Manns M, Patel K, Poynard T, Lindsay KL, Trepo C, et al. Adherence to combination therapy enhances sustained response in genotype-1-infected patients with chronic hepatitis C. Gastroenterology. 2002;**123**(4):1061-1069

[20] Manns MP, Wedemeyer H, Cornberg M. Treating viral hepatitis C: Efficacy, side effects, and complications. Gut. 2006;**55**(9):1350-1359

[21] Perales C, Quer J, Gregori J, Esteban JI, Domingo E. Resistance of hepatitis C virus to inhibitors: Complexity and clinical implications. Virus. 2015;**7**(11):5746-5766

[22] Tsai SM, Kao JT, Tsai YF. How hepatitis C patients manage the treatment process of pegylated interferon and ribavirin therapy: A qualitative study. BMC Health Services Research. 2016;**16**:247

[23] Group GBOHCW. Global burden of disease (GBD) for hepatitis C. Journal of Clinical Pharmacology. 2004;**44**(1):20-29

[24] Pontali E, Angeli E, Cattelan AM, Maida I, Nasta P, Verucchi G, et al. Cytopenias during treatment of HIV-HCV-coinfection with pegylated interferon and ribavirin: Safety analysis of the OPERA study. Antiviral Therapy. 2015;**20**(1):39-48

[25] Slim J, Afridi MS. Managing adverse effects of interferon-alfa and ribavirin in combination therapy for HCV. Infectious Disease Clinics of North America. 2012;**26**(4):917-929

[26] Hézode C. Management of anaemia and other treatment complications. Digestive and Liver Disease. 2013;**45**(Suppl 5):S337-S342

[27] Fortune BE, Francis S, Forman LM, Hepatitis C. Virus therapy-related skin manifestations. Gastroenterol Hepatol (N Y). 2010;**6**(5):326-328

[28] Veluru C, Atluri D, Chadalavada R, Burns E, Mullen KD. Skin rash during chronic hepatitis C therapy. Gastroenterol Hepatol (N Y). 2010;**6**(5):323-325

[29] Chopra A, Klein PL, Drinnan T, Lee SS. How to optimize HCV therapy in genotype 1 patients: Management of side-effects. Liver International. 2013;**33**(Suppl 1):30-34

[30] Baik SJ, Kim TH, Yoo K, Moon IH, Cho MS. Ischemic colitis during interferon-ribavirin therapy for chronic hepatitis C: A case report. World Journal of Gastroenterology. 2012;**18**(31):4233-4236

[31] Lucaciu LA, Dumitrascu DL. Depression and suicide ideation in chronic hepatitis C patients untreated and treated with interferon: Prevalence, prevention, and treatment. Annals of Gastroenterology. 2015;**28**(4):440-447

[32] Lotrich F. Management of psychiatric disease in hepatitis C treatment candidates. Current Hepatitis Reports. 2010;**9**(2):113-118

[33] Payen JL, Pillard F, Mascarell V, Rivière D, Couzigou P, Kharlov N. Is physical activity possible and beneficial for patients with hepatitis C receiving pegylated interferon and ribavirin therapy? Gastroentérologie Clinique et Biologique. 2009;**33**(1 Pt 1):8-14

[34] Rodis JL, Kibbe P. Evaluation of medication adherence and quality of life in patients with hepatitis C virus receiving combination therapy. Gastroenterology Nursing. 2010;**33**(5):368-373

[35] Manos MM, Ho CK, Murphy RC, Shvachko VA. Physical, social, and psychological consequences of treatment for hepatitis C : A community-based evaluation of patient-reported outcomes. Patient. 2013;**6**(1):23-34

[36] Zickmund S, Hillis SL, Barnett MJ, Ippolito L, LaBrecque DR. Hepatitis C virus-infected patients report communication problems with physicians. Hepatology. 2004;**39**(4):999-1007

[37] Gujral H, Viscomi C, Collantes R. The role of physician extenders in managing patients with chronic hepatitis C. Cleveland Clinic Journal of Medicine. 2004;**71**(Suppl 3):S33-S37

[38] Grogan A, Timmins F. Patients' perceptions of information and support received from the nurse specialist during HCV treatment. Journal of Clinical Nursing. 2010;**19**(19-20):2869-2878

[39] Silberbogen AK, Ulloa E, Mori DL, Brown K. A telehealth intervention for veterans on antiviral treatment for the hepatitis C virus. Psychological Services. 2012;**9**(2):163-173

[40] Evon DM, Simpson K, Kixmiller S, Galanko J, Dougherty K, Golin C, et al. A randomized controlled trial of an integrated care intervention to increase eligibility for chronic hepatitis C treatment. The American Journal of Gastroenterology. 2011;**106**(10):1777-1786

[41] Yee HS, Chang MF, Pocha C, Lim J, Ross D, Morgan TR, et al. Update on the management and treatment of hepatitis C virus infection: Recommendations from the Department of Veterans Affairs Hepatitis C Resource Center Program and the National Hepatitis C Program Office. The American Journal of Gastroenterology. 2012;**107**(5):669-689 quiz 90

[42] Alexopoulou A, Karayiannis P. Interferon-based combination treatment for chronic hepatitis C in the era of direct acting antivirals. Annals of Gastroenterology. 2015;**28**(1):55-65

[43] Stedman C. Sofosbuvir, a NS5B polymerase inhibitor in the treatment of hepatitis C: A review of its clinical potential. Therapeutic Advances in Gastroenterology. 2014;**7**(3):131-140

[44] Lawitz E, Matusow G, DeJesus E, Yoshida EM, Felizarta F, Ghalib R, et al. Simeprevir plus sofosbuvir in patients with chronic hepatitis C virus genotype 1 infection and cirrhosis: A phase 3 study (OPTIMIST-2). Hepatology. 2016;**64**(2):360-369

[45] Afdhal N, Reddy KR, Nelson DR, Lawitz E, Gordon SC, Schiff E, et al. Ledipasvir and sofosbuvir for previously treated HCV genotype 1 infection. The New England Journal of Medicine. 2014;**370**(16):1483-1493

[46] Afdhal N, Zeuzem S, Kwo P, Chojkier M, Gitlin N, Puoti M, et al. Ledipasvir and sofosbuvir for untreated HCV genotype 1 infection. The New England Journal of Medicine. 2014;**370**(20):1889-1898

[47] Cousien A, Tran VC, Deuffic-Burban S, Jauffret-Roustide M, Dhersin JS, Yazdanpanah Y. Hepatitis C treatment as prevention of viral transmission and liver-related morbidity in persons who inject drugs. Hepatology. 2016;**63**(4):1090-1101

[48] Khoo A, Tse E. A practical overview of the treatment of chronic hepatitis C virus infection. Australian Family Physician. 2016;**45**(10):718-720

[49] Panel. AIHG. Recommendations for Testing, Managing, and Treating Hepatitis C. 2016. Available from: http://www.hcvguidelines.org/

[50] Ly KN, Xing J, Klevens RM, Jiles RB, Ward JW, Holmberg SD. The increasing burden of mortality from viral hepatitis in the United States between 1999 and 2007. Annals of Internal Medicine. 2012;**156**(4):271-278

[51] EASL recommendations on treatment of hepatitis C 2016. Journal of Hepatology. 2017; **66**(1):153-194

[52] Poynard T, McHutchison J, Manns M, Trepo C, Lindsay K, Goodman Z, et al. Impact of pegylated interferon alfa-2b and ribavirin on liver fibrosis in patients with chronic hepatitis C. Gastroenterology. 2002;**122**(5):1303-1313

[53] Sise ME, Bloom AK, Wisocky J, Lin MV, Gustafson JL, Lundquist AL, et al. Treatment of hepatitis C virus-associated mixed cryoglobulinemia with direct-acting antiviral agents. Hepatology. 2016;**63**(2):408-417

[54] Ford N, Swan T, Beyer P, Hirnschall G, Easterbrook P, Wiktor S. Simplification of antiviral hepatitis C virus therapy to support expanded access in resource-limited settings. Journal of Hepatology. 2014;**61**(1 Suppl):S132-S138

[55] Dore GJ, Ward J, Thursz M. Hepatitis C disease burden and strategies to manage the burden (Guest Editors Mark Thursz, Gregory Dore and John Ward). Journal of Viral Hepatitis. 2014;**21**(Suppl 1):1-4

[56] Gane E, Kershenobich D, Seguin-Devaux C, et al. Strategies to manage hepatitis C virus (HCV) infection disease burden. Journal of Viral Hepatitis. 2015;46-73

Chapter 17

The Molecular Basis of Anti-HCV Drug Resistance

Shaina M. Lynch and George Y. Wu

Additional information is available at the end of the chapter

http://dx.doi.org/10.5772/intechopen.70775

Abstract

Hepatitis C virus (HCV) is a significant medical problem and has become one of the leading causes of chronic liver disease. HCV replicates at a high rate, and due to inherently inaccurate nucleotide incorporation and lack of proofreading and post-replication repair, mutations are inevitable. In the era of direct acting antivirals (DAAs), treatment for HCV has become highly effective, but there are still about 5–10% of treated patients who do not achieve sustained virological response (SVR). There are many factors that affect SVR rates including the absorption and metabolism of DAAs, genetic make-up, the presence or absence of cirrhosis, and severity and resistance of HCV to DAAs. An important factor influencing treatment failure is HCV resistance. The majority of treatment failures while on DAAs are not due to on-treatment failures, but due to relapses. The exact mechanism for mutation-associated relapse is unclear, but possible theories include persistent intrahepatocytic viral replication and/or differences in the levels of host immune response.

Keywords: HCV, molecular, treatment, drug resistance, mutation

1. Introduction

Hepatitis C virus (HCV) is an important medical problem, affecting millions of people worldwide [1]. HCV is one of the leading causes of chronic liver disease with one third of those affected eventually developing liver cirrhosis or hepatocellular carcinoma [2]. Additionally, HCV infection is asymptomatic in the majority of cases, and persons often do not receive necessary medical care as they are unaware of their infection. [3] Worldwide, HCV-related complications are responsible for about 350,000 deaths annually [2, 4].

HCV is an enveloped, positive-strand RNA virus and encodes a single polyprotein. This single polyprotein is cotranslationally and post-translationally processed by host and viral proteases to create 10 viral proteins: N terminus, Core, E1, E2, p7, NS2, NS3, NS4A, NS4B,

NS5A, NS5B, C-terminus. Of these, NS3, NS4A, NS4B, NS5A, and NS5B are nonstructural proteins that are the major players in RNA viral replication (**Figure 1**). The life cycle and replication of HCV is similar to other positive-strand RNA viruses. First, the virus enters the hepatocyte by receptor-mediated endocytosis, and after fusion and uncoating of the virion, it is released into the cytoplasm. The viral genome is then used as mRNA for translation of the viral polyprotein. After cleavage and processing of the viral polyprotein, the nonstructural proteins involved in replication (NS3-NS5B) are incorporated into a membranous web to make replication complexes. Replication occurs by the synthesis of a negative-strand RNA from the positive-strand RNA, from which multiple copies of positive-strand RNA are synthesized. Infectious viral particles are then assembled by combining the structural proteins and positive-strand viral RNA. The infectious viral particles are then able to be transported out of the cell using the host VLDL-secretory pathway [1].

The high rate of HCV replication and low fidelity of the HCV polymerase results in heterogeneous virus populations [5]. Due to these factors, mutations are inevitable and the genomic composition is constantly changing. For RNA viruses, the mutation rate is about 10^{-3}–10^{-5} per nucleotide copied. The low fidelity of HCV RNA polymerases is due to the inherent inaccuracy in nucleotide incorporation and lack of proofreading and post-replication repair [6, 7].

With the advent of direct acting antivirals (DAAs), treatment for HCV has become highly effective. However, even with these new treatments, still about 5–10% of people with HCV fail treatment [1, 3]. Treatment success is measured based on sustained virological response (SVR), which is defined as an undetectable level of HCV RNA at 12 weeks or 24 weeks after the completion of treatment. For those who do not achieve SVR, there are many types of treatment failures that are described. Null responders are persons who fail to suppress HCV RNA by at least two logs by completion of treatment, whereas partial responders refer to those who achieve a decrease in HCV RNA levels by ≤2 logs, but never become undetectable. There are also treatment failures whose HCV RNA becomes undetectable, but then reappears in the serum. Of these, viral breakthrough refers to HCV RNA reemerging in the serum while still on treatment reappearance of HCV RNA in the serum occurs after treatment completion is referred to as virological relapse [8].

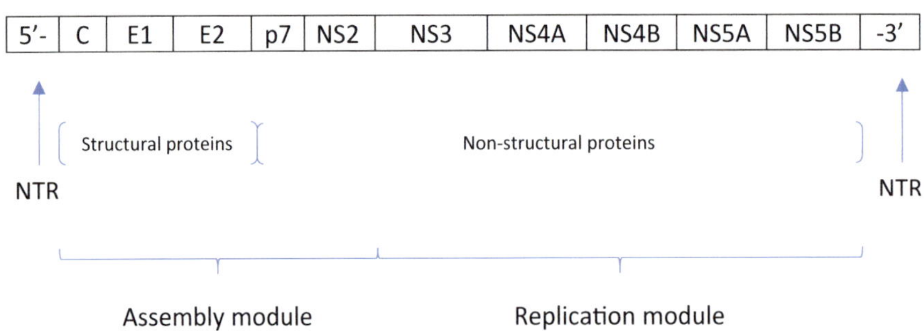

Figure 1. Hepatitis C viral genome configuration. The 5'- and 3'- designations indicate nontranslational regions (NTRs), and the 5'-region contains the internal ribosome entry site (IRES). The structural proteins (C, E1, E2) along with p7 and NS2 encompass the assembly module. The remainder of the nonstructural proteins makes up the replication complex.

http://dx.doi.org/10.5772/intechopen.70775

The ability to achieve SVR depends on a combination of viral and host genetic factors. [5] Until recently, little evidence was available to explain host differences associated with chronic HCV infection. The discovery of a human polymorphism at the IL28B gene, a variation in a single nucleotide polymorphism (SNP) on chromosome 19 that is associated with the poor interferon response, has been crucial in distinguishing responders and nonresponders to interferon-based antiviral therapy [5, 9].

The DAAs currently target the proteins involved in HCV RNA replication, specifically NS3, NS5A, and NS5B (**Table 1**) [1]. Given high mutation rate, HCV is predisposed to the development of resistance to DAAs. Large numbers of genetically distinct HCV viral variants are generated daily in infected individuals. Collectively, these variants can create unique "quasispecies," possibly resulting in reduced susceptibility to DAAs if polymorphisms are created in drug-targeted genes [7].

Viral resistance is an important factor associated with HCV treatment failure. Resistant variants may be selected or enriched, and drug resistance may emerge during HCV antiviral treatment. While viral resistance is a consequence of treatment failure, it is not always the cause. Resistant variants occur naturally and often exist before antiviral drug treatment [10]. The prevalence of intrinsically resistant variants is partially related to replicative fitness. In viral quasispecies, a dominant variant is usually identified along with other less fit variants, which exist at lower frequencies. These small groups of resistance-associated substitutions (RASs) apparent before the initiation of treatment can become dominant in the presence of selective treatment with DAAs. This, in turn, may affect treatment outcomes, leading to virological breakthrough or more commonly, relapse after treatment cessation [7, 11].

Of note, there is a discrepancy in the term used to describe amino acid substitutions that reduce susceptibility of a virus to a drug or drug class, or the viral variants that carry the substitution resulting in reduced susceptibility. The term resistance-associated variants (RAVs) have been used previously to describe these mutants. Some investigators have stated that this term should be replaced by a different term, resistance-associated substitutions (RASs), to refer to the amino acid substitutions that confer resistance [11].

NS3	NS5A	NS5B
Boceprevir	Daclatasvir	Sofosbuvir
Telaprevir	Ledipasvir	Dasabuvir
Simeprevir	Ombitasvir	Beclabuvir
Asunaprevir	Elbasvir	
Paritaprevir	Velpatasvir	
Grazoprevir	Pibrentasvir	
Glecaprevir		

Table 1. Primary targets for DAAs for the treatment of HCV.

2. Identification of mutations

To identify barriers to resistance of experimental antiviral drugs, *in vitro* resistance selection studies are utilized. Many tests have been developed to identify HCV resistance including replicon systems in hepatoma cell lines, *in vitro* cell-free biochemical assays, and structural studies. However, these *in vitro* studies are not necessarily predictive of clinical resistance [7].

2.1. Replicon systems

Cell culture systems were developed to identify specific HCV mutations and how they affect drug resistance. The first cell culture replicon system was described in 1999 and is now available for the majority of HCV genotypes. This replicon system supports HCV replication in Huh7 hepatoma cells. Some replicons are unable to support the production of infectious virus particles, while more recent models are. The HCV pseudoparticle system, a cell culture replicon assay, was developed in 2003. This system works by creating a retrovirus coated with HCV envelope glycoproteins E1 and E2, which allows investigators to follow the steps of the specific HCV entry pathway. With this method, the entry of the virus can be monitored either visually or quantitatively by integrating reporter genes. In 2005, the first cell culture-infectious clone was introduced using the genotype 2a JFH1 isolate. With this method, the entire HCV viral life cycle is replicated in cell culture [1].

2.2. Cell-free biochemical assays

Cell-free assays are useful to examine the susceptibility of HCV to treatment with DAAs. This method can detect the effects of individual and complex substitutions on HCV enzyme activity under the influence of an investigational drug [7]. One such test is the NS3/4a enzyme assay, which uses a purified NS3 protease *in vitro*. In this assay, the NS3/4A fragment is cloned into an *Escherichia coli* expression plasmid for protein synthesis [7]. The protease activity is compared to various drug concentrations, and resistance is measured as inhibitory concentrations of either 50 and 90% (IC50 and IC90, respectively), drug concentrations that inhibit by 50 and 90%, respectively. [7]

Enzyme-based assays can be expensive and time consuming. These tests are based on coupled *in vitro* transcription/translation systems and have a turnaround time of about 10 hours. Several tools have been developed to study HCV replication, which evaluate viral enzyme efficacy and resistance to an RdRp inhibitor. The RdRp enzyme catalyzes the synthesis of both positive- and negative-strand RNAs. As for NS3/4A assays, the IC50 and IC90 can be calculated [7].

Studies have shown that some mutations reduce affinity for NS5A and decrease replication because NS5A regulates RdRp activity, although NS5A has no intrinsic enzyme activity [7].

2.3. Structural studies

Structural studies used to determine the structure of HCV proteins, and interactions with potential drugs include X-ray crystallography, nuclear magnetic resonance (NMR) spectroscopy, and computational methods [7].

X-ray crystallography was used to examine the conformational flexibility and interaction of the investigational drug with conserved or mutated viral structures. By using crystallography, insight can be obtained into the cross-resistance of drugs in relation to a specific viral protein as well as the genetic barrier to resistance can be measured [7].

The NMR spectroscopy method provides data on proteins in solution without requiring protein crystallization and, therefore, allows for structural and functional studies. For unstable disordered proteins such as NS5, this is a particularly useful method [7].

Computational methods involve creating a software-based structural modeling analysis that analyze the X-ray structures of mutated NS3 or NS5B proteins. Using wild-type structures obtained from the Protein Data Bank, three-dimensional analyses of drug-binding sites and the impact of varying amino acid substitutions can be determined [7].

It is the data from structural studies that led to the modeling and understanding of structure–function relationships that ultimately led to development of highly effective DAAs with few side effects. However, the factors involved in clinical resistance could only be identified by clinical studies.

3. Clinical resistance studies

Samples from treatment failure patients have been sequenced and compared to known mutations identified from cell culture phenotypic analysis. In this way, mutations and amino acid substitutions known to impact drug susceptibility have been correlated [5, 11]. The RdRp and NS5B proteins have high barriers, whereas NS5A inhibitors and NS34A protease inhibitors have low barriers to resistance [11]. Information on the prevalence of RASs at baseline has been heterogeneous. This is not only due to differences in methods but also because studies generally select which RASs to study and which can affect their clinical significance [11]. Furthermore, most studies have been performed on HCV genotype 1 with very little data on other genotypes.

3.1. NS3/NS4A

The HCV NS3/NS4A protease cleaves four sites along the encoded protein. Rapid development of resistance due to NS3/NS4A mutations is common in patients on treatment with protease inhibitor therapy. In patients with genotype 1 infection, the most frequent substitution noted was Q80K, which was found in 13.6% of cases [11]. The R155K mutation, which is seen in genotype 1a virus, causes resistance against nearly all protease inhibitors. In genotype 1b, various resistance mutations can arise based on the protease inhibitor class to which the patient has been exposed. In response to ketoamide protease inhibitors, A156, V36, T54, and V36 + A155 mutations have been observed. When macrocyclic inhibitors were used, however, mutations in R155K and D168A were seen. Given this information, even though NS3/NS4A inhibitors have been very effective in the treatment of HCV, it is evident that drug resistance challenges the success of these agents [5].

The majority of drug-resistant mutations in the NS3/NS4A protease occur at the active site, as alterations in these areas can modify drug binding while also having minimal impact on substrate binding and viral fitness. Danoprevir, simeprevir, and boceprevir, all project from the substrate envelope in areas known to have resistant mutations, leading to multi-drug-resistant variants. For instance, the large P2 moieties of danoprevir and simeprevir bind at the S2 subsite resulting in high interaction rates with the R155, D168, and A156 residues. It is not completely understood how these molecular alterations reduce inhibitor binding without affecting the binding of viral substrates [5] (**Figure 2**).

3.2. NS5A/NS5B

Substitutions in NS5B affecting efficacy of nucleoside analogs and non-nucleoside RdRp Palm-1 inhibitors are rare at baseline, while NS5A RASs are often detected in treatment naïve

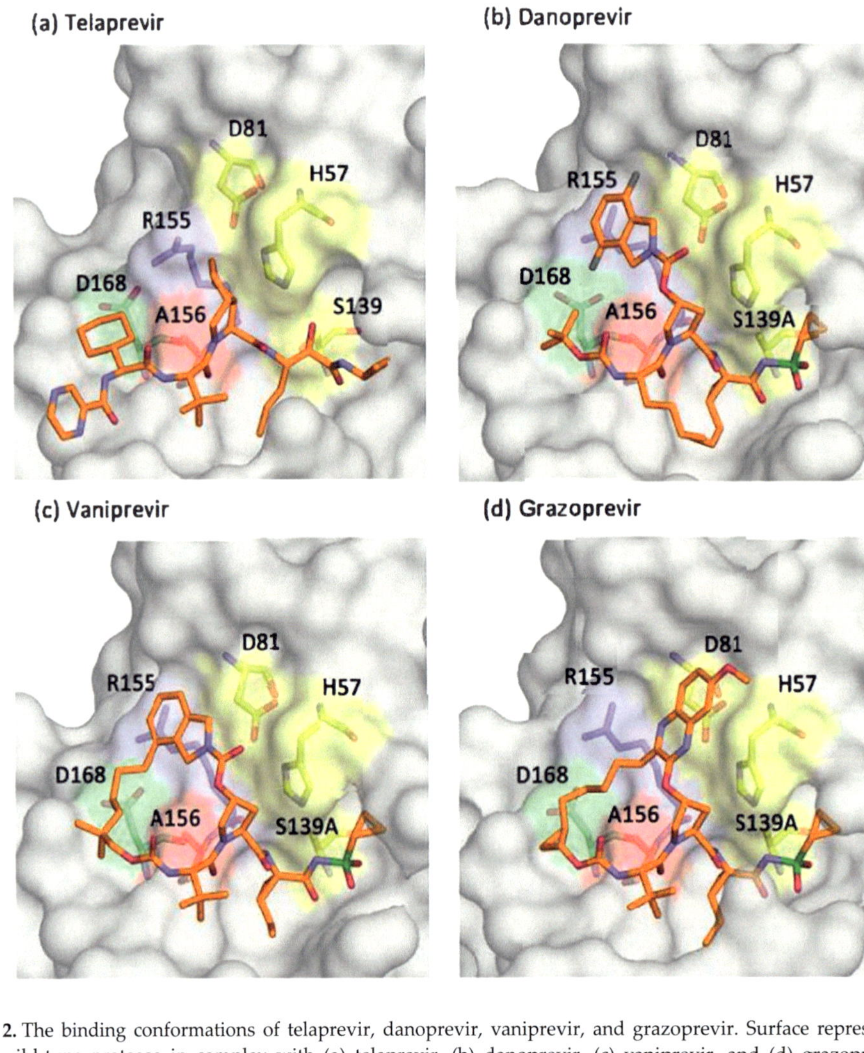

Figure 2. The binding conformations of telaprevir, danoprevir, vaniprevir, and grazoprevir. Surface representations of the wild-type protease in complex with (a) telaprevir, (b) danoprevir, (c) vaniprevir, and (d) grazoprevir. The catalytic triad consists of D81, H57, and S139A. The R155, A156, and D168 side chains are also labeled for each binding conformation. (Adapted from Romano et al. [5]).

patients. By using a 15% clinically relevant cutoff in patients with genotype 1a, one or more RASs were found in 13, 14, 7, and 16% of cases in North America, Europe, Asia-Pacific, and Oceania, respectively [11].

4. Clinical trial results

In patients treated with sofosbuvir/ledipasvir for genotype 1 infection, resistance has been examined in the ION 1–3 and ELECTRON studies. The presence of NS3-4A protease RASs at baseline did not affect the clinical response to treatment. NS5A RASs had no effect on the SVRs in naïve patients with or without cirrhosis and with or without ribavirin. They did, however, lead to a high level of resistance to ledipasvir. This resulted in a low SVR for treatment-experienced patients infected with genotype 1a. It was noted that all patients who relapsed had this RAS leading to reduced susceptibility to ledipasvir with an SVR of only 72%. Adding ribavirin improved SVR from 88 to 94% in cirrhotic patients treated for 12 weeks and from 85 to 100% for patients treated for 24 weeks. Ribavirin appears to reduce the effects of pre-existing NS5A RASs [11, 12].

A phase 2 study with combination of ombitasvir, paritaprevir, and ritonavir (ombitasvir/paritaprevir/ritonavir) plus dasabuvir showed that patients with HCV genotype 1a infection with RASs at baseline had an SVR of 86% compared to 92% to those without RASs [13]. Researchers have reported SVR in HCV genotype 1-infected patients with and without cirrhosis who had baseline RASs. Treatment consisted of combinations of ombitasvir/paritaprevir/ritonavir plus dasabuvir with or without ribavirin for 12 or 24 weeks. Patients treated with HCV genotype 1b without ribavirin had 100% SVR. However, this was a small study with only four patients. The RAS region in these patients was NS3 protease- and paritaprevir-specific, which may explain the efficacy without ribavirin. The patients without baseline RASs treated with ombitasvir/paritaprevir/ritonavir had an SVR of 97% in all treatment groups [11].

In phase 2 and 3 studies of sofosbuvir plus daclatasvir with or without ribavirin in patients infected with HCV genotype 1, both treatment naïve and experienced, an SVR of 100% was seen in patients with baseline RASs. In patients with genotype 3 infections treated with sofosbuvir plus daclatasvir without ribavirin for 12 weeks, SVR in noncirrhotics was 97% for treatment naïve patients and 94% for treatment-experienced patients, and for patients with cirrhosis, 58% for treatment-naive patients and 69% for treatment-experienced patients. In patients with baseline NS5A RASs with cirrhosis treated for only 12 weeks, a reduced rate of SVR was seen [11, 14]. Although the sample size was small, and the treatment lacked ribavirin, this may suggest a benefit of prolonging treatment in genotype 3 patients with baseline NS5A RRASs and cirrhosis.

In patients treated with sofosbuvir plus simeprevir without ribavirin for 12 weeks, a phase 2 study showed an SVR rate of 95% for genotype 1b, 88% for genotype 1a with Q80K present, and 94% for genotype 1a without the Q80K variant [15]. In a phase 3 study, SVR rates were studied in patients who were either treatment naïve or had been treated with pegylated-INF-based regimens with or without cirrhosis. In patients without cirrhosis, SVR rates of 97% in genotype 1b, 96% genotype 1a with Q80K, and 97% in genotype 1a without Q80K were seen. In patients with cirrhosis, the SVR was 84% in genotype 1b, 74% genotype 1a with Q80K, and 92% genotype 1a without Q80K [16]. This suggested a decreased rate of SVR in genotype 1a in cirrhotic patients who had the Q80K RAS [11].

In phase 2 and 3 trials on patients treated with grazoprevir/elbasvir, the NS3 protease RAS was found not to affect SVR. However, the presence of NS5A RASs did affect the SVR in patients with genotype 1a. Patients without the elbasvir-specific NS5A RAS had an SVR of 98% compared to 58% in those with the RAS. NS5A RASs did not affect SVR in patients with genotype 1b. This effect was not observed with the addition of ribavirin and prolonging treatment to 16–18 weeks. The SVR was 94 and 100% with and without the NS5A RAS in genotype 1b, respectively. [11]

The combination of sofosbuvir/velpatasvir was studied in three phase 3 trials and the presence of NS5A RAS at baseline did not affect SVR in patients with genotypes 1a, 1b, 2, 4, 5 or 6. In patients with genotype 3 without the NS5A RAS at baseline, SVR was 97% compared to 88% in those with the RAS. Another phase 3 trial studied sofosbuvir/velpatasvir treatment in patients with decompensated cirrhosis (Child-Pugh B) and genotypes 1 to 6 HCV infections. Patients were treated for 12 weeks with ribavirin or 24 weeks without ribavirin. In patients with genotype 1 infection with and without baseline NS5A RAS, SVRs were 80% versus 96% for 12 weeks without ribavirin, 100% versus 98% for 12 weeks with ribavirin, and 90% versus 98% for 24 weeks without ribavirin. [11, 17] This suggests that adding ribavirin reduced the effect of NS5A RAS more than extending the duration of treatment [17–19]. Although asunaprevir plus daclatasvir has not been approved in the United Stated or Europe, it is used in Asia and the Middle East. Studies have suggested that patients with HCV genotype 1b with a NS5A RASs at positions 31 or 93 should not use this treatment regimen [11, 20].

In compliant patients, most treatment failures are relapses. The relapse rate has been described in several trials. One phase 3 trial studied treatment with sofosbuvir plus simeprevir in patients without cirrhosis and found a relapse rate of 17% and 3% at 8 and 12 weeks, respectively. In patients treated with grazoprevir/elbasvir, the relapse rate was 2.3% in HIV co-infected patients. A phase 3 trial studied sofosbuvir/velpatasvir and found that 20 patients with Child-Pugh B had relapse and 19 of these patients had NS5A RASs. Alternatively, 2 of 625 patients with genotype 1a, 1b, 4, 5, 6 without cirrhosis or with compensated cirrhosis experienced relapse and they both were found to have the NS5A substitution. In patients with genotype 3 and NS5A RASs, 10/277 had a relapse [11].

4.1. Retreatment studies

Retreatment strategies with DAAs in patients who have failed an interferon-free regimen can lead to SVR in the majority of patients including patients with known RASs. Studies suggested that sofosbuvir in combination with 1–3 other DAAs can be considered for retreatment. In addition, prolonging treatment to 24 weeks and/or adding ribavirin may also be considered [11]. These recommendations were based mainly on small scale studies. One study investigated 15 patients who failed a daclatasvir-based regimen. They were retreated with sofosbuvir and simeprevir without ribavirin for 12 weeks and achieved an SVR of 87%. In a study on retreatment with sofosbuvir, ombitasvir/paritaprevir/ritonavir and dasabuvir

http://dx.doi.org/10.5772/intechopen.70775

with or without ribavirin, 92% of noncirrhotic patients with genotype 1a achieved SVR after 12 weeks with ribavirin and 100% achieved SVR after 24 weeks with ribavirin in patients with cirrhosis. In cirrhotics with genotype 1b, SVR without ribavirin achieved 100% after 12 weeks. Variants resistant to sofosbuvir were rarely selected and appeared not to affect retreatment with sofosbuvir possibly because sofosbuvir-resistant variants tend to be poorly fit and to disappear rapidly after treatment is stopped. In contrast, variants associated with NS5A RASs tend to persist which can affect re-treatment. [11].

5. Conclusions

In the era of DAAs, about 90–95% of persons treated for HCV to achieve SVR. While these new treatment regimens have significantly and dramatically improved SVR rates, about 5–10% of patients fail to achieve SVR [1]. Factors that influence SVR rates include the absorption and metabolism of the DAA, the immune response of the patient, the presence or absence of cirrhosis, and the severity and resistance of HCV to DAAs. [11] HCV resistance plays an important role in treatment failure. Most of the treatment failures on DAA treatment regimens are not due to on-treatment failures, but due to relapses. The persistence and development of resistant variants post treatment depend on the DAA class used [7].

There are several possible mechanisms of mutation-associated relapse. It seems most likely that relapse involves persistent intrahepatocytic viral replication. Treatment with DAAs is known to be biphasic with a rapid initial response followed by a slower second phase. The first phase is dependent on drug potency, exposure, and susceptibility. The second phase, which can be accelerated by ribavirin, is dependent on drug potency, host genetic features, and the severity of immune response [11]. During treatment, drug-sensitive HCV is suppressed in the blood, and the virus remains undetectable. Due to differences in host-specific hepatocyte factors or aggressiveness of the host immune system, the level of resistant variants in the hepatocytes may be higher in relapsers compared to responders.

Acknowledgements

The support of a grant from Alexion Corporation, and the Herman Lopata Chair in hepatitis Research are gratefully acknowledged.

Abbreviations

DAAs	direct acting antivirals
HCV	hepatitis C virus
SVR	sustained virological response

HIV human immunodeficiency virus

HBV hepatitis B virus

RdRp RNA-dependent RNA polymerase

SNP single nucleotide polymorphism

RASs resistance-associated substitutions

RAVs resistance-associated variants

NMR nucleic magnetic resonance

Author details

Shaina M. Lynch[1]* and George Y. Wu[2]

*Address all correspondence to: slynch@mcw.edu

1 Medical College of Wisconsin, Division of Gastroenterology and Hepatology, Milwaukee, USA

2 University of Connecticut, Division of Gastroenterology and Hepatology, Farmington, USA

References

[1] Kim S, Han KH, Ahn SH. Hepatitis C virus and antiviral drug resistance. Gut and Liver. 2016;**10**(6):890-895

[2] Esteban R, Nyberg L, Lalezari J, Ni L, Doehle B, Kanwar B, Brainard D, Subramanian M, Symonds WT, McHutchinson JG, Rodriguez-Torres M, Zeuzem S. Successful retreatment with sofosbuvir-containing regimens for HCV genotype 2 or 3 infected patients who failed prior sofosbuvir plus ribavirin therapy. Elsevier Science: Journal of Hepatology. 2014;**60**(1): Supplement, S4-S5

[3] Bartenschlager R, Lohmann V, Penin F. The molecular and structural basis of advanced antiviral therapy for hepatitis C virus infection. Nature Reviews. Microbiology. 2013;**11**(7):482-496

[4] Panel AIHG. Hepatitis C guidance: AASLD-IDSA recommendations for testing, managing, and treating adults infected with hepatitis C virus. Hepatology. 2015;**62**(3):932-954

[5] Romano KP, et al. The molecular basis of drug resistance against hepatitis C virus NS3/4A protease inhibitors. PLoS Pathogens. 2012;**8**(7):e1002832

[6] Perales C, et al. Resistance of hepatitis C virus to inhibitors: Complexity and clinical implications. Virus. 2015;**7**(11):5746-5766

[7] Fourati S, Pawlotsky JM. Virologic tools for HCV drug resistance testing. Virus. 2015;**7**(12): 6346-6359

[8] Ghany MG, et al. Diagnosis, management, and treatment of hepatitis C: An update. Hepatology. 2009;**49**(4):1335-1374

[9] Dienstag J. Chronic hepatitis C. In: Longo DL, Kasper DL, Jameson JL, Fauci AS, Hauser SL, Loscalzo J, editors. Harrison's Principles of Internal Medicine. McGraw Hill; New York, 2012. p. 2579-2585

[10] Rong L, et al. Rapid emergence of protease inhibitor resistance in hepatitis C virus. Science Translational Medicine. 2010;**2**(30):30ra32

[11] Pawlotsky JM. Hepatitis C virus resistance to direct-acting antiviral drugs in interferon-free regimens. Gastroenterology. 2016;**151**(1):70-86

[12] Sarrazin C. The importance of resistance to direct antiviral drugs in HCV infection in clinical practice. Journal of Hepatology. 2016;**64**(2):486-504

[13] Krishnan P, et al. Resistance analysis of baseline and treatment-emergent variants in hepatitis C virus genotype 1 in the AVIATOR study with paritaprevir-ritonavir, ombitasvir, and dasabuvir. Antimicrobial Agents and Chemotherapy. 2015;**59**(9):5445-5454

[14] Nelson DR, et al. All-oral 12-week treatment with daclatasvir plus sofosbuvir in patients with hepatitis C virus genotype 3 infection: ALLY-3 phase III study. Hepatology. 2015;**61**(4): 1127-1135

[15] Lawitz E, et al. Simeprevir plus sofosbuvir, with or without ribavirin, to treat chronic infection with hepatitis C virus genotype 1 in non-responders to pegylated interferon and ribavirin and treatment-naive patients: The COSMOS randomised study. Lancet. 2014;**384**(9956):1756-1765

[16] Kwo P, et al. Simeprevir plus sofosbuvir (12 and 8 weeks) in hepatitis C virus genotype 1-infected patients without cirrhosis: OPTIMIST-1, a phase 3, randomized study. Hepatology. 2016;**64**(2):370-380

[17] Curry MP, et al. Sofosbuvir and velpatasvir for HCV in patients with decompensated cirrhosis. The New England Journal of Medicine. 2015;**373**(27):2618-2628

[18] Feld JJ, et al. Sofosbuvir and velpatasvir for HCV genotype 1, 2, 4, 5, and 6 infection. The New England Journal of Medicine. 2015;**373**(27):2599-2607

[19] Foster GR, et al. Sofosbuvir and velpatasvir for HCV genotype 2 and 3 infection. The New England Journal of Medicine. 2015;**373**(27):2608-2617

[20] McPhee F, et al. High sustained virologic response to daclatasvir plus asunaprevir in elderly and cirrhotic patients with hepatitis C virus genotype 1b without baseline NS5A polymorphisms. Advances in Therapy. 2015;**32**(7):637-649